Shoulder Fractures

The Practical Guide to Management

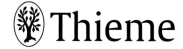

Shoulder Fractures
The Practical Guide to Management

Joseph D. Zuckerman, M.D.
Professor and Chairman
Department of Orthopaedic Surgery
NYU–Hospital for Joint Diseases
Walter A. L. Thompson Professor of Orthopaedic Surgery
New York University School of Medicine
New York, New York

Kenneth J. Koval, M.D.
Professor
Department of Orthopaedics
Dartmouth Hitchcock Medical Center
Lebanon, New Hampshire

Thieme
New York • Stuttgart

Thieme Medical Publishers, Inc.
333 Seventh Ave.
New York, NY 10001

Consulting Editor: Esther Gumpert
Associate Editor: Owen Zurhellen IV
Vice President, Production and Electronic Publishing: Anne T. Vinnicombe
Production Editor: Print Matters, Inc.
Sales Manager: Ross Lumpkin
Chief Financial Officer: Peter van Woerden
President: Brian D. Scanlan
Compositor: Compset
Printer: The Maple-Vail Book Manufacturing Group

Cover illustrations: Drawing of shoulder from: PROMETHEUS, Atlas of Anatomy; General Anatomy and Musculoskeletal System. By M. Shuenke, E. Schulte, U. Schumacher (authors), M. Voll, and K. Wesker (illustrators). Consulting Editors L. M. Ross and E. D. Lamperti. Thieme, 2005, p. 230 (illustration by K. Wesker). By permission of the publisher. Scans courtesy of J. Zuckerman.

Library of Congress Cataloging-in-Publication Data

Zuckerman, Joseph D. (Joseph David), 1952–
Shoulder fractures: the practical guide to management/Joseph D. Zuckerman, Kenneth J. Koval.
    p. cm.
   Includes bibliographical references and index.
   ISBN 1-58890-310-9 (US)—ISBN 3-13-140341-1 (GTV)
    1. Shoulder—Fractures—Surgery. 2. Shoulder—Fractures—Treatment. 3. Orthopedics. I. Koval, Kenneth J. II. Title.
  RD557.5.Z835 2005
  617.5′72044—dc22   2005041916

Important note: Medical knowledge is ever-changing. As new research and clinical experience broaden our knowledge, changes in treatment and drug therapy may be required. The authors and editors of the material herein have consulted sources believed to be reliable in their efforts to provide information that is complete and in accord with the standards accepted at the time of publication. However, in view of the possibility of human error by the authors, editors, or publisher of the work herein or changes in medical knowledge, neither the authors, editors, or publisher, nor any other party who has been involved in the preparation of this work, warrants that the information contained herein is in every respect accurate or complete, and they are not responsible for any errors or omissions or for the results obtained from use of such information. Readers are encouraged to confirm the information contained herein with other sources. For example, readers are advised to check the product information sheet included in the package of each drug they plan to administer to be certain that the information contained in this publication is accurate and that changes have not been made in the recommended dose or in the contraindications for administration. This recommendation is of particular importance in connection with new or infrequently used drugs.

Some of the product names, patents, and registered designs referred to in this book are in fact registered trademarks or proprietary names even though specific reference to this fact is not always made in the text. Therefore, the appearance of a name without designation as proprietary is not to be construed as a representation by the publisher that it is in the public domain.

Printed in the United States

5 4 3 2 1

TMP ISBN 1-58890-310-9
GTV ISBN 3 13 140341 1

To Frederick A. Matsen III, M.D., and Robert H. Cofield, M.D., the two individuals who taught me the most about the shoulder and have always supported my efforts through the years.

And to my wife, Janet, and my sons, Scott and Matthew, the joys of my life.

Joseph D. Zuckerman

To my wife, Mary, and my three children, Courtney, Michael, and Lauren.

Kenneth J. Koval

Contents

Acknowledgments

This book would not have been possible without the combined efforts of many individuals. It is therefore only appropriate that we acknowledge the contributions of all those involved. We would particularly like to acknowledge our contributors who assisted in the preparation of each chapter. Their work was outstanding and, equally as important, always timely. We would also like to acknowledge the contributions of our colleagues on the Shoulder Service and the Fracture Service at the NYU–Hospital for Joint Diseases Department of Orthopaedic Surgery. Drs. Andrew Rokito, Robert Meislin, Young Kwon, Laith Jazrawi, Nirmal Tejwani, and Toni McLaurin were extremely helpful in identifying many of the cases that were used to illustrate the different treatment approaches utilized. We were also able to obtain additional illustrative cases from Evan Flatow, M.D., Chief of the Shoulder Service at Mount Sinai Medical Center in New York. He contributed the cases of percutaneous pinning in Chapter 7. We also acknowledge the contribution of Anthony Miniaci, M.D., Chief of Sports Medicine at the Cleveland Clinic, who contributed the humeral head allograft case that was included in Chapter 8.

The figures utilized in this text were prepared by the Medical Graphics Department at the Hospital for Joint Diseases. Hugh Nachamie prepared all of the drawings and was assisted by Elliot Friedman. Frank Martucci, our medical photographer, was responsible for obtaining all intraoperative photographs as well as for photographing the hundreds of x-rays that we submitted to him. We have worked on multiple textbooks with Mr. Nachamie and Mr. Martucci over the past 15 years, and it seems that their contributions only increase with each project.

It is also important to recognize those individuals who work in our offices and assisted in the typing of the manuscripts, and the inevitable editing that follows. Jim Madden and Rosine DeCarolis were particularly helpful in this area. In addition, Robyn Smolen, and Migdalia Figueroa were invaluable in tracking down patients and their x-rays for inclusion in the text.

We also acknowledge the support provided by Thieme, particularly editor Esther Gumpert, who supported the project from its initial proposal. Associate editor Owen Zurhellen was meticulous in his editing, as was the production staff, including Anne Vinnicombe, Becky Dille, and Richard Rothschild.

Most importantly, we would like to acknowledge our colleagues in the NYU–Hospital for Joint Diseases Department of Orthopaedic Surgery both for contributing directly to this volume and for creating an environment of teaching and learning in which a project like this can be successfully completed.

Foreword

The authors have provided us with a uniquely comprehensive treatise on one of the most common and, simultaneously, most challenging of shoulder injuries: the spectrum of shoulder fractures. Ranging from the high-impact injury of the motorcycle rider to the fragility fracture of the 90-year-old, shoulder fractures vary as much as the overall health of the patients they affect. Such variability makes the systematic evaluation of the results of treatment highly complex. As the authors point out, attempts to assess efficacy and effectiveness are compromised further by the confusion of instruments used to assess the results of treatment. Our handle on the results is frustrated even more by the fact that proximal humeral fractures are usually cared for by practitioners who treat only a few such injuries each year. This means that few surgeons have mastered the steep learning curves of (1) matching patients, fractures, and procedures; (2) performing the techniques themselves; (3) optimizing postoperative care; and (4) contributing to our knowledge regarding outcomes of treatment.

In Chapter 1 the authors do an excellent job of reviewing the literature on outcomes assessment and pointing to the myriad of different treatments and the severe inadequacies of our knowledge of the effectiveness of various modes of treatment in even the best of hands. In Chapter 2 they set the basis for evaluation and management by reviewing the anatomy of the shoulder. In Chapter 3 they deal with the complex world of fracture classification. They point to the general consensus that these fractures have a tendency to occur in certain patterns, but also that the pattern of an individual fracture and thus the preoperative plan may be difficult to discern from plain radiographs alone.

Chapters 4 through 9 provide a thorough synthesis of the literature and the authors' recommendations for evaluation and management of one-, two-, three-, and four-part fractures as well as complications of fracture care. These chapters are superbly illustrated by both diagrams and radiographs, demonstrating both the wide variability of the injuries and the extensive experience of the authors. Chapter 10 provides a similarly complete treatise on fractures of the clavicle, and Chapter 11 does the same for fractures of the scapula.

Throughout the entire text, the exquisite attention to detail of the senior author shines through. One can easily envision his careful approach to each of his patients, his thoughtful assessment of their situation, his technically excellent surgery, and his concerned postoperative care and evaluation. We are fortunate to have this synthesis of current knowledge. I hope it can serve as a stimulus for the key next step: a rigorous attempt to establish a comprehensive national database on the results of treatment of shoulder fractures using a simple outcome measure that does not place an unacceptable burden on the patient or the surgeon. If anyone can make this happen, it is Drs. Zuckerman and Koval.

Frederick A. Matsen III, M.D.

Preface

When I joined the faculty at the Hospital for Joint Diseases in 1984, Victor Frankel, M.D., the chairman of the department, gave me the task of establishing the Shoulder Service, both to emphasize the clinical care of shoulder disorders as well as to enhance the education of our residents. At that time we were treating a significant volume of proximal humeral fractures, which immediately became an area of interest for us. When Dr. Koval joined the faculty in 1989, our interest expanded as the Fracture Service and the Shoulder Service collaborated on an increasing number of clinical and laboratory studies related to fractures about the shoulder. In 1997, when the Hospital for Joint Diseases and the New York University Medical Center Departments of Orthopaedic Surgery merged to become the NYU–Hospital for Joint Diseases Department of Orthopaedic Surgery, we became responsible for providing care at Bellevue Hospital Center, the primary trauma center in New York City. With this integration, the volume and variety of cases of fractures about the shoulder were expanded further and added to our growing experience in the care of fractures in this area. The decision to write a textbook on this topic was a natural extension of our almost 20-year experience with the care of these injuries.

This book is devoted to the evaluation and management of fractures about the shoulder including the proximal humerus, clavicle, and scapula. Although we feel this book provides comprehensive coverage, we recognize that every day new information becomes available concerning techniques for the evaluation and management of these injuries. That is exactly how it should be—an ever-expanding base of knowledge and experience that enhances our ability to optimize the outcomes following these injuries.

Fractures about the shoulder represent the full spectrum of injury—from the most simple to the most complex. By following a systematic approach to the evaluation of these fractures and selecting treatment based on a careful assessment of the fracture factors and patient factors that make each injury unique, a treatment approach can be developed. It is our feeling that by developing this systematic approach, each clinician will be able to determine the optimal treatment plan for each patient.

Although we have learned a lot over the past 20 years about fractures of the proximal humerus, scapula, and clavicle, preparing this textbook has only further enhanced our understanding of these injuries. It is our hope that those who use this textbook will find that their ability to care for these interesting and often complex injuries will also be enhanced.

Joseph D. Zuckerman, M.D.

Contributors

Andrew L. Chen, M.D.
Chief Orthopaedic Resident
NYU–Hospital for Joint Diseases
Department of Orthopaedic Surgery
New York University School
  of Medicine
New York, New York

Kenneth A. Egol, M.D.
Chief, Fracture Service
NYU–Hospital for Joint Diseases
Department of Orthopaedic Surgery
Associate Professor of Orthopaedic Surgery
New York University School
  of Medicine
New York, New York

Stephen A. Hunt, M.D.
Chief Orthopaedic Resident
NYU–Hospital for Joint Diseases
Department of Orthopaedic Surgery
New York University School
  of Medicine
New York, New York

Gerard K. Jeong, M.D.
Chief Orthopaedic Resident
NYU–Hospital for Joint Diseases
Department of Orthopaedic Surgery
New York University School
  of Medicine
New York, New York

Kenneth J. Koval, M.D.
Professor
Department of Orthopaedics
Dartmouth Hitchcock Medical Center
Lebanon, New Hampshire

Erik N. Kubiak, M.D.
Orthopaedic Resident
NYU–Hospital for Joint Diseases
Department of Orthopaedic
  Surgery
New York University School
  of Medicine
New York, New York

Matthew I. Leibman, M.D.
Chief Orthopaedic Resident
NYU–Hospital for Joint Diseases
Department of Orthopaedic
  Surgery
New York University School
  of Medicine
New York, New York

Frank A. Liporace, M.D.
Orthopaedic Resident
NYU–Hospital for Joint Diseases
Department of Orthopaedic
  Surgery
New York University School
  of Medicine
New York, New York

Frederick A. Matsen III, M.D.
Professor and Chairman
Department of Orthopaedics and Sports Medicine
University of Washington School of Medicine
Seattle, Washington

Douglas Murray, M.D.
Peachtree Orthopaedic Clinic
Atlanta, Georgia

Samuel S. Park, M.D.
Orthopaedic Resident
NYU–Hospital for Joint Diseases
Department of Orthopaedic Surgery
New York University School of Medicine
New York, New York

Steven S. Shin, M.D.
Orthopaedic Resident
NYU–Hospital for Joint Diseases
Department of Orthopaedic Surgery
New York University School
    of Medicine
New York, New York

Joseph D. Zuckerman, M.D.
Professor and Chairman
NYU–Hospital for Joint Diseases
Department of Orthopaedic Surgery
Walter A. L. Thompson Professor of
    Orthopaedic Surgery
New York University School of Medicine
New York, New York

Shoulder Fractures

The Practical Guide to Management

1

Principles of Treatment and Outcomes Assessment

JOSEPH D. ZUCKERMAN AND SAMUEL S. PARK

The ultimate goal of any medical treatment is to improve, or at least maintain, the overall health and function of the patient. On a purely technical level, fracture care aims to restore anatomy and alignment to prevent deformity and disability. Traditionally, the success of orthopaedic fracture care has been based on clinical and radiographic evaluation utilizing objective measures, such as range of motion, strength, alignment, and fracture union; however, satisfactory clinical and radiographic results do not always translate into patient satisfaction and restoration of function. Recognition of this potential disparity has led to the current emphasis on patient-oriented outcome measures. In conjunction with general health status, factors that are important to the patient—comfort, ability to perform activities of daily living (ADL), social well-being, work ability, and quality of life—impact directly on the patient's functional recovery and form the basis for outcomes assessment; therefore, the success or failure of a treatment should be based on both measures of objective clinical evaluation and subjective patient assessment.

■ Outcomes Research

Daum et al[1] has described outcomes research as one of the three elements of quality health care, which also includes the utilization of practice guidelines and necessitates continuous quality improvement. Efficacy indicates whether a treatment or procedure works, and is usually investigated in a specific setting by select individuals.[2] Effectiveness, on the other hand, indicates whether an efficacious treatment or procedure works when utilized by the general population. Outcomes research seeks to determine the effectiveness of treatments in terms of

both objective clinical measures and patient-oriented outcomes. A treatment that is efficacious in a controlled setting may prove to be ineffective when used in the general population. Ideal treatments would always lead to optimal outcomes. Treatments that fall short of these optimal outcomes are identified by outcomes research, thereby allowing revision of treatments to improve the overall quality of health care.

Outcomes research is composed of several different methods. Large databases can be analyzed retrospectively to perform epidemiologic studies and limited outcomes analyses. An example is the currently available Medicare database, which provides information on mortality, length of hospital stay, complications, and reoperations.[3] Because these are claims data, however, they are subject to errors in diagnoses and procedures, and do not reflect changes in patient's comfort, function, and health status.[3,4] Other limitations include lack of information on severity of disease, difficulty differentiating between preexisting disease and complications, and lack of patient-based outcomes. The American Academy of Orthopaedic Surgeons (AAOS) attempted to establish an important initiative in the development of outcomes research by developing a national musculoskeletal database called the Musculoskeletal Outcomes Data Evaluation and Management System (MODEMS) Program, which consisted of the Lower Limb Instrument, the Spine Instrument, the Pediatrics Instrument, and an upper extremity instrument, which was called the Disability of the Arm, Shoulder, and Hand (DASH) Instrument. The goal was to use the database to present national statistics on outcomes data, allow comparison between individual practices, and help establish standards for treatment.[5] Unfortunately, widespread use was never realized, and the project has been discontinued.

A major event in the development of outcomes research was Wennberg and Gittelsohn's[6] demonstration of the wide variation in rates of surgical procedures from one geographic region to another. The method of small-area analysis they developed allowed the calculation of per capita rates of medical and surgical procedures for patients at different hospitals serving different regions.[7] Within orthopaedics, although hip fracture and polytrauma have low variation, almost every other condition or procedure has considerable variation of hospital and surgical use rates.[8] Variation in health care utilization may signify uncertainty regarding the effectiveness of treatments and surgical indications. An unusually low rate would indicate that patients in that region are underserved, whereas an unusually high rate would indicate that patients are receiving excessive medical care. One of the aims of outcomes research is to determine the appropriate rate for different treatments. Vitale et al[9] investigated the state-to-state variation in rates for total shoulder arthroplasty, humeral head replacement, and rotator cuff repair. The rates for these procedures varied from state to state by as much as tenfold. Humeral head replacement showed the least variation of the three procedures. All three procedures were performed less often in states that are more densely populated. No consistent, significant relationship was found between the population density of orthopaedic surgeons and shoulder specialists and the rates of any procedure.

Meta-analysis utilizes literature review by combining data from multiple studies to create a larger, more statistically significant pool of data for analysis. To be included, the studies must conform to a rigorous protocol with strict inclusion and exclusion criteria to minimize publication and detection bias. Ideally, only prospective, randomized clinical trials would be included in the analysis; however, because few orthopaedic studies have adhered to this study design, the criteria may be broadened to include other types of studies. In orthopaedics, meta-analyses have been published for such conditions as hip fracture and lumbar spine fusion.[10,11] An attempted meta-analysis of treatment outcomes for three- and four-part proximal humerus fractures by Misra et al[12] concluded that the data from the orthopaedic literature are inadequate for evidence-based decision making mainly due to the lack of randomized controlled trials and uniformity of reporting outcomes. Nevertheless, based on the literature available, they found that nonoperatively treated patients showed inferior results with regard to pain relief and range of motion compared with operatively treated patients. Pain relief and range of motion showed no difference between patients treated with hemiarthroplasty and patients treated with open reduction and internal fixation (ORIF). In 2002 the Cochrane Musculoskeletal Injuries Group completed a systematic review of the literature in an attempt to determine the appropriate treatments for proximal humerus fractures.[13] The group was able to find only 10 studies that met the inclusion criteria of randomized or quasi-randomized (not strict randomization, e.g., allocation of treatment based on hospital record number) studies.[14-23] The group concluded that there is insufficient evidence from randomized trials to determine which interventions are the most appropriate for the different types of proximal humerus fractures. The available data do not confirm that surgery leads to better outcomes for three- and four-part fractures. The group's conclusion stressed the need for future randomized controlled trials to define more clearly the role and most effective type of surgical intervention in the management of proximal humerus fractures.

Clinical research studies are the cornerstone of outcomes research. Prospective studies that allow the investigator to determine which outcomes to observe and record in a standardized fashion are preferred over retrospective studies, which rely on patients' memory and review of medical records that were not specifically set up for the purpose of the study. A control or alternative treatment group enhances the validity of the study and allows for direct comparisons of interventions. The ideal study design is the prospective, randomized controlled clinical trial. Unfortunately, few orthopaedic studies have adhered strictly to these recommendations.[2,3,5,13] Whatever the study design, the end results being studied need to be clearly defined. In orthopaedic clinical research, these end results should include both objective clinical measures and patient-oriented outcomes, including physical, psychological, and social function as well as quality of life and patient satisfaction.

Much of the emphasis for the development of outcomes research grew from government policy makers' reaction to the rapidly rising cost of health care. In addition to determining the effectiveness of a treatment or procedure, outcomes research seeks to determine the effectiveness as a function of the financial cost; that is, the cost-effectiveness. Because of the limited resources in health care, cost-effectiveness analysis adds a new dimension to the goal of determining the best overall treatment for a particular disease.

■ Outcomes Instruments

Emphasis has been placed on the design of outcomes instruments that accurately determine objective clinical and patient-oriented outcomes after treatments. These self-assessment questionnaires assess treatment effectiveness from the perspective of the patient. To be clinically useful, the outcomes instrument must be valid, reproducible or reliable, internally consistent, and responsive

TABLE 1–1 Validity of Outcomes Instruments

Content validity: The comprehensiveness of the items on an outcomes instrument and the extent to which the items meet the aims of the instrument. Can be assessed by patient and clinician review.
Criterion validity: Whether the outcomes instrument correlates with the "gold standard" measure or with established objective tests and clinical evaluations.
Construct validity: Used when there is no "gold standard" measure for comparison. Assessed by comparison with already validated outcomes instruments.

to change. Validity refers to whether the instrument measures what it is supposed to measure, and consists of content validity, criterion validity, and construct validity[1,5] (Table 1–1). Reproducibility refers to the ability of the instrument to yield the same result both on separate occasions and when rated by different observers; that is, the test-retest reliability and interobserver reliability. Internal consistency means that the instrument is able to measure a single outcome correctly, independent of other variables. Responsiveness to change indicates that the instrument is sensitive to clinically important changes.

There are two types of outcomes instruments: (1) instruments that are specific to a particular disease or region of the body, and (2) general health status instruments. Region-specific instruments, such as those for the shoulder, disease-specific instruments, such as those for glenohumeral arthritis, and general health status instruments do not always demonstrate equal responsiveness to change for all aspects of a particular disability or disease. Because they potentially convey different information, both types of instruments are needed in the complete evaluation of a disability or disease.[24]

■ Outcomes Instruments in Proximal Humerus Fractures

Many studies of outcomes in proximal humerus fractures use shoulder scoring instruments that were originally developed in the context of surgery for various other shoulder pathologies, such as degenerative joint disease and rotator cuff tears. Only later were these instruments adopted for general use in the evaluation of shoulder problems. To varying degrees, all shoulder outcomes instruments assess pain, function, range of motion, and strength. The main problem with these instruments is that each one emphasizes a different aspect of the shoulder evaluation. Some instruments emphasize pain, whereas others place more emphasis on function, and still others emphasize range of motion. Because of these differences, comparing the

instruments becomes difficult if not impossible, and no individual instrument has become universally accepted. To date, an outcomes instrument specifically designed to evaluate proximal humerus fractures has not been developed.

Neer's Shoulder Grading Scale

Originally developed to assess shoulder arthroplasty for glenohumeral degenerative joint disease, the Neer grading scale has been used widely to assess outcome following proximal humerus fracture (Table 1–2).[25] In the 100-point system, 35 points are for pain, 25 points for range of motion (flexion, extension, abduction, internal and external rotation), 30 points for function (10 activities including strength, reaching, and stability), and 10 points for reconstruction of the anatomy based on radiographic appearance. Neer considered pain relief to be the most important consideration, and functional recovery secondary. A final question asks if the patient feels better, the same, or worse after surgery. An excellent result is 90 points or more; satisfactory, 80 to 89; unsatisfactory, 70 to 79; and failure, less than 70. Unlike other assessment tools, the Neer grading scale incorporates radiographic findings into the evaluation. It takes only a few minutes to complete and has been used widely in both Europe and the United States. Most reports on outcomes of proximal humerus fractures using the Neer grading scale have adhered to this original scoring system because of the opportunity the system offers to quantify results on a 0- to 100-point scale.[26–40] Nonetheless, the grading

TABLE 1–2 Neer Scoring System

	Points
Pain	35
Function	
Strength	10
Reaching	
Top of head	2
Mouth	2
Belt buckle	2
Opposite axilla	2
Brassiere hook	2
Stability	
Lifting, throwing, pounding, pushing, hold overhead	10
Range of motion	
Flexion	6
Extension	3
Abduction (coronal plane)	6
External rotation	5
Internal rotation	5
Radiograph	10
Maximum score	100
Patient satisfaction with outcome	Yes/No

Data from Neer CS II. Displaced proximal humeral fractures. I. Classification and evaluation. J Bone Joint Surg Am 1970;52:1077–1089.

system was modified by Neer et al[41] and Cofield[42] in the scoring of pain and strength, each on a 0 to 5 scale, and assessment of range of motion, which focused on active elevation, external rotation, and internal rotation. The modified Neer system considers an outcome excellent if the patient has slight or no pain, is satisfied with the treatment, and has at least 140° of active elevation and at least 45° of external rotation.[43] The outcome is considered satisfactory if the patient has no, slight, or moderate pain with strenuous activity only; is satisfied with treatment; and has at least 90° of elevation and at least 20° of external rotation. The outcome is considered unsatisfactory if any of these criteria are not met or if the patient undergoes an additional operative procedure. Although the modified Neer system continues to stratify outcomes according to excellent, satisfactory, and unsatisfactory results, it no longer assigns point values to the overall outcome.

American Shoulder and Elbow Surgeons Standardized Shoulder Assessment and Shoulder Score Index

The American Shoulder and Elbow Surgeons (ASES) adopted the ASES Standardized Shoulder Assessment in an attempt to create a universal method for evaluating shoulder function (Table 1–3).[44] The ASES assessment is composed of a patient self-evaluation section and a physician assessment section. The patient self-evaluation contains 10-point visual analogue scales (VASs) for pain and instability and a 10-item questionnaire to assess ADL. ADL is evaluated on a 4-point ordinal scale that can be summed to determine a cumulative ADL index.

TABLE 1–3 American Shoulder and Elbow Surgeons (ASES) Score and Shoulder Score Index (SSI)

Pain
  Are you having pain in the shoulder? — Yes/No
  Do you have pain in the shoulder at night? — Yes/No
  Do you take narcotic pain medication? — Yes/No
  How many pills do you take each day? — Yes/No

How bad is your pain today (mark line)?

0						10
No pain		5				Pain as bad as it can be

Subjective instability
  Does your shoulder feel unstable
    (as if it is going to dislocate)? — Yes/No

How unstable is your shoulder (mark line)?

0						10
Very stable		5				Very unstable

	Right Arm	Left Arm
Put on a coat	0 1 2 3	0 1 2 3
Sleep on affected side	0 1 2 3	0 1 2 3
Wash back/do up bra	0 1 2 3	0 1 2 3
Toileting	0 1 2 3	0 1 2 3
Comb hair	0 1 2 3	0 1 2 3
Reach high shelf	0 1 2 3	0 1 2 3
Lift 10 lbs above shoulder	0 1 2 3	0 1 2 3
Throw ball overhand	0 1 2 3	0 1 2 3
Work	0 1 2 3	0 1 2 3
Sports	0 1 2 3	0 1 2 3

Cumulative ADL score: _____/30

Activity (0 = Unable; 1 = Very difficult; 2 = Somewhat difficult; 3 = Not difficult)

	Right Arm		Left Arm	
Range of Motion	Active	Passive	Active	Passive
Forward elevation	___°	___°	___°	___°
External rotation (arm at side)	___°	___°	___°	___°
External rotation (arm at 90° abduction)	___°	___°	___°	___°
Internal rotation:				
Cross-body adduction: _____				
Physical findings/signs: _____				

Strength (0 = no contraction; 1 = flicker; 2 = movement with gravity eliminated; 3 = movement against gravity; 4 = movement against some resistance; 5 = normal power)

	Right	Left
Testing affected by pain?	Yes/No	Yes/No
Forward elevation	___/5	___/5
Abduction	___/5	___/5
External rotation (arm at side)	___/5	___/5
Internal rotation (arm at side)	___/5	___/5

Objective instability (0 = none; 1 = mild [0–1 cm translation]; 2 = moderate [1–2 cm translation or translates to glenoid rim]; 3 = severe [>2 cm translation or over glenoid rim])

	Right	Left
Anterior translation	0 1 2 3	0 1 2 3
Posterior translation	0 1 2 3	0 1 2 3
Inferior translation (sulcus sign)	0 1 2 3	0 1 2 3
Anterior apprehension	0 1 2 3	0 1 2 3
Reproduces symptoms?	0 1 2 3	0 1 2 3
Voluntary instability?	0 1 2 3	0 1 2 3
Relocation test positive?	0 1 2 3	0 1 2 3
Generalized ligamentous laxity?	0 1 2 3	0 1 2 3

Shoulder Score Index = [(10 − Pain VAS) × 5] + [(5/3) × Cumulative ADL score]

Data from Richards R, An K-N, Bigliani L, et al. A standardized method for the assessment of shoulder function. J Shoulder Elbow Surg 1994;3:347–352.

The physician assessment takes about 10 to 15 minutes to complete and evaluates active and passive range of motion, and physical findings such as tenderness and impingement, strength, and stability. The combination of the VAS score for pain (50%) and cumulative ADL index (50%) constitutes the Shoulder Score Index, which can be used for quantitative comparisons between studies. The self-evaluation section has the added benefits of not requiring the presence of a physician and taking only a few minutes to complete. A deficiency of the ASES assessment is that it does not evaluate overall patient satisfaction or subjective improvement with treatment. Experience with the Shoulder Score Index has shown that it may not be as sensitive to some shoulder disorders (instability) as others.[45]

The Constant Scoring System

The Constant Scoring System[46] was designed to be a simple method to evaluate shoulder function and to be sensitive to most shoulder problems (Table 1–4). The subjective section allows 15 points for pain and 20 points for ADLs, whereas the objective section allows 40 points for range of motion and 25 points for strength. The developers of the Constant score have demonstrated its reliability and validated the instrument by comparing normal individuals with symptomatic patients.[46] The Constant score decreases with age and varies with gender, so the scores should be age- and sex-adjusted. The assessment takes only a few minutes to complete but requires a spring balance or dynamometer for strength testing, which may not be readily available in many clinical practices. An additional limitation is that the Constant score may be insensitive to shoulder instability.[47] It should be noted that 65% of the score is allocated to objective measures, which may diminish the patient-based contribution to the score. Although not utilized as widely in the United States, the Constant Scoring System is used widely in Europe and has been adopted by the European Society for Surgery of the Shoulder and Elbow.

The UCLA Shoulder Rating Scales

The UCLA Shoulder Assessment was created to assess the outcome for total shoulder arthroplasty.[48] A modification of this scoring system, the UCLA End-Result Score (UCLA score) was used to evaluate rotator cuff repair (Table 1–5).[49] Considered more detailed and easier to use in terms of assessment of range of motion and strength, the UCLA score is more widely accepted and utilized than its earlier version. Out of a possible 35 points, the score includes up to 10 points each for pain and function, and up to 5 points each for range of active forward elevation, strength of forward elevation,

TABLE 1–4 Constant Shoulder Scoring System

	Points
Pain	
None	15
Mild	10
Moderate	5
Severe	0
Activities of daily living	
Activity	
Work	Up to 4 points
Recreation/sports	Up to 4 points
Sleep	Up to 2 points
Positioning	
Up to waist	2
Up to xiphoid	4
Up to neck	6
Up to top of head	8
Above head	0
Active range of motion	
Forward elevation	
0–30°	0
31–60°	2
61–90°	4
91–120°	6
121–150°	8
151–180°	10
Lateral elevation	
0–30°	0
31–60°	2
61–90°	4
91–120°	6
121–150°	8
151–180°	10
External rotation	
Hand behind head with elbow flexed	2
Hand behind head with elbow held back	4
Hand on top of head with elbow held forward	6
Hand on top of head with elbow held back	8
Full elevation from on top of head	10
Internal rotation	
Dorsum of hand to lateral thigh	0
Dorsum of hand to buttock	2
Dorsum of hand to lumbosacral junction	4
Dorsum of hand to waist (third lumbar vertebra)	6
Dorsum of hand to twelfth dorsal vertebra	8
Dorsum of hand to interscapular region (seventh dorsal vertebra)	10
Power: _____ lbs	25
Maximum score	100

Data from Constant CR, Murley AH. A clinical method of functional assessment of the shoulder. Clin Orthop 1987;214:160–164.

and patient satisfaction. This scoring system primarily emphasizes pain and function. The overall score is stratified as excellent (34 to 35 points), good (29 to 33 points), or poor (28 points or less). The UCLA assessment is simple to use, takes only a few minutes to complete, and incorporates patient satisfaction into the evaluation; however, it does not test external and internal

TABLE 1–5 UCLA Shoulder Score

	Points
Pain	
Present all of the time and unbearable; strong medication frequently	1
Present all of the time but bearable; strong medication occasionally	2
None or little at rest, present during light activities; NSAIDs frequently	4
Present during heavy or particular activities only; NSAIDs occasionally	6
Occasional and slight	8
None	10
Function	
Unable to use limb	1
Only light activities possible	2
Able to do light housework or most ADLs	4
Most housework, shopping, and driving possible; able to do hair and dress and undress, including fastening brassiere	6
Slight restriction only; able to work above shoulder level	8
Normal activities	10
Active forward flexion	
150° or more	5
120 to 150°	4
90 to 120°	3
45 to 90°	2
30 to 45°	1
Less than 30°	0
Strength of forward flexion (manual muscle-testing)	
Grade 5 (normal)	5
Grade 4 (good)	4
Grade 3 (fair)	3
Grade 2 (poor)	2
Grade 1 (muscle contraction)	1
Grade 0 (nothing)	0
Satisfaction of the patient	
Satisfied and better	5
Not satisfied and worse	0
Overall score	___ (out of 35)

NSAIDs, nonsteroidal antiinflammatory drugs.
Data from Ellman H, Hanker G, Bayer M. Repair of the rotator cuff: end-result study of factors influencing reconstruction. J Bone Joint Surg Am 1986;68:1136–1144.

rotation range of motion or strength. Patient satisfaction is allotted only 5 of the possible 35 points, which underemphasizes this component of the assessment. Moreover, because the score is based on only 35 points, minor alterations in any of the parameters could disproportionately affect the overall score.

Shoulder Severity Index

The Shoulder Severity Index (SSI), also called the Severity Index for Chronically Painful Shoulders, was developed to assess patients with painful, chronic shoulder disabilities.[50] Through mathematical formulas, the SSI allocates 30 points to pain, 40 points to function, 15 points to strength, and 15 points to a VAS for daily handicap. Adjustments are then made for chronically painful

shoulders, and for elderly patients with limited activity or prosthetic replacement. The significance of the SSI is that it was one of the first outcomes instruments to evaluate pain in different situations of daily life, and assess function according to specific daily activities. This complicated system has largely been supplanted by simpler instruments.

Simple Shoulder Test

The Simple Shoulder Test (SST) was designed to be a quick and easy shoulder assessment instrument that is sensitive to a wide range of shoulder problems (Table 1–6).[4] The SST has proven useful in the assessment of primary glenohumeral degenerative joint disease, and has used to demonstrate the effectiveness of shoulder arthroplasty in treating this condition.[51,52] The SST consists of 12 "yes" or "no" questions derived from common complaints of patients presenting to the University of Washington Shoulder Service with a variety of shoulder problems. The limitations of the SST are that it provides little information on the severity of symptoms, it does not ask about overall patient satisfaction with treatment, and, because there is no scoring system, it makes comparisons among patients and treatments difficult. The creators of the SST advocate its use as a minimal data set of functional information that can be gathered quickly in any type of practice, as well as an efficient means of

TABLE 1–6 Simple Shoulder Test

(Answer "Yes" or "No" to each)
1. Is your shoulder comfortable with your arm at rest by your side?
2. Does your shoulder allow you to sleep comfortably?
3. Can you reach the small of your back to tuck in your shirt with your hand?
4. Can you place your hand behind your head with the elbow straight out to the side?
5. Can you place a coin on a shelf at the level of your shoulder without bending your elbow?
6. Can you lift 1 pound (say, a full pint container) to the level of your shoulder without bending your elbow?
7. Can you lift 8 pounds (say, a full gallon container) to the level of the top of your head without bending your elbow?
8. Can you carry 20 pounds (say, a bag of potatoes) at your side with the affected extremity?
9. Can you toss a softball underhand 10 yards or more with the affected extremity?
10. Can you throw a softball overhand 20 yards or more with the affected extremity?
11. Can you wash the back of your opposite shoulder with the affected extremity?
12. Would your shoulder allow you to work full-time at your regular job?

Data from Matsen F III, Smith K. Effectiveness evaluation and the shoulder. In: Harryman D II, ed. The Shoulder, 2nd ed. Philadelphia: WB Saunders, 1998:1313–1341.

follow-up for patients who can perform the evaluation by themselves. Additional questions tailored to the individual patient may then be asked by the clinician.

Disabilities of the Arm, Shoulder, and Hand Instrument

The Disabilities of the Arm, Shoulder, and Hand (DASH) Instrument began as a joint initiative of the AAOS, the Council of Musculoskeletal Specialty Societies (COMSS), and the Institute for Work and Health (Toronto, Ontario, Canada) (Table 1–7).[53,54] The DASH instrument is a validated questionnaire intended to measure upper extremity symptoms and functional status during the preceding week, with a focus on physical function.[54,55] The main component of the DASH instrument is the disability/symptom section, which consists of 30 questions, each with five response choices that range from "no difficulty" or "no symptom" (0 points) to "unable to perform activity" or "very severe symptom" (5 points). The scores for all items are then used to calculate a scaled disability/symptom score ranging from 0 (no disability) to 100 (severest disability) (Table 1–7). Two optional modules, each consisting of four questions, can be used to identify specific difficulties that athletes/artists or other groups of workers might experience but that may remain undetected by the disability/symptom section because these limitations may not affect their ADLs. The DASH is the upper extremity module of the MODEMS program, which was intended to establish a national database for outcomes research. The DASH is intended to be used by clinicians in daily practice. The questionnaire can be self-administered, and takes about 15 minutes to complete.

■ Other Outcomes Instruments

Hawkins et al[56–58] has evaluated functional outcome after proximal humerus fractures by measuring the ability to perform 11 different ADLs. For each ADL, the patient assigns a value from 0 to 4 in decreasing order of difficulty: 0 indicates an inability to perform the task, whereas 4 indicates normal ability. The total score is then averaged for the 11 tasks. A good outcome is an average score of 3.5 or more; a fair outcome, 2.5 to 3.4; and a poor outcome, less than 2.5.

The Hospital for Special Surgery (HSS) shoulder scoring system was designed to evaluate outcomes in patients with rheumatoid arthritis after total shoulder arthroplasty, although it has never been validated for this purpose.[59] The HSS score assesses pain, function, power, and range of motion on a 100-point scale.

Outcomes are stratified as follows: an excellent outcome is a score from 85 to 100 points; a good outcome, 70 to 84; a fair outcome, 50 to 69; and failure, less than 50 points.

Koval et al[60] devised their own outcomes assessment to evaluate 104 patients with one-part proximal humerus fractures treated nonoperatively with a period of sling immobilization and early range of motion. Pain was graded in increasing severity on a 0 to 4 scale, with 0 indicating no pain and 4 indicating totally disabling pain. Functional ability was assessed by determining the degree of difficulty with 15 ADLs. Each task was graded on a 0 to 4 scale, with 4 indicating complete independence with the task and 0 indicating complete dependence on another individual to perform the task; the total functional score was then divided by 60 (the total possible points) to establish a percentage of function. Assessment of range of motion in forward elevation, internal rotation, and external rotation, was expressed as a percentage by comparison to the range of motion of the uninjured shoulder.

■ General Health Status Instruments

General health status instruments assess all domains of human activity, including physical, psychological, social, and role functioning. They assess the patient as a whole from the patient's perspective. They do not refer to the specific disability or disease that is causing compromised health. The four most common general health status instruments are the Short Form-36, the Sickness Impact Profile, the Nottingham Health Profile, and the Quality of Well-Being Scale (a part of the Quality Adjusted Life Years methodology). All have been validated and are reproducible, internally consistent, and sensitive to changes in health status over time. Unfortunately, studies on outcomes of proximal humerus fractures have universally not included general health status as part of the evaluation. However, more recently, inclusion of general health status assessment has become more commonplace.

Short Form-36

The Short Form-36 (SF-36) is the most widely used general health status instrument.[61] It measures eight aspects of health: comfort or pain, energy or fatigue, physical function, physical role function, psychological role function, social role function, mental health, and general health perceptions (Table 1–8). Two summary measures can then be constructed: the physical component summary and the mental component summary. Each parameter is scored individually out of 100 points. The instrument takes

TABLE 1–7 Disabilities of the Arm, Shoulder, Hand (DASH) Questionnaire

This questionnaire asks about your symptoms as well as your ability to perform certain activities. Please answer every question, based on your condition in the last week, by circling the appropriate number. If you did not have the opportunity to perform an activity in the past week, please make your best estimate on which response would be the most accurate. It doesn't matter which hand or arm you use to perform the activity; please answer based on your ability regardless of how you perform the task.

Please rate your ability to do the following activities in the past week by circling the number below the appropriate response:

	No Difficulty	Mild Difficulty	Moderate Difficulty	Severe Difficulty	Unable
1. Open a tight or new jar	1	2	3	4	5
2. Write	1	2	3	4	5
3. Turn a key	1	2	3	4	5
4. Prepare a meal	1	2	3	4	5
5. Push open a heavy door	1	2	3	4	5
6. Place an object on a shelf above your head	1	2	3	4	5
7. Do heavy household chores (e.g., wash walls, wash floors)	1	2	3	4	5
8. Garden or do yard work	1	2	3	4	5
9. Make a bed	1	2	3	4	5
10. Carry a shopping bag or briefcase	1	2	3	4	5
11. Carry a heavy object (over 10 lbs)	1	2	3	4	5
12. Change a light bulb overhead	1	2	3	4	5
13. Wash or blow-dry your hair	1	2	3	4	5
14. Wash your back	1	2	3	4	5
15. Put on a pullover sweater	1	2	3	4	5
16. Use a knife to cut food	1	2	3	4	5
17. Recreational activities that require little effort (e.g., card playing, knitting, etc.)	1	2	3	4	5
18. Recreational activities in which you take some force or impact through your arm, shoulder, or hand (e.g., golf, hammering, tennis, etc.)	1	2	3	4	5
19. Recreational activities in which you move your arm freely (e.g., playing Frisbee, badminton, etc.)	1	2	3	4	5
20. Manage transportation needs (getting from one place to another)	1	2	3	4	5
21. Sexual activities	1	2	3	4	5
	Not at All	Slightly	Moderately	Quite a Bit	Extremely
22. During the past week, to what extent has your arm, shoulder, or hand problem interfered with your normal social activities with family, friends, neighbors or groups?	1	2	3	4	5
	Not Limited at All	Slightly Limited	Moderately Limited	Very Limited	Unable
23. During the past week, were you limited in your work or other daily activities as a result of your arm, shoulder, or hand problem?	1	2	3	4	5
	None	Mild	Moderate	Severe	Extreme
24. Arm, shoulder, or hand pain	1	2	3	4	5
25. Arm, shoulder, or hand pain when you perform any specific activity	1	2	3	4	5
26. Tingling (pins and needles) in your arm, shoulder, or hand	1	2	3	4	5
27. Weakness in your arm, shoulder, or hand	1	2	3	4	5
28. Stiffness in your arm, shoulder, or hand	1	2	3	4	5

TABLE 1–7 *(Continued)*

	No Difficulty	Mild Difficulty	Moderate Difficulty	Severe Difficulty	Unable
29. During the past week, how much difficulty have you had sleeping because of the pain in your arm, shoulder, or hand?	1	2	3	4	5

	Strongly Disagree	Disagree	Neither Agree nor Disagree	Agree	Strongly Agree
30. I feel less capable, less confident, or less useful because of my arm, shoulder, or hand problem	1	2	3	4	5

Disability/symptom score = [(sum of *n* responses)/*n* – 1] × 25, where *n* = number of completed response.

A DASH score may *not* be calculated if there are more than three missing items.

Work Module (Optional)

The following questions ask about the impact of your arm, shoulder, or hand problem on your ability to work (including homemaking if that is your main work role).

Please indicate what your job/work is: _____

I do not work. (You may skip this section.)

Please circle the number that bests describes your physical ability in the past week. Did you have any difficulty:

	No Difficulty	Mild Difficulty	Moderate Difficulty	Severe Difficulty	Unable
1. Using your usual technique for your work?	1	2	3	4	5
2. Doing your usual work because of arm, shoulder, or hand pain?	1	2	3	4	5
3. Doing your work as well as you would like?	1	2	3	4	5
4. Spending your usual amount of time doing your work?	1	2	3	4	5

Work disability score = [(sum of responses/4) – 1] × 25

An optional module score may *not* be calculated if there are any missing items.

Sports/Musical Instrument Module (Optional)

The following questions relate to the impact of your arm, shoulder, or hand problem on playing your musical instrument or sport or both. If you play more than one sport or instrument (or play both), please answer with respect to the activity that is most important to you.

Please indicate the sport or instrument that is most important to you: _____

I do not play a sport or instrument. (you may skip this section.)

Please circle the number that best describes your physical ability in the past week. Did you have any difficulty:

	No Difficulty	Mild Difficulty	Moderate Difficulty	Severe Difficulty	Unable
1. Using your usual technique for playing your instrument or sport?	1	2	3	4	5
2. Playing your usual musical instrument or sport because of arm, shoulder, or hand pain?	1	2	3	4	5
3. Playing your usual musical instrument or sport as well as you would like?	1	2	3	4	5
4. Spending your usual amount of time practicing or playing your instrument or sport?	1	2	3	4	5

Sports/musical instrument disability score = [(sum of responses/4) – 1] × 25

An optional module score may *not* be calculated if there are any missing items.

Data from Hudak PL, Amadio PC, Bombardier C. Development of an upper extremity outcome measure: the DASH (disabilities of the arm, shoulder and hand) [corrected]. The Upper Extremity Collaborative Group (UECG). Am J Ind Med 1996;29:602–608.

TABLE 1–8 The MOS 36-Item Short-Form Health Survey

1. In general, would you say your health is:	Excellent		1
	Very good		2
	Good		3
	Fair		4
	Poor		5
2. *Compared with 1 year ago*, how would you rate your health in general now?	Somewhat better now than 1 year ago		2
	About the same		3
	Somewhat worse now than 1 year ago		4
	Much worse now than 1 year ago		5

3. The following questions are about activities you might do during a typical day. Does your health limit you in these activities? If so, how much?

	Yes, Limited a Lot	Yes, Limited a Little	No, Not Limited at All
a. Vigorous activities, such as running, lifting heavy objects, participating in strenuous sports	1	2	3
b. Moderate activities, such as moving a table, pushing a vacuum cleaner, bowling, or playing golf	1	2	3
c. Lifting or carrying groceries	1	2	3
d. Climbing several flights of stairs	1	2	3
e. Climbing one flight of stairs	1	2	3
f. Bending, kneeling, or stooping	1	2	3
g. Walking more than one mile	1	2	3
h. Walking several blocks	1	2	3
i. Bathing and dressing yourself	1	2	3

4. During the *past month*, have you had any of the following problems with your work or other regular daily activities *as a result of your physical health*?

	Yes	No
a. Cut down on the amount of time you spent on work or other activities	1	2
b. Accomplished less than you would like	1	2
c. Were limited in the kind of work or other activities	1	2
d. Had difficulty performing the work or other activities (e.g., it took extra effort)	1	2

5. During the *past month*, have you had any of the following problems with your work or other regular daily activities as a result of any emotional problems (e.g., feeling depressed or anxious)?

	Yes	No
a. Cut down on the amount of time you spent on work or other activities	1	2
b. Accomplished less than you would have liked	1	2
c. Didn't do work or other activities as carefully as usual	1	2

6. During the *past month*, to what extent have your physical health or emotional problems interfered with your normal social activities with family, friends, neighbors, or groups?	Not at all	1
	Slightly	2
	Moderately	3
	Quite a bit	4
	Extremely	5
7. How much *body* pain have you had during the *past month*?	None	1
	Very mild	2
	Mild	3
	Severe	4
	Very severe	5
8. During the past month, how much did pain interfere with your normal work (including work both outside the home and housework)?	Not at all	1
	A little	2
	Moderately	3
	Quite a bit	4
	Extremely	5

TABLE 1–8 *(Continued)*

9. These questions are about how you feel and how things have been with you *during the past month*. For each question, please indicate the one answer that comes closest to the way you have been feeling. How much of the time *during the past month*:

	All of the Time	Most of the Time	A Good Bit of the Time	Some of the Time	A Little of the Time	None of the Time
a. Did you feel full of pep?	1	2	3	4	5	6
b. Have you been a very nervous person?	1	2	3	4	5	6
c. Have you felt so down in the dumps nothing could cheer you up?	1	2	3	4	5	6
d. Have you felt calm and peaceful?	1	2	3	4	5	6
e. Did you have a lot of energy?	1	2	3	4	5	6
f. Have you felt downhearted and blue?	1	2	3	4	5	6
g. Did you feel worn out?	1	2	3	4	5	6
h. Have you been a happy person?		1	2	3	4	5
i. Did you feel tired?	1	2	3	4	5	6
j. Has your health limited your social activities (like visiting your friends or close relatives)?	1	2	3	4	5	6

10. Please choose the answer that best describes how true or false each of the following statements is for you.

	Definitely True	Mostly True	Not Sure	Mostly False	Definitely False
a. I seem to get sick a little easier than other people	1	2	3	4	5
b. I am as healthy as anybody I know	1	2	3	4	5
c. I expect my health to get worse	1	2	3	4	5
d. My health is excellent	1	2	3	4	5

11. Please answer YES or NO for each question.

	Yes	No
a. In the past year, have you had 2 weeks or more during which you felt sad, blue, or depressed; or when you lost all interest or pleasure in things you usually care about or enjoyed?	1	2
b. Have you had 2 years or more in your life when you felt depressed or sad most days, even if you felt okay sometimes?	1	2
c. Have you felt depressed or sad much of the time in the past year?	1	2

Data from Ware JE Jr, Sherbourne CD. The MOS 36-item short-form health survey (SF-36). I. Conceptual framework and item selection. Med Care 1992;30:473–483.

about 5 to 10 minutes to complete and can be self-administered by the patient (in the office or at home), or administered by an interviewer in person or by telephone, increasing the yield of responses. Based on results from population-based control groups, the SF-36 parameters decrease with age, so results must be age-adjusted. The SF-36 has been used to study the effects of various shoulder conditions on patients' perceptions of their general health status. Because of its wide use, the SF-36 can also be used to compare the impact of orthopaedic conditions on general health perception with the impact of other medical conditions. Gartsman et al[62] demonstrated a significant decrease in general health status using the SF-36 in five common shoulder conditions (anterior instability, rotator cuff tear, adhesive capsulitis, glenohumeral degenerative joint disease, and impingement). Interestingly, the impact of these shoulder conditions on general health perception ranks in severity with that for hypertension, congestive heart failure, acute myocardial infarction,

diabetes mellitus, and depression. The SF-36 has also been used to assess the effects of treatments on general health status.[52] Unfortunately, unless patients have used the SF 36 for unrelated medical problems, those who suffer proximal humerus fractures usually do not have the opportunity to use the SF-36 before their unexpected injury. The SF-36 does not correlate well with shoulder-specific instruments for various shoulder disorders, which confirms the need to use both shoulder-specific and general health status instruments to evaluate patients with shoulder disorders.[24]

■ Other General Health Status Instruments

The Sickness Impact Profile (SIP) is a 136-item questionnaire containing 12 domains with "yes" or "no" responses.[63] The 12 domains are scored separately and combined into physical and psychological subscales. It has been used in musculoskeletal trauma.[64] It is best administered by trained interviewers and takes about 25 to 35 minutes to complete. The Nottingham Health Profile (NHP) consists of a 38-item questionnaire measuring subjective general health status and a list of seven statements with "yes" or "no" responses to measure the influence of health problems on daily life.[65] It has been used successfully to assess functional outcomes of limb salvage versus early amputation for complex lower extremity injuries.[66] It is administered by an interviewer and takes about 10 minutes to complete. Forming the basis for the Quality Adjusted Life Years (QALY) methodology, the Quality of Well-Being Scale (QWB) was developed to measure the effectiveness of treatments, which may then be used for policy analysis and resource allocation.[67] Administered over 6 days, the QWB involves questions regarding physical activity, mobility, social activity, and the one problem that has bothered the patient the most on the day the questionnaire is administered. Each session of questions takes about 10 to 15 minutes to complete. Using population data multiplied by years of life expectancy and cost per intervention, the QALY or cost per year of well life expectancy is calculated. The QALY can be viewed as a quantification of the benefit of a medical treatment relative to its cost, and can be used to compare treatments with a range of financial costs for a given disease. Compared with other medical treatments, shoulder and hip arthroplasty have performed well in the analysis.[45]

■ Review of Outcomes Literature for the Treatment of Proximal Humerus Fractures

The factors that affect outcome after proximal humerus fracture include the age of the patient, the type of fracture, and the type of treatment provided. The type of fracture is most commonly described using the classification described by Neer; the AO/Association for the Study of Internal Fixation (ASIF) classification is used less commonly. In the discussion that follows the outcome measure used for each study cited will be italicized. This will provide a sense of the different measures used.

Minimally Displaced (One-Part) Proximal Humerus Fractures

Approximately 85% of proximal humerus fractures are minimally displaced and are treated nonoperatively with good functional outcomes. Young and Wallace[68] utilized a *qualitative instrument* to evaluate outcomes in patients with proximal humerus fractures. Patients who were pain free,

satisfied with their shoulder function, able to place the hand above the head and behind the neck, and able to abduct above 110° were classified as having good outcomes. Patients who had the same characteristics but could only abduct to 60° were classified as having acceptable outcomes. Finally, patients with any degree of pain and dissatisfaction were classified as having poor outcomes. Ninety-seven percent of patients (33 of 34 patients) with minimally displaced fractures had good or acceptable outcomes at 6 months with nonoperative treatment and physical therapy; one patient had a poor outcome because of limited range of motion but was pain free. The authors noted that good outcomes are more likely when physical therapy is started early. Kristiansen and Christensen[26] reported excellent or good outcomes in 45 of 48 patients with minimally displaced fractures at an average of 2 years using *Neer's scoring system.* Using *their own instrument,* Koval et al[60] reported excellent or good results in 80 of 104 patients at an average of 41 months. The authors suspected that the inferior outcomes in their study might have been due to the use of a more detailed assessment of functional outcome than had been used in previous investigations. Despite the lower overall scores, 90% of patients still had mild or no pain; functional recovery averaged 94%; and patients regained 88% range of motion compared with the uninjured shoulder. The percentage of good and excellent outcomes was significantly greater in patients who had started supervised physical therapy less than 14 days after the injury.

Two-Part Proximal Humerus Fractures

Using an outcomes assessment involving an *18-point scale* that factors in pain, subjective opinions of the patient and physician, and range of motion, Jaberg et al[69] reported 62% excellent or good results at an average of 3 years' follow-up in a cohort of 48 patients with two-part surgical neck fractures treated with closed reduction and percutaneous pinning. The fair results were due predominantly to the patients' subjective symptoms and decreased range of motion. Cuomo et al,[70] using *their own measure,* evaluated pain, patient satisfaction, range of motion, and strength to assess functional outcome in 14 patients at an average of 3.3 years following two-part surgical neck fractures treated with limited ORIF using interfragmentary sutures or wire with the addition of Enders nails if comminution was present. They reported excellent or good results in 71% of patients. Using the same criteria to assess outcome in patients with two-part greater tuberosity fractures, the same authors reported excellent or good outcomes at an average of 5 years' follow-up in a small series of 12 patients treated with ORIF with heavy, nonabsorbable suture, rotator cuff repair, and early passive motion.[71] All patients had mild or no pain. Moda et al[27] reported on six two-part surgical neck fractures treated with blade plates made from modified AO semitubular plates. All patients achieved excellent or satisfactory *Neer scores*. In a series of 97 patients at least 50 years old with displaced two-part surgical neck fractures, Court-Brown et al[28] found that outcome using the *Neer score* was significantly correlated with age of the patient and degree of initial displacement of the fracture; poorer outcomes occurred in older patients and in those with greater initial displacement. The average Neer score at 1 year of follow-up was 78.9. It was interesting that in the subgroup of patients with at least 67% displacement/translation, there was no difference in Neer score between patients treated operatively and nonoperatively. In patients younger than 50 years, the Neer score was uniformly satisfactory to excellent.

Three- and Four-Part Proximal Humerus Fractures and Fracture-Dislocations

Most reports on treatment outcomes of three- and four-part proximal humerus fractures discuss operative results; however, Zyto[72] in 1998 reported the outcomes of nonoperative treatment in 12 elderly patients with a minimum of 10 years' follow-up. The mean *Constant scores* for the three- and four-part fracture groups were 59 and 47, respectively. Despite these low functional scores, all patients reported mild or no pain and all but four patients had mild or no disability. One patient developed severe osteoarthritis and two developed osteonecrosis. All patients in this small series were accepting of their shoulder condition. In a prospective, randomized trial of 40 patients comparing nonoperative treatment to tension-band wiring in three- and four-part fractures, Zyto et al[23] reported comparable results in terms of pain, range of motion, power, and ADLs. Mean *Constant scores* were 65 for the nonoperatively treated patients and 60 for those who underwent ORIF; however, only the operative group developed complications (one case each of osteonecrosis and nonunion). Comparing nonoperative treatment, ORIF, and hemiarthroplasty for three- and four-part fractures, Zyto et al[29] reported a discrepancy between *Neer and Constant scores*. Patients tended to score better using the Constant system compared with the Neer system. Thirty-four patients had mild or no disability according to the Constant score but only 19 had excellent or satisfactory outcomes according to the Neer score; on the other hand, 16 patients were classified as unsatisfactory or failures according to the Neer score, but only one patient had moderate to severe disability according to the Constant score. Comparing the scores with the opinions of the patients, the authors found that the Constant score more accurately assessed the subjective outcome and considered the Constant score to be more useful in elderly patients because it takes into account age and sex of the patient. In a similar study, Schai et al[73] reported that functional outcome

utilizing the *Constant score* in patients with three-part fractures was superior with operative treatment than nonoperative treatment, that four-part fracture outcomes were better following arthroplasty than nonoperative treatment or ORIF, and that three-part fracture outcomes were better than those of four-part fractures. Patients with three-part fractures treated with minimal internal fixation or ORIF had Constant scores of 83 and 91, respectively, while those with four-part fractures treated with hemiarthroplasty or ORIF had Constant scores of 74 and 52, respectively. Nonoperative treatment resulted in Constant scores of 78 for three-part fractures and 54 for four-part fractures.

Using *his own outcomes instrument,* Neer reported 63% excellent or satisfactory results in a cohort of 30 patients following three-part fractures treated with ORIF; this number increased to 86% when only patients treated with suture fixation of the tuberosities and cuff repair were included.[31] Four-part fractures treated with ORIF uniformly failed in 13 patients, but those treated with hemiarthroplasty resulted in excellent or satisfactory outcomes in 31 of 32 patients.

Using *his own outcome measure,* which included pain, functional recovery with ADLs, range of motion, and strength, Stableforth[21] prospectively compared the results of nonoperative treatment and hemiarthroplasty for four-part fractures. At a minimum of 18 months' follow-up, unsatisfactory outcomes were common following nonoperative treatment due to persistent pain in nine of 16 patients, functionally inadequate range of motion in eight patients, and difficulty with ADLs in nine patients. Patients fared better after hemiarthroplasty, with 11 out of 16 patients having mild or no pain, 14 being independent with ADLs, and most regaining functional range of motion and strength. In Willem and Lim's[30] series of 10 patients with four-part fractures treated with hemiarthroplasty, at an average of 2.5 years all but one patient was pain-free but only four had excellent or satisfactory *Neer scores*. Poor outcomes were usually due to limited range of motion, and the authors stressed the importance of postoperative rehabilitation. Using the *HSS scoring system,* Moeckel et al[74] reported excellent or good outcomes in 20 of 24 patients at an average of 3 years after hemiarthroplasty for three-part, four-part, and head-splitting fractures. Both age and the interval from the injury to surgery correlated inversely with outcome. Using the *UCLA rating scale* to evaluate two patients with three-part and 18 patients with four-part fractures treated with hemiarthroplasty, Hawkins and Switlyk[57] reported excellent and good outcomes in only eight cases. Despite these low outcome scores, 18 patients had good pain relief and 16 patients were satisfied with their treatment at an average of 40 months following surgery. Poor results were documented in patients who were noncompliant with postoperative rehabilitation and had poor rotator cuff integrity and limited active range of motion.

Goldman et al[75] evaluated the outcome of hemiarthroplasty in 22 patients with three- and four-part fractures using the *ASES assessment instrument*. Sixteen patients had slight or no pain, all patients had good to normal strength, and 20 patients had normal stability. Age over 70 years, female sex, and four-part fractures correlated with poor range of motion. Lifting, carrying a weight, and using the hand at or above shoulder level were the most common functional limitations. The authors concluded that hemiarthroplasty for three- and four-part fractures can be expected to result in pain-free shoulders, but recovery of range of motion and function were less predictable. Dimakopoulos et al[32] reported similar outcomes for pain relief following hemiarthroplasty in 38 patients, but reported better range of motion and function at 1 year utilizing continuous stretching and strengthening exercises. Zyto et al[76] reported disappointing *Constant scores* after hemiarthroplasty for three- and four-part fractures. At an average of 39 months' follow-up, the median Constant scores were 51 and 46, respectively. Nine of the 17 patients had moderate or severe pain, and eight had moderate or severe disability. Movin et al[77] reported similar disappointing results with hemiarthroplasty or total shoulder arthroplasty for both acute and late three- and four-part fractures in 29 patients. The mean *Constant score* at an average of 3 years following surgery was 38. Patients who underwent surgery within 3 weeks of injury had the same Constant score as those who were operated on later; the grouping of patients as long as 3 weeks postinjury into the acute group may have adversely affected the Constant score.

Becker et al[33] looked at both the *Neer and Constant scores* to assess outcome at a minimum of 1 year after hemiarthroplasty for four-part fractures in 27 patients. Most deductions were due to limited range of motion; because the Constant score places considerable emphasis on range of motion, the patients had a low mean Constant score of 45. The Neer score, on the other hand, places greater emphasis on pain; because 23 of the 27 patients had mild or no pain, the mean Neer score was a relatively high 89 points. Only four patients were dissatisfied with treatment because of intermittent pain and limited range of motion, demonstrating that the overall outcome of this particular study seemed to be better represented by the Neer score than the Constant score. The authors found that a delay in surgery worsened the outcome. In their series of 39 patients at an average of 42 months following hemiarthroplasty for three- and four-part fractures, Bosch et al[78] reported excellent or good results in 20%, 28%, 48%, and 72% of patients using the *UCLA, Constant, HSS, and VAS scores*, respectively; mean scores were 24, 54, 67, and 74, respectively. Eighty percent of patients, however, were satisfied

with the outcome, and all had satisfactory pain relief. The VAS scores correlated most closely with patient satisfaction. The authors stressed that early surgery resulted in much better outcomes, especially for range of motion.

In three-part fractures and in four-part fractures that occur in young patients, reduction and fixation of the fracture is usually preferred over hemiarthroplasty. Savoie et al[34] reported excellent and satisfactory *Neer scores* at an average of 2 years' follow-up in all nine of their patients with three-part fractures treated with ORIF using AO/ASIF buttress plating. All patients had mild or no pain and seven returned to work. Esser[79] treated three- and four-part fractures with ORIF using a modified cloverleaf plate. Twenty-four of 26 patients had good to excellent results based on evaluation with the *ASES assessment*. All patients were satisfied with the result and were pain free. Using the *Hawkins outcomes instrument,* Cornell et al[58] reported good outcomes at an average of 20 months' follow-up in 10 of 13 patients with two- and three-part fractures treated with a screw and tension band technique. All patients had mild or no pain. Using a blade plate for rigid internal fixation, Hintermann et al[80] utilized *their own outcomes criteria* to evaluate treatment of three- and four-part fractures. Excellent outcomes involved no pain and no limitation in ADLs; good outcomes involved mild or occasional pain, and slight limitation in ADLs; fair outcomes involved moderate or frequent pain and moderate limitation in ADLs; and poor outcomes involved severe or nearly constant pain and severe limitation in ADLs. According to these criteria, 24 of 31 patients with three-part fractures and six of seven patients with four-part fractures had good or excellent outcomes at an average of 3.4 years. Despite these good results, mean *Constant scores* for three- and four-part fractures were only 75 and 69, respectively. Pain was usually mild, and range of motion and power were acceptable to almost all of the patients. Osteonecrosis developed in two patients. In a review of 97 patients treated with ORIF, Szyszkowitz et al[35] reported 70% excellent and satisfactory *Neer scores* at an average of 42 months for three-part fractures, and 22% for four-part fractures. Patients treated with Kirschner wires (K-wires) or screws and cerclage wires had better outcomes than did those treated with plate fixation.

Using K-wires and tension band reinforcement, Darder et al[36] had excellent and satisfactory *Neer scores* in 21 of 33 patients with four-part fractures at an average of 7 years' follow-up. Despite 12 unsatisfactory outcomes based on the Neer score, all patients had good pain relief, and all except two returned to their usual daily activities and work. All cases of fracture-dislocation resulted in unsatisfactory or poor outcomes, and patients over 75 years of age obtained the worst results. Ko and

Yamamoto[37] reported excellent or satisfactory *Neer scores* at an average of 3.8 years in 14 of 16 patients treated with heavy suture or wire fixation combined with either threaded pins or external fixation for 12 three-part and 4 four-part fractures. Resch et al[81] performed percutaneous reduction and screw fixation in 9 three-part and 18 four-part fractures. At an average of 2 years' follow-up, all patients with three-part fractures had good to excellent outcomes, with an average *Constant score* of 91. Two cases of four-part fractures required revision to prostheses because of osteonecrosis and redisplacement of the fracture, respectively. In the remaining 16 cases, the outcomes were good, with an average Constant score of 87. Thirteen of the four-part fractures, however, were valgus impacted patterns, which have better prognoses. Hessmann et al[38] retrospectively reviewed a cohort of 98 patients consisting of 50 two-part, 37 three-part, and 6 four-part proximal humerus fractures, and 5 three- or four-part fracture-dislocations, treated with indirect reduction and buttress plate fixation. Based on the *Neer, Constant, and UCLA scores,* this cohort of patients respectively had 59%, 69%, and 76% good to excellent outcomes at a minimum of 2 years. Eighty-five percent of the patients were satisfied with their result, while the remainder were unsatisfied because of either pain or loss of range of motion secondary to various complications.

Special consideration should be given to valgus impacted proximal humerus fractures because of their different prognoses, treatment, and functional outcome. In Jakob et al's[39] series of 19 patients with four-part valgus impacted fractures, 74% of patients had excellent or satisfactory *Neer scores* after either closed reduction or limited ORIF. Osteonecrosis occurred in 26% of the cases and accounted for all of the poor outcomes. Union occurred in all patients. In a later review of 125 patients with AO B1.1 valgus impacted fractures treated nonoperatively with 2 weeks of immobilization, Court-Brown et al[40] reported 81% excellent or satisfactory *Neer scores* at an average follow-up of 1 year. The average Neer score for B1.1 valgus impacted fractures that were minimally displaced was 90.3, whereas average Neer scores for those associated with displacement of the greater tuberosity, surgical neck, or both, were 88.4, 84.3, and 81.3, respectively, suggesting worse functional outcome with more severe fractures. The authors recommended nonoperative treatment for all valgus impacted fractures. They did not report the incidence of osteonecrosis.

■ Summary of Outcomes Instruments in Proximal Humerus Fractures

As is evident from this literature review, currently utilized outcome scores contain shortcomings that may misrepresent patient perceptions of treatment

outcomes. In Zyto's[72] 1998 study on outcomes of nonoperative treatment in three- and four-part fractures, despite having low mean *Constant scores* of 59 and 47, respectively, all patients had mild or no pain, eight of 12 patients had mild or no disability, and all patients were accepting of their disability. Based on pain relief and ability to carry out ADLs, Hintermann et al[80] reported good or excellent subjective outcomes in 24 of 31 patients treated with ORIF for three-part and six of seven patients with four-part fractures, despite low mean *Constant scores* of 75 and 69, respectively. Although Hawkins and Switlyk[57] reported excellent and good *UCLA scores* in only eight of 20 patients treated with hemiarthroplasty for three- and four-part fractures, 18 out of the 20 patients had good pain relief and 16 patients were still satisfied with their treatment. In Darder et al's[36] study of tension-band wiring of four-part fractures, 12 patients had unsatisfactory *Neer scores,* yet all 33 patients in the study had good pain relief and all except two returned to usual daily activities and work. Patients may lack full range of motion and strength—objective measures that are often weighed heavily in outcomes instruments—yet remain satisfied with a pain-free shoulder and restoration of a functional range of motion. These examples demonstrate how currently utilized outcomes scores do not always correlate with patient perceptions of treatment outcomes.

Disparity exists among the various outcomes instruments because each one emphasizes different aspects of the evaluation; for example, one instrument may emphasize pain; another, range of motion; still another, functional capacity with ADLs. This disparity is particularly evident in studies that report multiple scoring systems. In Zyto et al's[29] comparison of nonoperative treatment, ORIF, and hemiarthroplasty for three- and four-part fractures, patients tended to score better using the *Constant system* compared with the *Neer system.* Thirty-four patients had mild or no disability according to the Constant score, but only 19 had excellent or satisfactory outcomes according to the Neer score. Furthermore, 16 patients were categorized as unsatisfactory or failures by the Neer system, but only one patient had moderate to severe disability according to the Constant system. Moreover, the authors found that the Constant score more closely reflected the subjective outcomes of the patients and concluded that the Constant score was more useful in elderly patients. In contrast to these results, Becker et al[33] found that the *Neer score* better represented the overall patient satisfaction than the *Constant score* in their study of hemiarthroplasty for four-part fractures. Although 23 of 27 patients had good pain relief, many had restricted range of motion, accounting for most of the deductions. Because the Constant score places considerable emphasis on range of motion, patients had a low mean Constant score of 45. On the other hand, because the Neer score places greater emphasis on pain, the Neer score was a relatively high 89 points. This result supports the premise that patients are frequently satisfied by good pain relief and restoration of at least a functional range of motion, despite having mild limitations in overall range of motion or strength. Using the *Neer score* to assess outcome following indirect reduction and internal fixation for two-, three-, and four-part fractures and fracture-dislocations, Hessmann[38] et al reported good to excellent results in only 59% of patients; when assessed with the *Constant and UCLA scores,* the percentage of good to excellent outcomes rose to 69% and 76%, respectively. Even greater disparities among outcome scores were found by Bosch et al[78] in their reporting of outcomes following hemiarthroplasty for three- and four-part fractures. Utilization of the *Constant and UCLA scores* resulted in good to excellent outcomes in only 28% and 20% of patients. When assessed with the *HSS and VAS scores,* the percentage of excellent or good outcomes rose to 48% and 72%, respectively. The disparity in outcomes of the four instruments reinforces the point that emphasis is placed on different aspects of the shoulder evaluation in each of the four instruments. These inherent differences in the various outcome measures contribute to their limited ability to make comparisons between studies and derive definitive conclusions regarding treatments.

■ Case Reports

Case 1

The patient is a 74-year-old right-hand dominant woman who complains of right shoulder pain after slipping in her bathroom and falling onto an outstretched right hand. On physical examination the patient was found to have moderate swelling and ecchymosis about her right shoulder. Palpation revealed tenderness around her proximal humerus. Range of motion was limited in all directions due to pain. Manipulation revealed slight crepitus of the shoulder. Neurologic examination revealed intact sensation in the axillary, radial, median, and ulnar nerve distributions. Motor examination demonstrated firing of the lateral deltoid. Radiographs demonstrated a surgical neck fracture of the right proximal humerus with 10° of varus angulation and 4 mm of medial translation. The patient was treated initially in a shoulder sling. At 12 days following the injury, the patient was started on a regimen of supervised physical therapy consisting of active range of motion exercises for the elbow, wrist, and hand, in combination with assisted passive range of motion exercises for the injured shoulder. The patient attended physical therapy sessions

twice each week and performed the exercises three times daily at home. At 5 weeks following the injury there was clinical and radiographic evidence of fracture union and the sling was discontinued. Active shoulder range of motion exercises and isometric deltoid and rotator cuff strengthening exercises were then begun. At 9 weeks following the injury, after achievement of good active shoulder motion, isotonic deltoid and rotator cuff strengthening exercises were initiated, followed by a more vigorous stretching program at 12 weeks.

Supervised physical therapy was continued for the next 2 months, and the patient was encouraged to continue with her exercises at home after this time. At 3 years following her injury, the patient was pain free and had no symptoms of instability; however, she continued to be unable to sleep on the affected shoulder. She had mild difficulty with reaching high on a shelf, clasping/unclasping her bra, combing her hair, and throwing a ball overhead. Examination of active and passive range of motion revealed forward elevation to 130°, external rotation at the side to 40°, and internal rotation to T12. Strength in all shoulder motions was 5/5, and she was able to hold a 10-pound weight with her affected shoulder in 90° of abduction. Radiographs demonstrated slight residual angulation but full union. Tables 1–9, 1–10, and 1–11 illustrate the patient's Neer, Constant, and ASES scores. With the Neer score weighing heavily pain and function, the patient scored an excellent outcome (90 points). In contrast, with its emphasis on the objective measures of range of motion and strength, her Constant score (73 points) reflected fair outcome. The shoulder score index of the ASES

TABLE 1–9 Neer Score of Case 1

		Points
Pain	None	35/35
Function		
Strength	Good	8/10
Reaching		
Top of head		1/2
Mouth		2/2
Belt buckle		2/2
Opposite axilla		2/2
Brassiere hook		1/2
Stability		
Lifting, throwing, pounding, pushing, hold overhead		10/10
Range of motion		
Flexion	130°	4/6
Extension	30°	2/3
Abduction (coronal plane)	140°	4/6
External rotation	40°	5/5
Internal rotation	T12	4/5
Radiograph	Union, no malunion	10/10
Overall score	Excellent	90/100
Patient satisfaction with outcome:		Yes

TABLE 1–10 Constant Score of Case 1

		Points
Pain	None	15/15
ADL		
Activity		
Work	Mild limitation	3/4
Recreation/sport	Mild limitation	3/4
Sleep	Unaffected	0/2
Positioning:		
behind head		8/10
Range of motion		
Forward elevation	130°	8/10
Lateral elevation	140°	8/10
External rotation:		8/10
hand behind head		
with elbow held back		
Internal rotation	T12	8/10
Power	10 pounds	10/25
Overall score	Fair	73/100

score weighs only the subjective measures of pain and function, and the patient scored a good outcome (83 points). Overall, the patient was satisfied with her treatment.

Case 2

The patient is a 58-year-old right-hand-dominant man who complains of right shoulder pain after falling off his bicycle during an amateur race. On physical exam, considerable swelling and ecchymosis was noted about his right shoulder and point tenderness over the proximal aspect of his right arm. There was crepitus on attempted range of motion, which was limited by pain and guarding. The patient had no neurologic deficits, and active firing of the deltoids could be elicited. Radiographs demonstrated a surgical neck fracture of the right proximal humerus with 50° of varus angulation and 2 cm of medial displacement, along with a greater tuberosity fracture with 1 cm of displacement. Closed reduction was attempted under conscious sedation in the emergency room, but residual angulation and displacement was noted on postreduction radiographs. At this point, the patient was taken to the operating room and open reduction with tension-band wiring was performed under general anesthesia. Intraoperative fluoroscopic imaging demonstrated anatomic reduction. Postoperatively, the patient was discharged with sling immobilization until the following day, when supervised active range of motion of the elbow, wrist, and hand and passive range of motion of the affected shoulder were started with a supervised physical therapy program. At 6 postoperative weeks, radiographs demonstrated fracture union and the sling was discontinued. Isometric deltoid and rotator cuff strengthening was then begun, along with active shoulder range of motion exercises. Good active shoulder motion was achieved at 9 weeks, at

TABLE 1–11 ASES Score and Shoulder Score Index (SSI) of Case 1

		Points
Pain:	None	VAS score: 0/10
Pain score: 0/10		
Subjective instability	Very stable	VAS score: 0/10
ADL		
Put on a coat	Not difficult	3/3
Sleep on affected side	Unable	0/3
Wash back/do up bra	Somewhat difficult	2/3
Toileting	Not difficult	3/3
Comb hair	Somewhat difficult	2/3
Reach high shelf	Somewhat difficult	2/3
Lift 10 lbs above shoulder	Somewhat difficult	2/3
Throw ball overhand	Somewhat difficult	2/3
Work	Somewhat difficult	2/3
Sports	Somewhat difficult	2/3
Cumulative ADL score: 20/30		
Active range of motion		
Forward elevation	130°	
External rotation (arm at side)	40°	
External rotation (arm at 90° abduction)	40°	
Internal rotation	T12	
Cross-body adduction	Opposite shoulder	
Passive range of motion		
Forward elevation	130°	
External rotation (arm at side)	40°	
External rotation (arm at 90° abduction), head with elbow held back	40°	
Internal rotation	T12	
Cross-body adduction	Opposite shoulder	
Physical findings/signs	Mild crepitus	
Strength		
Forward elevation		5/5
Abduction		5/5
External rotation (arm at side)		5/5
Internal rotation (arm at side)		5/5
Objective instability	None	

Shoulder Score Index = [(10 − Pain VAS) × 5] + [(5/3) × cumulative ADL score] = 50 + 33 = 83

which time resistive strengthening exercises were initiated and stretching was progressed. After the completion of supervised physical therapy sessions, the patient continued to perform his exercises at a gym near his home.

At the 3-year follow-up visit the patient was pain free and had no instability symptoms. With the exception of mild difficulty with such overhead sports as throwing, the patient had no difficulties with ADL, work, or other

TABLE 1–12 Neer Score of Case 2

		Points
Pain	None	35/35
Function		
Strength	Good	8/10
Reaching		
Top of head		2/2
Mouth		2/2
Belt buckle		2/2
Opposite axilla		2/2
Brassiere hook		2/2
Stability		
Lifting, throwing, pounding, pushing, hold overhead		10/10
Range of motion:		
Flexion	150°	4/6
Extension	35°	2/3
Abduction (coronal plane)	160°	4/6
External rotation	50°	3/5
Internal rotation	T10	4/5
Radiograph	Union, no malunion	10/10
Overall score	Excellent	90/100
Patient satisfaction with outcome	Yes	

recreational activities. Examination of active and passive range of motion revealed forward elevation to 150°, external rotation at the side to 50°, and internal rotation to T10. The patient was able to lift the full 25-pound weight with the affected arm abducted to 90° during strength testing for the Constant score, although strength was slightly less compared with the unaffected shoulder. X-rays demonstrated no malunion or osteonecrosis. Tables **1–12, 1–13,** and **1–14** show the Neer, Constant, and ASES scores for this patient at the most recent follow-up. In contrast to the patient in Case 1, who had an excellent Neer score but only a good Constant score and shoulder score index, the patient in Case 2 was rated an excellent result on all three scoring systems: Neer score 90 points, Constant score 91 points, and ASES shoulder score index 95 points. The higher Constant score compared with Case 1 can be attributed to the emphasis of the objective measure of strength,

TABLE 1–13 Constant Score of Case 2

		Points
Pain	None	15/15
ADL		
Activity:		
Work	Unaffected	4/4
Recreation/sport	Mild limitation	3/4
Sleep	Unaffected	2/2
Positioning	Above head	10/10
Range of motion:		
Forward elevation	150°	8/10
Lateral elevation	150°	8/10
External rotation: Hand behind head with elbow held back		8/10
Internal rotation	T10	8/10
Power:	25 pounds	25/25
Overall score	Excellent	91/100

TABLE 1–14 ASES Score and Shoulder Score Index (SSI) of Case 2

		Points
Pain	None	VAS score: 0/10
Pain score: 0/10		
Subjective instability	Very stable	VAS score: 0/10
ADL:		
Put on a coat	Not difficult	3/3
Sleep on affected side	Not difficult	3/3
Wash back/do up bra	Not difficult	3/3
Toileting	Not difficult	3/3
Comb hair	Not difficult	3/3
Reach high shelf	Somewhat difficult	2/3
Lift 10 lbs above shoulder	Not difficult	3/3
Throw ball overhand	Somewhat difficult	2/3
Work	Not difficult	3/3
Sports	Somewhat difficult	2/3
Cumulative ADL score: 27/30		
Active range of motion		
Forward elevation	150°	
External rotation (arm at side)	50°	
External rotation (arm at 90° abduction)	50°	
Internal rotation	T10	
Cross-body adduction	Opposite shoulder	
Passive range of motion:		
Forward elevation	150°	
External rotation (arm at side)	50°	
External rotation (arm at 90° abduction), head with elbow held back	50°	
Internal rotation	T10	
Cross-body adduction	Opposite shoulder	
Physical findings/signs	Scar	
Strength		
Forward elevation	5/5	
Abduction	5/5	
External rotation (arm at side)	5/5	
Internal rotation (arm at side)	5/5	
Objective instability	None	

Shoulder Score Index = [(10 − Pain VAS) × 5] + [(5/3) × cumulative ADL score] = 50 + 45 = 95

which was full for this patient. The additional 10 points elevated this patient's Constant score to excellent. The ability to perform ADLs explains the excellent ASES shoulder score index. Overall, he was quite satisfied with his outcome.

Case 3

A 69-year-old left-hand dominant woman presents with left shoulder pain and an inability to move her left shoulder after slipping and falling on her kitchen floor. Physical exam revealed an anterior prominence

TABLE 1–15 Neer Score of Case 3

		Points
Pain	Slight	30/35
Function		
Strength	Fair	6/10
Reaching		
Top of head		1/2
Mouth		2/2
Belt buckle		2/2
Opposite axilla		1/2
Brassiere hook		0/2
Stability		
Lifting, throwing, pounding, pushing, hold overhead		10/10
Range of motion		
Flexion	100°	2/6
Extension	20°	1/3
Abduction (coronal plane)	100°	2/6
External rotation	30°	3/5
Internal rotation	L2	3/5
Radiograph	Prosthesis well aligned, no radiolucencies	10/10
Overall score	Unsatisfactory	73/100
Patient satisfaction with outcome	Yes	

TABLE 1–16 Constant Score of Case 3

		Points
Pain	Mild	10/15
ADL		
Activity		
Work	Mild limitation	2/4
Recreation/sport	Mild limitation	2/4
Sleep	Unaffected	8/2
Positioning: top of head		6/10
Range of motion:		
Forward elevation	100°	6/10
Lateral elevation	100°	6/10
External rotation: hand on top of head with elbow held forward		6/10
Internal rotation	L2	6/10
Power	5 pounds	5/25
Overall score	Poor	51/100

and squaring-off of the posterolateral acromion. There was tenderness to palpation in the left proximal humerus and pain with attempted motion. Neurologic examination revealed decreased sensation in the lateral aspect of the shoulder. Radiographs demonstrated a four-part anterior fracture-dislocation of the proximal humerus. Under conscious sedation, an attempt at closed reduction was made in the emergency room but was unsuccessful. The decision was made to take the patient to the operating room, where she underwent hemiarthroplasty of the injured shoulder 36 hours after her initial injury. At the time of surgery, the long head of the biceps was found to be interposed between the fracture fragments. The patient wore a shoulder sling and on postoperative day 1 was started on a supervised physical therapy regimen involving active range of motion of the elbow, wrist, and hand, along with pendulum exercises for the affected shoulder. Passive assisted range of motion exercises were continued until union of the tuberosities was evident 6 weeks after the procedure. At this point, the sling was discontinued, active assisted range of motion exercises and isometric deltoid and rotator cuff exercises were initiated. Isotonic deltoid and rotator cuff strengthening was begun at 10 weeks postoperative, in combination with a more aggressive stretching program. Supervised physical therapy continued for the next 4 months, after which time the patient continued her exercises unsupervised at home.

At the 3-year follow-up visit, the patient reported only intermittent pain with heavy lifting or strenuous activity.

She had difficulty with ADLs, particularly involving overhead activity and lifting, but was able to remain independent in most activities. She had no subjective complaints of instability. Examination of active and passive range of motion revealed forward elevation to 100°, external rotation at the side to 30°, and internal rotation to L2. She had supraspinatus tenderness and a positive impingement sign. Strength testing demonstrated that she could hold a 5-pound weight while holding her shoulder in 90° of abduction. Radiographs demonstrated good alignment of the prosthesis and no evidence of loosening. Tables **1–15, 1–16,** and **1–17** show that the patient scored an unsatisfactory Neer score (73 points), a poor Constant score (51 points), and poor ASES shoulder score index (65 points). Despite these low functional scores, the patient accepted her mild degree of pain and, overall, was satisfied with her outcome. The scores of these three case examples are summarized in Table **1–18.**

■ Conclusion

Clinical assessment using objective measures, such as range of motion, strength, and radiographic union alone, often does not accurately reflect treatment outcome. Subjective, patient-oriented assessments must be added to the evaluation to obtain a full impression of the outcome. Outcomes research involves many methodologies to determine the effectiveness of treatments, but it relies most heavily on clinical research studies with clearly defined patient-oriented outcome measures. The ideal research tool is the prospective, randomized, controlled clinical trial with clearly defined end points for measurement and comparison. Unfortunately, few orthopaedic studies have adhered to this study design. This is particularly true in the area of proximal humerus fractures.

TABLE 1–17 ASES Score and Shoulder Score Index (SSI) of Case 3

		Points
Pain	None	VAS score: 2/10
Pain score: 2/10		
Subjective instability	Very stable	VAS score: 0/10
ADL		
Put on a coat	Somewhat difficult	2/3
Sleep on affected side	Somewhat difficult	2/3
Wash back/do up bra	Very difficult	1/3
Toileting	Somewhat difficult	2/3
Comb hair	Somewhat difficult	2/3
Reach high shelf	Very difficult	1/3
Lift 10 lbs above shoulder	Very difficult	1/3
Throw ball overhand	Unable	0/3
Work	Somewhat difficult	2/3
Sports	Somewhat difficult	2/3
Cumulative ADL score: 15/30		
Active range of motion		
Forward elevation	100°	
External rotation (arm at side)	30°	
External rotation (arm at 90° abduction)	30°	
Internal rotation	L2	
Cross-body adduction	Mid-chest	
Passive range of motion:		
Forward elevation	100°	
External rotation (arm at side)	30°	
External rotation (arm at 90° abduction), head with elbow held back	30°	
Internal rotation	L2	
Cross-body adduction	Mid-chest	
Physical findings/signs	Supraspinatus tenderness, impingement, mild crepitus, scar	
Strength		
Forward elevation	4+/5	
Abduction	4+/5	
External rotation (arm at side)	4+/5	
Internal rotation (arm at side)	5/5	
Objective instability	None	

Shoulder Score Index = [(10 – Pain VAS) × 5] + [(5/3) × cumulative ADL score] = 40 + 25 = 65

Based on the literature, the treatment of minimally displaced proximal humerus fractures is clear: nonoperative treatment involving brief immobilization and early range of motion; however, the treatment of displaced, unstable proximal humerus fractures is not as clearly defined. One method of outcomes research, meta-analysis, utilizes a comprehensive literature review to pool data from multiple studies to gain stronger statistical power for analysis. Because of the lack of well-designed, prospective randomized studies, however, attempts at meta-analysis to determine the most effective treatments for unstable proximal

TABLE 1–18 Summary of Outcomes Assessment of Three Case Examples

Case	*Neer Score*	*Constant Score*	*ASES Shoulder Score Index*
1	90 (Excellent)	73 (Fair)	83 (Excellent)
2	90 (Excellent)	91 (Excellent)	95 (Excellent)
3	73 (Unsatisfactory)	51 (Poor)	65 (Poor)

humerus fractures have failed to determine definitive treatment recommendations. To eliminate bias and produce the most valid results, future orthopaedic research should strive to adhere to the prospective, randomized, controlled design.

It is evident from the literature review on the treatment of proximal humerus fractures that currently used outcome scores do not always correlate with patient perceptions of the results of treatment. For example, it was not infrequent that patients had low outcome scores based on limited range of motion, yet were still pain free and satisfied with the outcome. Furthermore, disparity exists among the various outcomes instruments because each one emphasizes different aspects of the evaluation; for example, some instruments emphasize pain; others, range of motion; still others, functional capacity with ADLs. This is particularly evident in studies that report multiple scoring systems. As a result, comparison between studies becomes difficult if not impossible. The ASES has created an assessment intended to be a standardized shoulder outcomes instrument. The ASES instrument is relatively simple to use yet comprehensive enough to evaluate most shoulder disorders accurately. Moreover, calculation of the SSI allows comparison of shoulder disorders, treatments, and research studies.

General health status impacts directly on the functional recovery of the patient. General health status instruments assess all domains of human activity and, more importantly, assess the patient as a whole from the patient's perspective. Unfortunately, studies on outcomes of proximal humerus fractures have universally failed to include general health status as part of the evaluation. General health status and region-specific instruments provide different information, and evaluating only one gives an incomplete assessment of the patient. To evaluate the patient fully and arrive at definitive conclusions, efforts to include general health status instruments should be standard in clinical evaluation and future research.

REFERENCES

1. Daum WJ, Brinker MR, Nash DB. Quality and outcome determination in health care and orthopaedics: evolution and current structure. J Am Acad Orthop Surg 2000;8:133–139

2. Keller RB, Rudicel SA, Liang MH. Outcomes research in orthopaedics. Instr Course Lect 1994;43:599–611

3. Keller RB. Outcomes research in orthopaedics. J Am Acad Orthop Surg 1993;1:122–129

4. Matsen F III, Smith K. Effectiveness evaluation and the shoulder. In: Harryman D II, ed. The Shoulder, 2nd ed. Philadelphia: WB Saunders, 1998:1313–1341

5. Simmons BP, Swiontkowski MF, Evans RW, Amadio PC, Cats-Baril W. Outcomes assessment in the information age: available instruments, data collection, and utilization of data. Instr Course Lect 1999;48:667–685

6. Wennberg J. Gittelsohn A. Small area variations in health care delivery. Science 1973;182:1102–1108

7. Wennberg J, Gittelsohn A. Variations in medical care among small areas. Sci Am 1982;246:120–134

8. Keller RB, Soule DN, Wennberg JE, Hanley DF. Dealing with geographic variations in the use of hospitals. The experience of the Maine Medical Assessment Foundation Orthopaedic Study Group. J Bone Joint Surg Am 1990;72:1286–1293

9. Vitale MG, Krant JJ, Gelijns AC, et al. Geographic variations in the rates of operative procedures involving the shoulder, including total shoulder replacement, humeral head replacement, and rotator cuff repair. J Bone Joint Surg Am 1999;81:763–772

10. Lu-Yao GL, Keller RB, Littenberg B, Wennberg JE. Outcomes after displaced fractures of the femoral neck. A meta-analysis of one hundred and six published reports. J Bone Joint Surg Am 1994;76:15–25

11. Turner JA, Herron L, Deyo RA. Meta-analysis of the results of lumbar spine fusion. Acta Orthop Scand Suppl 1993;251:120–122

12. Misra A, Kapur R, Maffulli N. Complex proximal humeral fractures in adults–a systematic review of management. Injury 2001;32:363–372

13. Gibson JN, Handoll HH, Madhok R. Interventions for treating proximal humeral fractures in adults. Cochrane Database Syst Rev 2002:CD000434

14. Bertoft ES, Lundh I, Ringqvist I. Physiotherapy after fracture of the proximal end of the humerus. Comparison between two methods. Scand J Rehabil Med 1984;16:11–16

15. Kristiansen B, Kofoed H. Transcutaneous reduction and external fixation of displaced fractures of the proximal humerus. A controlled clinical trial. J Bone Joint Surg Br 1988;70:821–824

16. Kristiansen B, Angermann P, Larsen TK. Functional results following fractures of the proximal humerus. A controlled clinical study comparing two periods of immobilization. Arch Orthop Trauma Surg 1989;108:339–341

17. Livesley PJ, Mugglestone A, Whitton J. Electrotherapy and the management of minimally displaced fracture of the neck of the humerus. Injury 1992;23:323–327

18. Lungberg BJ, Svenungson-Hartwig E, Wikmark R. Independent exercises versus physiotherapy in nondisplaced proximal humeral fractures. Scand J Rehabil Med 1979;11:133–136

19. Revay S, Dahlstrom M, Dalen N. Water exercise versus instruction for self-training following a shoulder fracture. Int J Rehabil Res 1992;15:327–333

20. Rommens PM, Heyvaert G. [Conservative treatment of subcapital humerus fractures. A comparative study of the classical Desault bandage and the new Gilchrist bandage.] Unfallchirurgie 1993;19:114–118

21. Stableforth PG. Four-part fractures of the neck of the humerus. J Bone Joint Surg Br 1984;66:104–108

22. Hoellen IP, Bauer G, Holbein O. [Prosthetic humeral head replacement in dislocated humerus multi-fragment fracture in the elderly–an alternative to minimal osteosynthesis?] Zentralbl Chir 1997;122:994–1001

23. Zyto K, Ahrengart L, Sperber A, Tornkvist H. Treatment of displaced proximal humeral fractures in elderly patients. J Bone Joint Surg Br 1997;79:412–417

24. Beaton DE, Richards RR. Measuring function of the shoulder. A cross-sectional comparison of five questionnaires. J Bone Joint Surg Am 1996;78:882–890

25. Neer CS II. Displaced proximal humeral fractures. I. Classification and evaluation. J Bone Joint Surg Am 1970;52:1077–1089

26. Kristiansen B, Christensen SW. Proximal humeral fractures. Late results in relation to classification and treatment. Acta Orthop Scand 1987;58:124–127

27. Moda SK, Chadha NS, Sangwan SS, Khurana DK, Dahiya AS, Siwach RC. Open reduction and fixation of proximal humeral fractures and fracture-dislocations. J Bone Joint Surg Br 1990;72:1050–1052

28. Court-Brown CM, Garg A, McQueen MM. The translated two-part fracture of the proximal humerus. Epidemiology and outcome in the older patient. J Bone Joint Surg Br 2001;83:799–804

29. Zyto K, Kronberg M, Brostrom LA. Shoulder function after displaced fractures of the proximal humerus. J Shoulder Elbow Surg 1995;4:331–336

30. Willems WJ, Lim TE. Neer arthroplasty for humeral fracture. Acta Orthop Scand 1985;56:394–395

31. Neer CS II. Displaced proximal humeral fractures. II. Treatment of three-part and four-part displacement. J Bone Joint Surg Am 1970;52:1090–1103

32. Dimakopoulos P, Potamitis N, Lambiris E. Hemiarthroplasty in the treatment of comminuted intraarticular fractures of the proximal humerus. Clin Orthop 1997;341:7–11

33. Becker R, Pap G, Machner A, Neumann WH. Strength and motion after hemiarthroplasty in displaced four-fragment fracture of the proximal humerus: 27 patients followed for 1–6 years. Acta Orthop Scand 2002;73:44–49

34. Savoie FH, Geissler WB, Vander Griend RA. Open reduction and internal fixation of three-part fractures of the proximal humerus. Orthopedics 1989;12:65–70

35. Szyszkowitz R, Seggl W, Schleifer P, Cundy PJ. Proximal humeral fractures. Management techniques and expected results. Clin Orthop 1993;292:13–25

36. Darder A, Darder A Jr, Sanchis V, Gastaldi E, Gomar F. Four-part displaced proximal humeral fractures: operative treatment using Kirschner wires and a tension band. J Orthop Trauma 1993;7:497–505

37. Ko JY, Yamamoto R. Surgical treatment of complex fracture of the proximal humerus. Clin Orthop 1996;327:225–237

38. Hessmann M, Baumgaertel F, Gehling H, Klingelhoeffer I, Gotzen L. Plate fixation of proximal humeral fractures with indirect reduction: surgical technique and results utilizing three shoulder scores. Injury 1999;30:453–462

39. Jakob RP, Miniaci A, Anson PS, Jaberg H, Osterwalder A, Ganz R. Four-part valgus impacted fractures of the proximal humerus. J Bone Joint Surg Br 1991;73:295–298

40. Court-Brown CM, Cattermole H, McQueen MM. Impacted valgus fractures (B1.1) of the proximal humerus. The results of non-operative treatment. J Bone Joint Surg Br 2002;84:504–508

41. Neer CS II, Watson KC, Stanton FJ. Recent experience in total shoulder replacement. J Bone Joint Surg Am 1982;64:319–337

42. Cofield RH. Total shoulder arthroplasty with the Neer prosthesis. J Bone Joint Surg Am 1984;66:899–906

43. Sperling JW, Cofield RH, Rowland CM. Neer hemiarthroplasty and Neer total shoulder arthroplasty in patients fifty years old or less. Long-term results. J Bone Joint Surg Am 1998;80:464–473

44. Richards R, An K-N, Bigliani L, et al. A standardized method for the assessment of shoulder function. J Shoulder Elbow Surg 1994;3:347–352

45. Kuhn JE, Blasier RB. Measuring outcomes in shoulder arthroplasty. Semin Arthroplasty 1995;6:245–264

46. Constant CR, Murley AH. A clinical method of functional assessment of the shoulder. Clin Orthop 1987;214:160–164

47. Conboy VB, Morris RW, Kiss J, Carr AJ. An evaluation of the Constant-Murley shoulder assessment. J Bone Joint Surg Br 1996;78:229–232

48. Amstutz HC, Sew Hoy AL, Clarke IC. UCLA anatomic total shoulder arthroplasty. Clin Orthop 1981;155:7–20

49. Ellman H, Hanker G, Bayer M. Repair of the rotator cuff. End-result study of factors influencing reconstruction. J Bone Joint Surg Am 1986;68:1136–1144

50. Patte D. Directions for the use of the Index Severity for Painful and/or Chronically Disable Shoulders. Presented at the First Open Congress of the European Society for Surgery of the Shoulder and Elbow, 1987, Paris

51. Matsen FA III, Ziegler DW, DeBartolo SE. Patient self-assessment of health status and function in glenohumeral degenerative joint disease. J Shoulder Elbow Surg 1995;4:345–351

52. Matsen FA III. Early effectiveness of shoulder arthroplasty for patients who have primary glenohumeral degenerative joint disease. J Bone Joint Surg Am 1996;78:260–264

53. Hudak PL, Amadio PC, Bombardier C. Development of an upper extremity outcome measure: the DASH (disabilities of the arm, shoulder and hand) [corrected]. The Upper Extremity Collaborative Group (UECG). Am J Ind Med 1996;29:602–608

54. SooHoo NF, McDonald AP, Seiler JG III, McGillivary GR. Evaluation of the construct validity of the DASH questionnaire by correlation to the SF-36. J Hand Surg [Am] 2002;27:537–541

55. Beaton DE, Katz JN, Fossel AH, Wright JG, Tarasuk V, Bombardier C. Measuring the whole or the parts? Validity, reliability, and responsiveness of the Disabilities of the Arm, Shoulder and Hand outcome measure in different regions of the upper extremity. J Hand Ther 2001;14:128–146

56. Hawkins RJ, Bell RH, Gurr K. The three-part fracture of the proximal part of the humerus. Operative treatment. J Bone Joint Surg Am 1986;68:1410–1414

57. Hawkins RJ, Switlyk P. Acute prosthetic replacement for severe fractures of the proximal humerus. Clin Orthop 1993;289:156–160

58. Cornell CN, Levine D, Pagnani MJ. Internal fixation of proximal humerus fractures using the screw-tension band technique. J Orthop Trauma 1994;8:23–27

59. McCoy SR, Warren RF, Bade HA III, Ranawat CS, Inglis AE. Total shoulder arthroplasty in rheumatoid arthritis. J Arthroplasty 1989;4:105–113

60. Koval KJ, Gallagher MA, Marsicano JG, Cuomo F, McShinawy A, Zuckerman JD. Functional outcome after minimally displaced fractures of the proximal part of the humerus. J Bone Joint Surg Am 1997;79:203–207

61. Ware JE Jr, Sherbourne CD. The MOS 36-item short-form health survey (SF-36). I. Conceptual framework and item selection. Med Care 1992;30:473–483

62. Gartsman GM, Brinker MR, Khan M, Karahan M. Self-assessment of general health status in patients with five common shoulder conditions. J Shoulder Elbow Surg 1998;7:228–237

63. Bergner M, Bobbitt RA, Carter WB, Gilson BS. The Sickness Impact Profile: development and final revision of a health status measure. Med Care 1981;19:787–805

64. MacKenzie EJ, Burgess AR, McAndrew MP, et al. Patient-oriented functional outcome after unilateral lower extremity fracture. J Orthop Trauma 1993;7:393–401

65. Hunt SM, McEwen J, McKenna SP. Measuring health status: a new tool for clinicians and epidemiologists. J R Coll Gen Pract 1985;35:185–188

66. Georgiadis GM, Behrens FF, Joyce MJ, Earle AS, Simmons AL. Open tibial fractures with severe soft-tissue loss. Limb salvage compared with below-the-knee amputation. J Bone Joint Surg Am 1993;75:1431–1441

67. Williams A. Setting priorities in health care: an economist's view. J Bone Joint Surg Br 1991;73-B:365–367

68. Young TB, Wallace WA. Conservative treatment of fractures and fracture-dislocations of the upper end of the humerus. J Bone Joint Surg Br 1985;67:373–377

69. Jaberg H, Warner JJ, Jakob RP. Percutaneous stabilization of unstable fractures of the humerus. J Bone Joint Surg Am 1992;74:508–515

70. Cuomo F, Flatow E, Maday M, Miller S, McIlveen S, Bigliani L. Open reduction and internal fixation of two- and three-part displaced surgical neck fractures of the proximal humerus. J Shoulder Elbow Surg 1992;1:287–295

71. Flatow EL, Cuomo F, Maday MG, Miller SR, McIlveen SJ, Bigliani LU. Open reduction and internal fixation of two-part displaced fractures of the greater tuberosity of the proximal part of the humerus. J Bone Joint Surg Am 1991;73:1213–1218

72. Zyto K. Non-operative treatment of comminuted fractures of the proximal humerus in elderly patients. Injury 1998;29:349–352

73. Schai P, Imhoff A, Preiss S. Comminuted humeral head fractures: a multicenter analysis. J Shoulder Elbow Surg 1995;4:319–330

74. Moeckel BH, Dines DM, Warren RF, Altchek DW. Modular hemiarthroplasty for fractures of the proximal part of the humerus. J Bone Joint Surg Am 1992;74:884–889

75. Goldman RT, Koval KJ, Cuomo F, Gallagher MA, Zuckerman JD. Functional outcome after humeral head replacement for acute three- and four-part proximal humeral fractures. J Shoulder Elbow Surg 1995;4:81–86

76. Zyto K, Wallace WA, Frostick SP, Preston BJ. Outcome after hemiarthroplasty for three- and four-part fractures of the proximal humerus. J Shoulder Elbow Surg 1998;7:85–89

77. Movin T, Sjoden GO, Ahrengart L. Poor function after shoulder replacement in fracture patients. A retrospective evaluation of 29 patients followed for 2–12 years. Acta Orthop Scand 1998;69:392–396

78. Bosch U, Skutek M, Fremerey RW, Tscherne H. Outcome after primary and secondary hemiarthroplasty in elderly patients with fractures of the proximal humerus. J Shoulder Elbow Surg 1998;7:479–484

79. Esser RD. Treatment of three- and four-part fractures of the proximal humerus with a modified cloverleaf plate. J Orthop Trauma 1994;8:15–22

80. Hintermann B, Trouillier HH, Schafer D. Rigid internal fixation of fractures of the proximal humerus in older patients. J Bone Joint Surg Br 2000;82:1107–1112

81. Resch H, Povacz P, Frohlich R, Wambacher M. Percutaneous fixation of three- and four-part fractures of the proximal humerus. J Bone Joint Surg Br 1997;79:295–300

2

Anatomy of the Shoulder

ERIK N. KUBIAK, KENNETH J. KOVAL, AND JOSEPH D. ZUCKERMAN

The shoulder is a complex joint composed of four articulations, the sum of whose motions provide for its vast mobility. During the course of evolution, stability has been sacrificed for mobility, especially in higher primates where the upper extremity is no longer a primary weight-bearing appendage. The shoulder is described as having three degrees of freedom: flexion and extension in the paramedian plane, abduction and adduction in the coronal plane, and medial and lateral rotation. The clavicle, scapula, and humerus provide the shoulder's osseous scaffolding. They share three diarthrodial articulations: the sternoclavicular joint, the acromioclavicular joint, and the glenohumeral joint. The scapulothoracic joint is the fourth articulation of the shoulder; it is formed by the scapula as it rides over the posterior superior thorax on a bed of muscle and bursae. The three bones are manipulated and stabilized to the axial skeleton by 19 muscles. The muscles are divided into an intrinsic group that moves the humerus with respect to the scapula, and an extrinsic group that moves the pectoral girdle and humerus with respect to the axial skeleton.

◾ Osteology

A large flat bone, the scapula rests on the posterior superior thorax and acts primarily as a site of muscle attachment (Fig. 2–1). Almost the entire surface of the

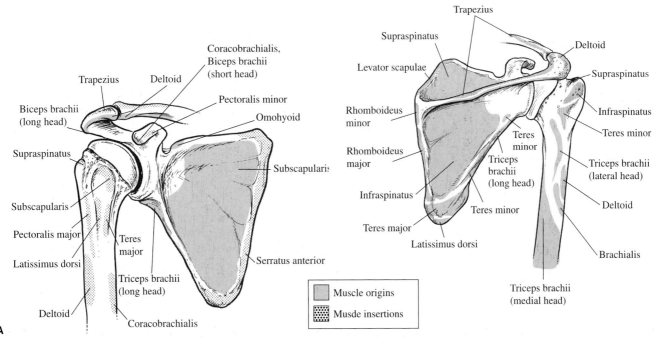

A

B

FIGURE 2–1 Interior **(A)** and posterior **(B)** views of the scapula, demonstrating that it is the origin or insertion site for almost all of the shoulder girdle muscles.

scapula is covered by muscle. Thus protected, the body of the scapula is rarely fractured and only by severe direct trauma. Most scapular fractures occur to the vulnerable processes of the scapula: the acromion, coracoid, and glenoid. The scapula articulates with the clavicle, the humerus, and the thorax. The costal surface of the scapula is covered by the subscapularis muscle, which lies in the concave subscapular fossa. Posteriorly, the surface of the scapula is divided by the scapular spine into the supraspinatus and infraspinatus fossae, which contain the supraspinatus and infraspinatus muscles, respectively. The superior border of the scapula is the site of attachment for the omohyoid muscle. This muscle is just medial to the scapular notch and the superior transverse scapular ligament. The medial border of the scapula serves as the attachment site for the levator scapulae. This medial border is perpendicular to the scapular spine and parallel to the spinal column. The minor and major rhomboids are attached to the medial border. The lateral border of the scapula extends from the inferior angle to the glenoid. From inferior to superior the following muscles attach to the lateral border of the scapula: the latissimus dorsi, teres major, teres minor, and long head of the triceps.

The predominant blood supply to the scapula derives from blood vessels that supply the muscles with scapular origins. The primary nutrient artery to the scapula enters in the lateral suprascapular fossa or infrascapular fossa. Scapular circulation is predominantly metaphyseal, with the subscapular, suprascapular, circumflex scapular, and acromial vessels contributing to the scapula's blood supply.

Readily palpable on the posterior surface of the scapula is the scapular spine, which arcs anterolaterally, becoming the acromion process. The acromion articulates with the clavicle and serves as the only ligamentous attachment of the scapula with the axial skeleton. The scapular spine serves as the site of attachment for the trapezius and deltoid. Additionally, the scapular spine suspends the acromion laterally and anteriorly, improving the leverage of the deltoid.

Overhanging the head of the humerus, the acromion is often implicated in impingement syndromes of the shoulder. In the anterior plane, there is 9 to 10 mm (6.6 to 13.8 mm in men and 7.1 to 11.9 mm in women) of space between the humeral head and the acromion.[1] This space is referred to as the supraspinatus outlet. Acromial epiphyseal nonunion, called os acromiale, has been found in 1.4 to 8.2%[2] of cadaveric specimens. This can be mistaken for acromial fracture in trauma patients but has not been implicated as a cause of impingement.[3]

Anterolaterally on the scapula, the coracoid process is an anterior projecting process of bone just medial to the glenoid and inferior to the suprascapular notch. Two ligaments, the coracoclavicular (divided into two bundles,

the conoid and trapezoid) and the coracohumeral attach to the coracoid. The coracoid is the origin of the coracobrachialis and short head of the biceps. Inserting into the coracoid at its inferomedial border is the pectoralis minor. At the medial base of the coracoid lies the suprascapular notch, which contains the suprascapular nerve.

The glenoid is the disk-shaped lateral process of the scapula inferior to the acromion and lateral to the coracoid. The long head of the biceps arises from the supraglenoid tubercle, a small bony prominence on the anterosuperior aspect of the glenoid. Covered by fibrocartilage, the glenoid articulates with the head of the humerus. Circumferential thickening of the articular cartilage around the outside rim of the glenoid forms the labrum. The labrum is composed of fibrocartilage, which is distinctly different from the hyaline cartilage that covers the articular surface of the glenoid. The articular surface of the glenoid is 6° retroverted with respect to the blade of the scapula.

The superior, medial, and inferior glenohumeral ligaments provide the primary ligamentous attachments of the humerus to the scapula, whereas the coracohumeral ligament is a secondary attachment. The superior glenoid tubercle is the origin for the long head of the biceps, and the inferior glenoid tubercle is the origin for the long head of the triceps.

■ Clavicle

Anchoring the scapula to the axial skeleton, the clavicle is an essentially straight bone in the anterior posterior plane but S-shaped in the transverse plane; it is convex anteriorly at its medial third and concave anteriorly at its lateral third (Fig. 2–2). The clavicle's medial anterior curve accommodates the trunks of the brachial plexus and the subclavian artery. The clavicle acts as a strut to the shoulder, optimizing the glenohumeral range of motion by keeping it lateral to the axial skeleton. The clavicle serves primarily as a site for muscle attachment, but also transfers the force generated by the trapezius to the scapula, resulting in scapular elevation. Scapular elevation maintains glenohumeral joint separation from the axial skeleton and maximizes glenohumeral range of motion.

The clavicle is the first bone to ossify during the fifth week of gestation by intramembranous ossification. The epiphyses (growth plates) of the clavicle are late to form and fuse; the proximal epiphysis of the clavicle appears at 18 to 20 years and fuses at about 25 years. The presence of this epiphysis makes differentiating physeal fractures from dislocations of the sternoclavicular joint difficult in the 18- to 25-year-old patient. A small epiphysis appears at the distal end of the clavicle at about 20 years and soon fuses with the shaft of the clavicle.[4]

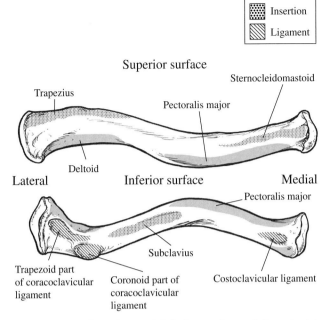

Superior surface

Trapezius

Sternocleidomastoid

Pectoralis major

Deltoid

Lateral   Inferior surface   Medial

Pectoralis major

Subclavius

Trapezoid part of coracoclavicular ligament

Coronoid part of coracoclavicular ligament

Costoclavicular ligament

Origin
Insertion
Ligament

FIGURE 2–2 Superior and inferior surface of the clavicle, showing the muscular origins and insertions and the sites of ligament attachments.

The clavicle has two diarthrodial articulations: one with the sternum and one with the scapula. The sternoclavicular joint is the only joint in the entire shoulder construct that articulates with the axial skeleton.

The clavicle is the insertion point for the subclavius, sternocleidomastoid, and the trapezius, whereas the pectoralis major and deltoid originate from the clavicle (Fig. 2–2). The costoclavicular ligament anchors the medial third of the clavicle to the first rib, whereas the trapezoid and conoid ligaments anchor the lateral third of the clavicle, leaving the middle third unsupported and prone to fracture.

■ Humerus

The proximal spherical head of the humerus articulates with the scapula via the glenoid (Fig. 2–3). On average, the radius of curvature of the head is 2.25 cm. The humeral head is generally described as retroverted 25° to 35° with respect to a line drawn through the medial and lateral epicondyles of the humerus. Edelson[2] has demonstrated humeral head retroversion to vary from −8° to 74°. The articular surface is covered with fibrocartilage, which terminates distally at the anatomic neck of the humerus. The borders of the anatomic neck are the greater tuberosity, the lesser tuberosity, the intertubercular groove, and the medial surface of the

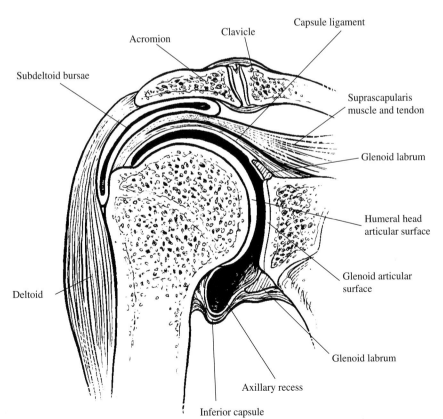

Subdeltoid bursae

Acromion

Clavicle

Capsule ligament

Suprascapularis muscle and tendon

Glenoid labrum

Humeral head articular surface

Glenoid articular surface

Deltoid

Glenoid labrum

Axillary recess

Inferior capsule

FIGURE 2–3 Coronal section of the glenohumeral joint, showing the spherical-shaped humeral head articulating with the relatively flat glenoid articular surface.

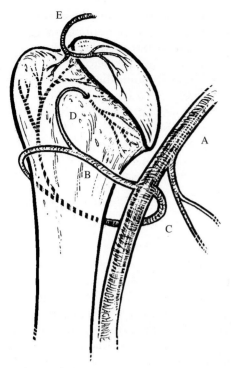

FIGURE 2–4 The blood supply to the humeral head originates with the axillary artery (A) and is derived from the anterior (B) and posterior (C) humeral circumflex arteries through the arcuate artery (D) and through the rotator cuff insertion (E).

The intertubercular groove lies ~1 cm lateral to the midline. The greater tuberosity is the insertion point for the supraspinatus, the infraspinatus, and the teres minor. The lesser tuberosity is the insertion point for the subscapularis. Between the tuberosities, the intertubercular groove contains the tendon of the long head of the biceps. This groove is roofed by the transverse humeral ligament. The intertubercular groove continues distally as the shallow bicipital groove. The lateral border of the bicipital groove is the insertion of the pectoralis major. The latissimus dorsi and teres major insert on the medial border and floor of the bicipital groove. The primary blood supply to the humeral head is via the anterior humeral circumflex artery, which enters the humeral head at the intertubercular groove or one of the tuberosities (Fig. **2–4**). On the lateral border of the humerus, at the mid-diaphyseal level, the deltoid inserts into the deltoid tuberosity.

■ Articulations

There are four articulations in the shoulder joint, each contributing to the overall shoulder motion. The glenohumeral, acromioclavicular, and sternoclavicular joints are diarthrodial joints, articulations composed of two cartilage-covered bone surfaces bathed in synovial fluid and contained within a fibrous capsule lined by synovium. The osseous architecture of these joints contributes little to their stability, and therefore they rely primarily on their ligamentous architecture and secondarily on the surrounding muscles for stability and support. The fourth articulation of the shoulder is the scapulothoracic joint. This joint consists of the scapula riding over the rib cage on a cushion of loose connective tissue; roughly one third of shoulder motion occurs at this joint.

humerus. This anatomic neck is easily visualized during arthroscopy as a ring of bone devoid of hyaline cartilage that varies from 1 cm wide medially to nonexistent superiorly, proximal to the insertions of the hyaline humeral ligaments and rotator cuff muscles. Distal to the tuberosities, the humerus narrows into an area called the surgical neck.

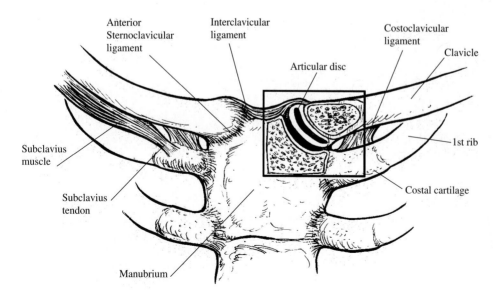

FIGURE 2–5 The sternoclavicular joint is a diarthrodial articulation that connects the shoulder complex to the axial skeleton.

Sternoclavicular Joint

The sternoclavicular joint is the only joint that directly connects the shoulder complex to the axial skeleton (Fig. **2–5**). This articulation of the proximal end of the clavicle with manubrium contains an intraarticular disk. The anterior and posterior sternoclavicular ligaments are the primary stabilizers of the joint, with the posterior ligament being the strongest and a restraint to inferior depression of the lateral end of the clavicle. Range of motion in this joint is 30° to 35° of upward elevation, 35° anterior-posterior, and 44° to 50° of rotation along the long axis of the clavicle. Elevation occurs after 30° to 90° of arm elevation, and rotation occurs after 70° to 80° of arm elevation.[5–8]

Acromioclavicular Joint

The acromioclavicular ligaments attach the clavicle to the scapula at the acromioclavicular joint (Fig. **2–6**). This is a diarthrodial joint, which, like the sternoclavicular joint, contains an intraarticular disk. There is 20° of rotation in this joint, which occurs during the first 20° and the last 40° of shoulder elevation.[7,8] The trapezoid and conoid ligaments attach to the clavicle adjacent to the acromioclavicular ligament and serve to anchor the distal clavicle to the coracoid process of the scapula.[9] The acromioclavicular ligaments are primary restraints to posterior displacement of the clavicle and

posterior axial rotation.[9,10] The conoid ligament is a primary restraint to anterior and superior rotation. It also resists anterior and superior displacement of the clavicle.[9–11]

Glenohumeral Joint

The glenohumeral joint is a polyaxial diarthrodial joint that links the humerus to the scapula. The articular surface of the humerus has roughly four times the surface area of the articular surface of the glenoid. The thin joint capsule provides little restraint to the glenohumeral joint except in abduction and lateral rotation. The capsule has three variable consolidations that form the glenohumeral ligaments: the superior glenohumeral ligament, middle glenohumeral ligament, and inferior glenohumeral ligament (Fig. **2–7A**). The glenohumeral ligaments and the coracohumeral ligament are the only ligamentous connections between the humerus and the scapula. The long head of the biceps passes within the joint as it arises from the supraglenoid tubercle. This joint lies beneath the coracoacromial arc, which is composed of the acromion, the coracoacromial ligament, and the coracoid process (Fig. **2–7B**). Superior dislocation of the humerus on the glenoid is blocked by the capsule, the long head of the biceps, the rotator cuff, and the coraco acromial arch. There are no inferior counterparts to these structures; therefore, the shoulder is prone to inferior dislocation. The subdeltoid

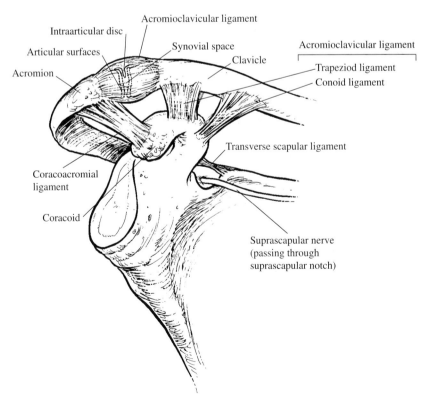

FIGURE 2–6 The acromioclavicular joint is a diarthrodial articulation that connects the clavicle to the scapula.

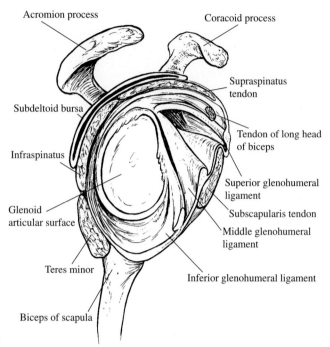

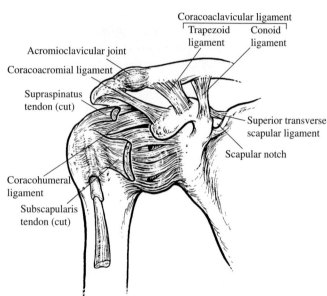

A

B

FIGURES 2–7 (A) The stability of the glenohumeral joint is provided by the glenohumeral ligaments (static stabilizers) and the rotator cuff musculature (dynamic stabilizers).

(B) The humeral head is located beneath the coracoacromial arch formed by the acromion, coracoacromial ligament, and the coracoid process.

and subacromial bursae reduce friction between the acromial arch and the rotator cuff as it overlies the humeral head; 90° to 120° of shoulder abduction glenohumeral in origin, whereas roughly 60° is scapulothoracic in origin.[12,13] For the arm to be brought vertical, the remaining motion must come from contralateral vertebral flexion.

■ Muscles

The muscles of the shoulder have been described in terms of layers (Fig. **2–8**) and functional groups (Table **2–1**, page 30). The extrinsic muscles of the shoulder are designated as those that move the pectoral girdle and humerus

in relationship to the axial skeleton. All originate from the axial skeleton and are divided into a superficial and deep layer. The superficial extrinsic muscles are the latissimus dorsi, trapezius, and pectoralis major. The deep extrinsics are the levator scapulae, rhomboids major and minor, serratus anterior, pectoralis minor, and subclavius. The intrinsic muscles of the shoulder move the humerus with respect to the scapula.

The intrinsic muscles of the shoulder are the deltoid, coracobrachialis, teres major, and the rotator cuff. The latter is composed of the subscapularis, supraspinatus, infrascapularis, and teres minor (Fig. **2–9**). All these muscles are innervated by the brachial plexus except for the trapezius, which is innervated by the spinal accessory nerve.

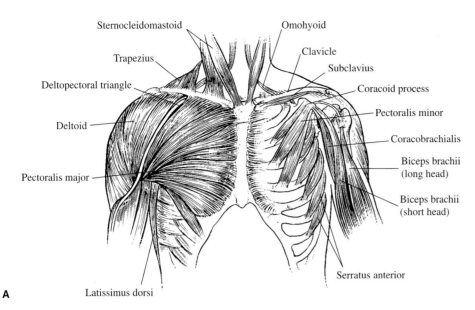

Sternocleidomastoid
Omohyoid
Trapezius
Clavicle
Deltopectoral triangle
Subclavius
Coracoid process
Deltoid
Pectoralis minor
Coracobrachialis
Biceps brachii (long head)
Pectoralis major
Biceps brachii (short head)
Serratus anterior
A
Latissimus dorsi

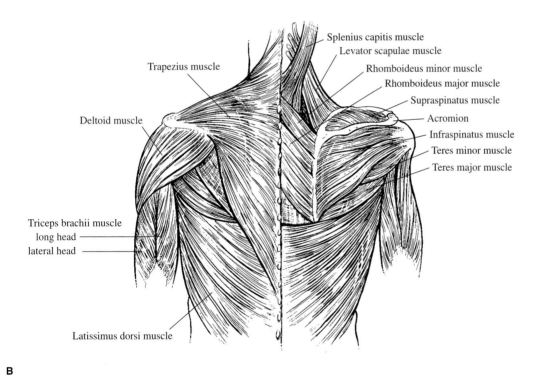

Splenius capitis muscle
Levator scapulae muscle
Trapezius muscle
Rhomboideus minor muscle
Rhomboideus major muscle
Supraspinatus muscle
Deltoid muscle
Acromion
Infraspinatus muscle
Teres minor muscle
Teres major muscle
Triceps brachii muscle
long head
lateral head
Latissimus dorsi muscle
B

FIGURE 2–8 Superficial and deep muscular anatomy of the shoulder. **(A)** Anterior view. **(B)** Posterior view.

TABLE 2–1 Muscles of the Shoulder Repair

Muscle	Origin	Insertion	Action	Innervation	Blood Supply
Scapulothoracic					
Levator scapulae	Transverse process C1-C4	Superomedial border scapula	Elevate, rotate scapula	Direct branches 3–4 cervical spinal nerves and dorsal scapular nerve	
Rhomboid major	Spinal process T2-T5	Medial border scapula	Adduct scapula	Dorsal scapular	Dorsal scapular
Rhomboid minor	Spinal process C7-T1	Medial border scapula	Adduct scapula	Dorsal scapular	Dorsal scapular
Serratus anterior	Rib 1–9	Medial border scapula	Protracts the scapula	Long thoracic	Lateral thoracic artery
Glenohumeral					
Deltoid	Acromion, clavicle	Deltoid tubercle of humerus	Abduction	Axillary	Axillary artery
Triceps, long head	Infraglenoid	Olecranon	Extends arm	Radial	Radial collateral artery
Triceps, medial head	Post humerus	Olecranon	Extends arm	Radial	Radial collateral artery
Triceps, lateral head	Post humerus	Olecranon	Extends arm	Radial	Radial collateral artery
Biceps, long head	Supraglenoid	Radial tuberosity	Supination, flexion	Musculocutaneous	Brachial artery
Biceps, short head	Coracoid	Radial tuberosity	Supination, flexion	Musculocutaneous	Brachial artery
Coracobrachialis	Coracoid	Mid-humerus medial	Flexion, adduction	Musculocutaneous	Brachial artery
Rotator cuff					
Subscapularis	Ventral scapula	Humerus lessor tuberosity	Internally rotate	Upper and lower subscapular	
Supraspinatus	Superior scapula	Humerus greater tuberosity	Abduction	Suprascapular	Suprascapular artery
Infraspinatus	Dorsal scapula	Humerus greater tuberosity	External rotation	Suprascapular	Suprascapular artery
Terres minor	Scapular dorsal lateral border	Humerus greater tuberosity	External rotation	Axillary	
Accessory					
Subclavius	Rib 1	Inferior clavicle	Depress clavicle	Upper trunk brachial plexus	Suprascapular artery
Trapezius	Spinal process C7-T12	Clavicle, acromion, spine of scapula	Rotate scapula	Cranial nerve XI	Dorsal scapula, superficial cervical
Pectoralis major	Sternum, ribs, clavicle	Humerus lateral intertubercular groove	Adduct, internally rotate arm	Medial and lateral pectoral nerve	Superior thoracic artery, lateral thoracic artery, pectoral branch thoracoacromial artery
Pectoralis minor	Ribs 3–5	Scapula	Protract scapula	Medial and lateral pectoral nerve	Superior thoracic artery, lateral thoracic artery, pectoral branch thoracoacromial artery
Latissimus dorsi	Spinal process T6-S5	Humerus intertubercular groove	Extend, adduct, internally rotate humerus	Thoracodorsal	Thoracodorsal art, dorsal scapula
Terres major	Inferior scapula	Humerus medial intertubercular groove	Adduct, internally rotate, extend	Lower subscapular nerve	

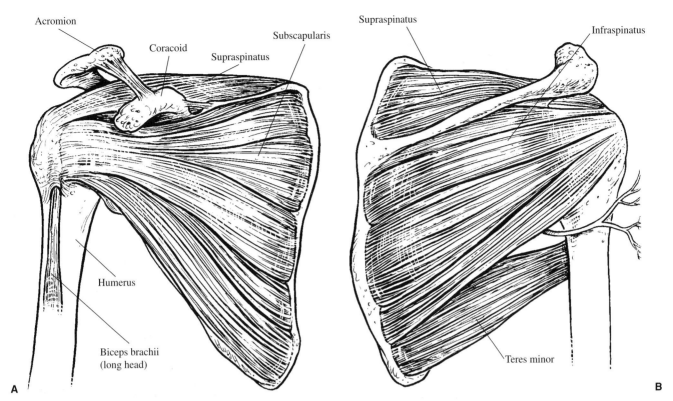

FIGURE 2–9 Anterior **(A)** and posterior **(B)** representations of the rotator cuff musculature and the relationship of the gleno-humeral joint.

■ Neurovascular Structures

The neurovascular anatomy of the shoulder region focuses on the brachial plexus and the vascular structures that lie in close proximity (Fig. **2–10**). The brachial plexus arises from the anterior rami of C5-T1 (C4 contributes to the brachial plexus in 28 to 62% of patients[14,15]), which are the roots of the brachial plexus. The prevertebral fascia continues laterally with the roots of the plexus as it passes between the anterior and middle scalene muscles. It encloses both the axillary artery and plexus as it passes through the axilla; this sheath is known as the interscalene sheath, and it allows the transmission and containment of local anesthetic when performing a scalene block. The brachial plexus enters the axillary space as it passes between the anterior and middle scalene muscles. The plexus passes behind the clavicle at the cord level. The roots combine to form the three trunks of the plexus (superior, middle, and inferior), which separate into anterior and posterior divisions. The anterior division supplies the flexor compartment, and the posterior division supplies the extensor compartment of the upper extremity. The posterior divisions combine to form the posterior cord, and the anterior divisions combine into the medial and lateral cords. The cords divide into the terminal branches of the brachial plexus. The posterior cord becomes the axillary nerve and the radial nerve. The lateral cord becomes the musculocutaneous nerve (which enters the coracobrachialis 5 to 6 cm [range 1.5 to 9 cm] from the tip of the coracoid) and the median nerve. The medial cord becomes the ulnar nerve.

Several terminal branches of the brachial plexus are particularly vulnerable to trauma, both accidental and surgical, secondary to their anatomic location and fixed nature. The most proximal of these is the suprascapular nerve, which arises from the upper trunk at Erb's point, 2 to 3 cm above the clavicle behind the posterior edge of the sternocleidomastoid muscle and passes behind the scapula through the suprascapular notch. The nerve is fixed in the notch below the transverse scapular ligament. The musculocutaneous nerve enters the coracobrachialis muscle 5 to 6 cm (range 1.5 to 9 cm) below the coracoid and is vulnerable to traction injury during anterior approaches to the shoulder. The axillary nerve is the last branch of the posterior cord. It passes between the subscapularis muscle and the teres major accompanied by the posterior humeral circumflex artery through the quadrilateral space. It divides into a posterior branch, which innervates the teres minor, and an anterior branch,

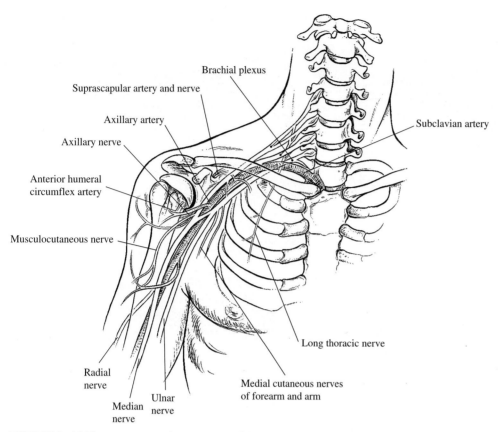

FIGURE 2–10 The neurovascular anatomy of the shoulder region from the base of the neck to the arm.

which innervates the deltoid and lies 4 to 8 cm below the acromion angle or tip.[16]

The eleventh cranial nerve or the spinal accessory nerve arises from roots in the medulla, ascends through the foramen magnum, and exits the base of the skull through the jugular foramen, innervating the sternocleidomastoid muscle. It then crosses the posterior triangle of the neck and innervates the trapezius. Other nerves of note are the intercostal brachial nerve, which innervates the medial arm above the elbow, and the supraclavicular nerves, which are branches of the C3-C4 spinal roots and innervate the skin over the clavicle.

The blood supply to the shoulder arises from the subclavian artery, which becomes the axillary artery at the lateral border of the first rib. It has five branches: (1) the vertebral artery, (2) the internal thoracic or mammary artery, (3) the thyrocervical artery with its transverse cervical branch that supplies the trapezius and the rhomboids, (4) the costocervical artery, and (5) the dorsal scapular artery. The suprascapular artery branches off the thyrocervical artery and passes over the transverse scapular ligament to supply the supraspinatus. The dorsal scapular artery supplies the rhomboids, latissimus, and trapezius, branching from the transverse cervical artery of the subclavian artery.

The axillary artery, vein, and branches of the brachial plexus are contained with the axillary sheath within the axilla. The subclavian artery becomes the axillary artery as it crosses the first rib and becomes the brachial artery at the lower border of the teres major. The artery is divided into three parts as it passes behind the pectoralis minor: the first part is above the muscle, the second part lies behind the muscle, and the third part is below the muscle. Six branches arise from the axillary artery. The first part gives off the superior thoracic artery, the second part gives off the thoracoacromial artery and the long lateral thoracic artery, and the third part gives off the subscapular artery and the two humeral circumflex arteries. The thoracoacromial artery has branches to the pectoral muscles, the deltoid, the acromion, and the clavicle. The subscapular artery arises from the axillary artery at the inferior border of the subscapularis and follows the inferior angle of the scapula, giving rise to the circumflex scapular artery that passes through the triangular space supplying the infraspinatus fossa before continuing on as the thoracodorsal artery.

The posterior humeral circumflex artery descends into the quadrilateral space (Fig. 2–11) with the axillary nerve passing 4 to 5 cm below the acromion and supplying two thirds of the deltoid and most of the overlying

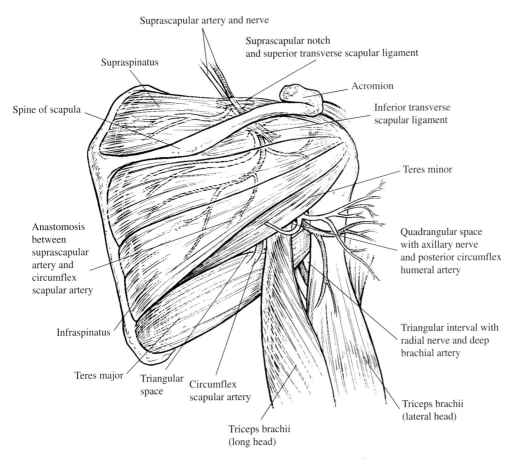

Suprascapular artery and nerve

Suprascapular notch
and superior transverse scapular ligament

Supraspinatus

Spine of scapula

Acromion

Inferior transverse
scapular ligament

Teres minor

Anastomosis
between
suprascapular
artery and
circumflex
scapular artery

Quadrangular space
with axillary nerve
and posterior circumflex
humeral artery

Infraspinatus

Triangular interval with
radial nerve and deep
brachial artery

Teres major   Triangular   Circumflex
space   scapular artery

Triceps brachii
(lateral head)

Triceps brachii
(long head)

FIGURE 2–11 Posterior neurovascular anatomy of the shoulder region.

skin. The last branch is the anterior circumflex humeral artery, which supplies the humeral head crossing the subscapularis tendon anteriorly.

REFERENCES

1. Petersson CJ, Redlund-Johnell I. The subacromial space in normal shoulder radiographs. Acta Orthop Scand 1984;55:57–58
2. Edelson G. Variations in the retroversion of the humeral head. J Shoulder Elbow Surg 1999;8:142–145
3. Neer CS II. Impingement lesions. Clin Orthop 1983;173:70–77
4. Rosse C, Gaddum-Rosse P, eds. Hollinshead's Textbook of Anatomy. Philadelphia: Lippincott-Raven, 1997:193–237
5. Fung M, Kato S, Barrance PJ, et al. Scapular and clavicular kinematics during humeral elevation: a study with cadavers. J Shoulder Elbow Surg 2001;10:278–285
6. Hogfors C, Peterson B, Sigholm G, Herberts P. Biomechanical model of the human shoulder joint. II. The shoulder rhythm. J Biomech 1991;24:699–709
7. Lucas DB. Biomechanics of the shoulder joint. Arch Surg 1973; 107:425–432
8. van der Helm FC. Analysis of the kinematic and dynamic behavior of the shoulder mechanism. J Biomech 1994;27:527–550
9. Debski RE, Parsons IM III, Fenwick J, Vangura A. Ligament mechanics during three degree-of-freedom motion at the acromioclavicular joint. Ann Biomed Eng 2000;28:612–618
10. Lee KW, Debski RE, Chen CH, Woo SL, Fu FH. Functional evaluation of the ligaments at the acromioclavicular joint during anteroposterior and superoinferior translation. Am J Sports Med 1997;25:858–862
11. Costic RS, Jari R, Rodosky MW, Debski RE. Joint compression alters the kinematics and loading patterns of the intact and capsule-transected AC joint. J Orthop Res 2003;21:379–385
12. Inman VT, Saunders JB, Abbott LC. Observations of the function of the shoulder joint. Clin Orthop 1996;330:3–12
13. Kapandji IA. The shoulder. Clin Rheum Dis 1982;8:595–616
14. Urbanowicz Z. [Brachial plexus roots in man] Ann Univ Mariae Curie Sklodowska [Med] 1994;49:47–55
15. Yan J, Horiguchi M. The communicating branch of the 4th cervical nerve to the brachial plexus: the double constitution, anterior and posterior, of its fibers. Surg Radiol Anat 2000;22:175–179
16. Vathana P, Chiarapattanakom P, Ratanalaka R, Vorasatit P. The relationship of the axillary nerve and the acromion. J Med Assoc Thai 1998;81:953–957

3

Proximal Humeral Fractures: Clinical Evaluation and Classification

MATTHEW I. LEIBMAN AND JOSEPH D. ZUCKERMAN

Fractures of the proximal humerus are potentially complex injuries that can be challenging to diagnose and treat. A comprehensive evaluation of the entire shoulder girdle is an essential component of the management of these injuries. Imaging of the proximal humerus can be difficult. An accurate radiographic evaluation must be obtained, however. Classification systems have evolved over time, and their ability to reliably predict outcome and guide treatment have greatly improved. This chapter focuses on the clinical and radiographic evaluation of the patient who sustains a proximal humerus fracture, and describes the classification systems that are currently in use.

■ Epidemiology

Proximal humerus fractures are relatively common, representing 4 to 5% of all fractures.[1] They are considered to be an osteoporosis-related fracture based on an increased incidence in elderly women and this location in metaphyseal bone.[2,3] Approximately 75% of proximal humerus fractures occur in elderly postmenopausal women, and they are most commonly associated with simple falls.[1] Lind et al[4] demonstrated this female predominance (3:1), as well as a low-energy injury pattern in an epidemiologic study of 730 proximal humerus fractures.[4] Like other osteoporosis-related fractures, a unipolar age distribution exists, with the highest incidence occurring in octogenarian woman.[3] Fractures of the proximal humerus tend to occur most commonly in the subset of the elderly population that is relatively healthy and physically fit. Court-Brown et al[3] evaluated 1027 proximal humerus fractures in Edinburgh over a 5-year period, and found that less than 10% of these

fractures occurred in institutionalized patients and more than two thirds of the patients were living independently at the time of fracture.

A large epidemiologic study from Sweden demonstrated a steady and significant increase in the incidence of proximal humerus fractures over the last 30 years.[5] Other investigators have reported similar results and have partially attributed these findings to the increased average life span.[4] All epidemiologic data confirm that fractures of the proximal humerus are primarily an osteoporosis injury. As our population ages, these fractures will represent an increasingly significant socioeconomic problem and source of morbidity in the elderly population.[1,6,7]

■ Clinical Evaluation

History and Physical Examination

When evaluating a patient with a proximal humerus fracture, it is essential to obtain a detailed history and perform a comprehensive examination. The history should include the mechanism of injury, to determine if a high- or low-energy event occurred. It is critical to determine whether a fall was secondary to a syncopal episode and if the patient sustained a head injury. If either occurred, full medical and neurologic evaluation is necessary. The patient's handedness, occupation, and health status should be determined. It is also important to inquire about previous injuries to the shoulder or preexisting loss of function. The patient's overall psychological well-being should be assessed during the initial interview, as well as the patient's expectations of treatment. The patient's own assessment of the impact of the injury may very well impact the ultimate outcome.[8,9]

The physical examination of the injured extremity requires visualization of the entire shoulder region and upper extremity. Proximal humerus fractures usually result in varied degrees of swelling, which may make it difficult to palpate specific bony landmarks. Significant ecchymosis can develop 24 to 48 hours after the injury, frequently with extension to the chest wall flank and distally into the arm, elbow, and forearm (Fig. **3–1**). It is important to instruct patients to remove any jewelry from the ipsilateral extremity, as tendon swelling of the wrist and hand can also develop within 24 to 48 hours. Palpation of the proximal humerus area is anticipated to be painful, and attempts to initiate active motion will also be painful and possibly associated with crepitance.[10]

Careful inspection of the contours of the shoulder is important. Although swelling may obscure these landmarks, a significant deformity should raise a suspicion for fracture dislocation. Anterior prominence, posterior flattening, and the prominence of the posterolateral acromion should suggest an anterior dislocation component. Conversely, posterior prominence, prominent coracoid process, and anterior flattening should suggest a posterior dislocation.[10,11]

The chest wall should be carefully examined because rib fractures may occur in association with the fall. More significant associated thoracic injury, although rare, can occur with proximal humerus fractures and especially with fracture dislocations. Pneumothorax and intrathoracic penetration of the humeral head have been reported. These more significant injuries usually occur in association with fracture dislocations.[12,13]

The stability of the fracture should be assessed during the physical exam. Gentle rotation of the humeral shaft is performed while palpating its proximal portion (Fig. **3–2**). If the humerus moves as a unit, some degree of fracture stability is present. If the humerus does not move as a unit or if crepitance is present, the fracture is unstable. It is important to note that fracture stability

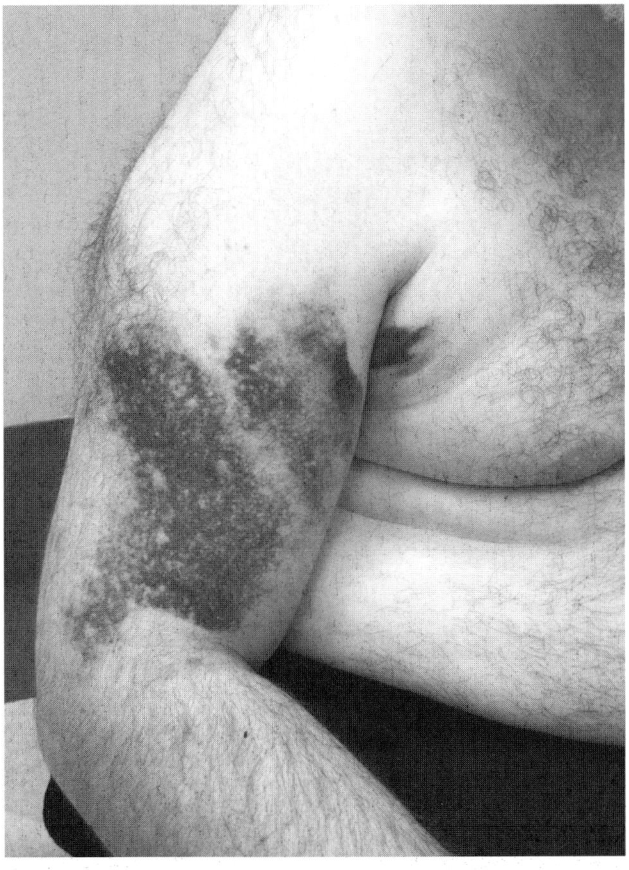

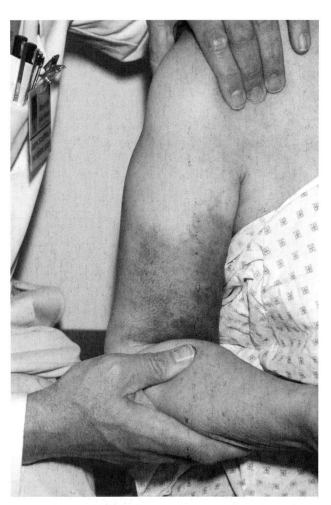

FIGURE 3–1 Ecchymosis of the arm down to the elbow is evident in this 58-year-old man less than 48 hours after sustaining a one-part fracture.

FIGURE 3–2 The stability of the fracture can be most easily assessed by gently rotating the humeral shaft while palpating its proximal portion to determine if the humerus "moves as a unit."

and adequate alignment are different issues. A stable fracture pattern may be significantly malaligned but impacted, providing some stability.[7]

A detailed neurovascular examination must be done and documented at the time of the initial examination. The close proximity to the brachial plexus and axillary artery makes them susceptible to injury. Distal pulses must be documented; however, the presence of a distal pulse does not preclude an arterial injury.[14–16] A thorough sensory exam is essential. The axillary nerve is most commonly injured, followed by the suprascapular nerve. Nerve injuries have a reported prevalence of 5 to 30%.[17] These injuries are typically neuropraxias and occur with displaced fractures. It is difficult to assess deltoid activity due to pain inhibition; however, the sensory component of the axillary nerve can easily be assessed by examination of the lateral aspect of the deltoid.[10] If a complete and reliable neurologic exam cannot be obtained at the time of the initial assessment, it should be repeated as symptoms subside.

Deltoid atony may occur after a proximal humerus fracture or in a postoperative setting. This condition results in inferior subluxation of the humeral head, which is visualized on the anteroposterior (AP) radiograph (Fig. 3–3). This condition must be differentiated from an axillary nerve injury. The inferior subluxation associated

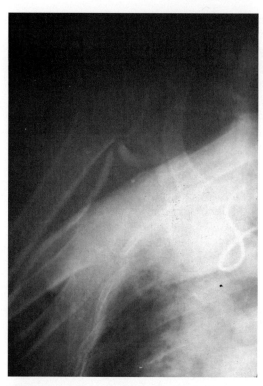

FIGURE 3–4 Following closed reduction of a displaced surgical neck fracture, diminished distal pulses were noted in this 68-year-old patient. Angiogram showed the axillary artery to be caught in the fracture site, requiring vascular repair and fracture stabilization.

with deltoid atony usually resolves within 3 to 4 weeks of injury as deltoid function improves.[18]

The axillary artery injuries are much less common than neurologic injuries. Excellent collateral circulation exists around the shoulder, which may mask a thrombosis or laceration. Injury to the vasculature can occur as a result of direct impingement by fracture fragments or by entrapment of the vessel in the fracture site (Fig. 3–4). Distal pulses may still be present in the setting of a vascular injury. An expanding hematoma may be the only clinical sign suggesting a vascular injury. An associated brachial plexus deficit should raise the suspicion of a possible vascular injury.[15,16]

Mechanism of Injury

Proximal humerus fractures most commonly result from a fall onto an outstretched hand from a standing position.[4,6] The fracture results from an indirect force that is transmitted to the proximal humerus as the patient attempts to cushion the fall with the outstretched arm. Two alternative injury mechanisms include: (1) a direct lateral blow to the shoulder, or (2) an axial load transmitted through the elbow.[11] Codman described an additional mechanism of injury that involved excessive rotation of the arm in an abducted position that leads

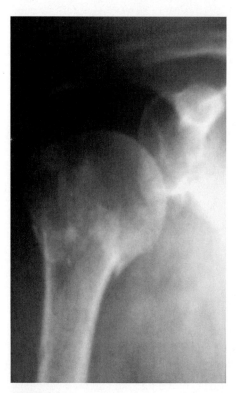

FIGURE 3–3 Inferior subluxation ("pseudosubluxation") may be evident following proximal humerus fractures as a result of pain inhibition of the deltoid ("deltoid atony").

to impingement of the humerus on the acromion.[10] Electrical shock or seizure activity can lead to violent and powerful muscle contractions around the shoulder girdle, resulting in fracture, dislocation, or fracture-dislocation.[19–22] Proximal humerus fractures in young adults typically represent injuries in polytrauma. When a very low energy injury results in a proximal humerus fracture, a pathologic etiology should be considered.

Radiographic Evaluation

A critical aspect of evaluating proximal humerus fractures is determining the position of the fracture fragments and the degree of displacement. The radiographic imaging of the glenohumeral joint can be difficult due to the fact that it lies between the sagittal and coronal planes of the body.[23] Therefore, anteroposterior and lateral views oriented to the body do not provide true images of the glenohumeral joint. Overlapping osseous and soft tissue shadows in combination with multiple fracture lines further increases the difficulty of interpreting radiographs. Nonetheless, accurate radiographic evaluations are essential to determine the appropriate treatment plan.

Trauma Series

The trauma series is considered the gold standard for the radiographic evaluation of proximal humerus fractures. Fracture classification and treatment decisions are typically based on these views, which include AP and lateral views of the plane of the scapula and an axillary lateral view[24,25] (Fig. 3–5). By orienting the projection of the x-ray to the scapula instead of to the body, a view of in the plane of the glenohumeral joint can be obtained. These three radiographs allow for evaluation of the fracture in three distinct orthogonal planes.[26]

The scapula AP view provides a general overview of the fracture and is typically evaluated first (Fig. 3–6). It can be obtained easily with the injured extremity maintained in a sling for comfort. Because the scapula lies posterior and somewhat lateral on the thorax (angulated 45° from the frontal plane), the true plane of the glenohumeral joint lies in this 45° plane, not in the plane of the thorax. The x-ray must be angled 45° from medial to lateral to demonstrate the glenohumeral joint in profile. This view avoids the overlap of the humeral head and the glenoid; that is, there should be clear separation of the glenoid from the humeral head.[24,26] When an x-ray is taken in the plane of the thorax, an oblique view of the glenohumeral joint will be obtained. In this situation, overlap of the humeral head and glenoid can obscure the details of the fracture.

The axillary view is obtained with the patient supine and the arm abducted 30° to 90°. The beam is directed into the axilla angulated toward the coracoid in an inferior to superior direction. The x-ray cassette is placed on the superior aspect of the shoulder. The patient's head is tilted to the opposite side so that the plate could be placed medially.[27] This view is excellent for visualizing dislocations and fractures involving the articular surface (Fig. 3–7). Positioning of the patient for the axillary view is more difficult because of the need for shoulder abduction. Proper positioning usually requires the physician to gently abduct the arm, and at times hold the arm in position while the x-ray is obtained.

The scapula lateral, like the scapula AP view, can be obtained with the arm in a sling. It does not require manipulation of the arm and is less painful for the patient. The x-ray beam is directed parallel to the spine of the scapula. A true lateral projection of the scapula forms the letter Y in which the upper arms of the Y are formed by the coracoid process anteriorly and the scapula spine posteriorly. The vertical portion of the Y is formed by the scapula body. All three limbs of the Y intersect in the position of the glenoid and the humeral head (Fig. 3–8). It should be visualized overlapping this point.[14,22] This view assists in delineating the position of the humeral head relative to the glenoid and demonstrates anteriorly and posteriorly displaced fragments.[28,29]

A study by Sidor et al[25] evaluated the relative contributions of the axillary and scapula lateral views to the fracture classification using the Neer system. Each x-ray of the trauma series in 50 proximal humerus fractures was evaluated by four orthopaedic surgeons and one musculoskeletal radiologist using different sequences: scapula AP, axillary view and scapula lateral versus scapula AP, scapula lateral, and axillary view. They found that the combination of the axillary and AP view was just as effective in determining fracture classification as the entire trauma series. The axillary view had a much greater impact on fracture classification than the scapula lateral view.

Additional Radiograph Views

Inadequate x-rays are probably the most common problem encountered when evaluating proximal humerus fractures. The three views of the trauma series should be obtained first using proper technique so they will provide as much information as possible. Other views have been described that may provide additional information to augment the trauma series. The Velpeau axillary view is a modification of the axillary view that was designed for the acutely injured patient because it allows the x-ray to be taken with the arm adducted in the sling (Fig. 3–9). The patient sits or stands near the x-ray table and leans back 20° to 30°. The x-ray cassette is placed in the table slot directly

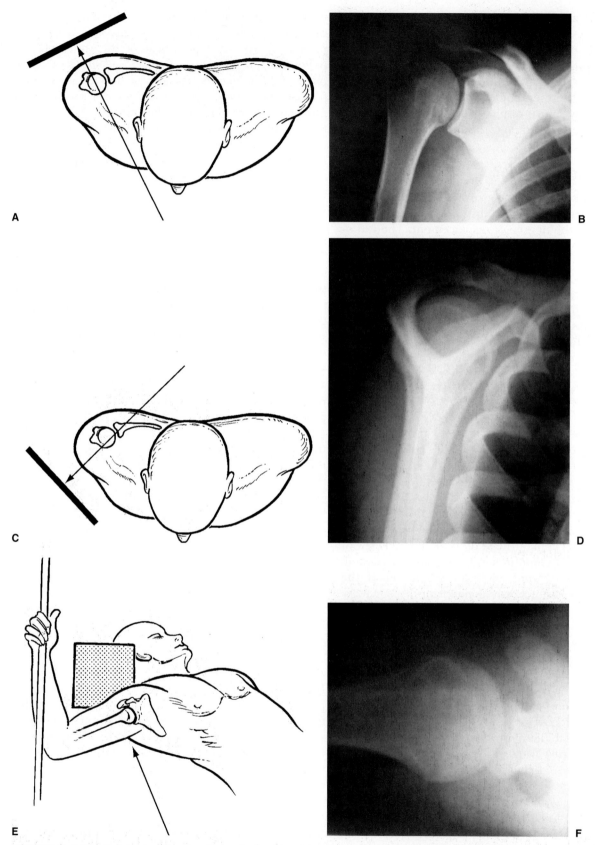

FIGURE 3–5 The trauma series of radiographs consists of anteroposterior **(A,B)** and lateral views **(C,D)** in the scapular plane and an axillary view **(E,F)**.

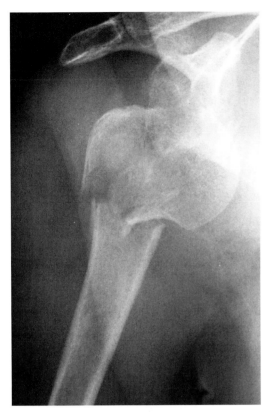

FIGURE 3–6 The anteroposterior (AP) view generally provides important information about the fracture pattern, especially when the surgical neck and greater tuberosity are involved. It also shows the presence of an anterior dislocation.

beneath the patient's shoulder. The beam passes vertically from superior to inferior through the shoulder.[30] This radiograph results in a magnified view of the glenohumeral joint and is helpful for identifying anterior/posterior dislocations. Our experience has been

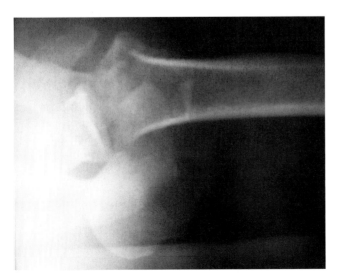

FIGURE 3–7 The axillary view can delineate humeral head dislocations, angulation of surgical neck fractures, and displacement of the tuberosities.

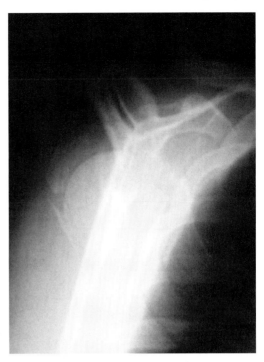

FIGURE 3–8 The scapular lateral view also provides information about dislocation as well as shaft displacement in the sagittal plane.

that it does not provide the details of fracture anatomy, and a properly positioned supine standard axillary and lateral view is preferred. Other modifications of the axillary view have been described such as the stripp axial.[31]

Some surgeons have chosen to add a fourth view to the trauma series and obtain a scapula AP with the arm at 20° of external rotation. This additional x-ray provides a clearer view of the greater tuberosity;[10] however, achieving 20° of external rotation in the acutely injured shoulder can be difficult.

Other Imaging Studies

Computed tomography (CT) has been used frequently in the evaluation of proximal humeral fractures (Fig. **3–10**), although its benefits other than for specific fracture patterns remain unclear. It is helpful in the evaluation of fracture dislocations, glenoid fractures, posterior displacement of the greater tuberosity, and anterior displacement of the lesser tuberosity. It is extremely helpful in the evaluation of chronic dislocations to evaluate the size of the impression fracture and the degree of secondary glenoid changes (Fig. **3–11**). To obtain the most information, the CT scan should include 3 mm cuts from the top of the acromion to the inferior aspect of the glenoid.[10]

It was initially believed that CT scans would provide additional information that allowed more accurate

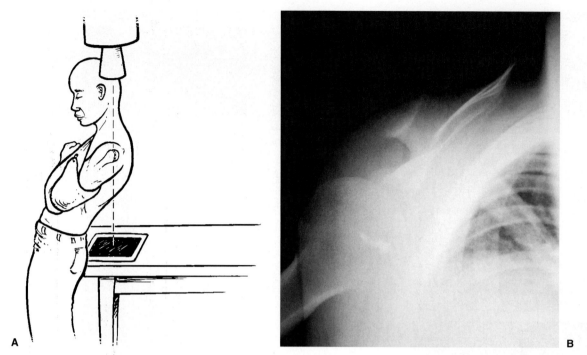

FIGURE 3–9 (A) The Velpeau axillary view can be obtained without moving the injured shoulder and maintaining the extremity in a sling. **(B)** It is helpful in identifying the relationship of the humeral head to the glenoid.

understanding of the pathoanatomy of the fracture.[32,33] Despite the potential usefulness of CT scans, the literature has not supported this concept. Sallay et al[34] found that CT scans did not improve the reliability or reproducibility of the Neer fracture classification. Two studies by Sjoden et al[35,36] found that CT scans did not improve reproducibility of the Neer and AO/Association for the Study of Internal Fixation (ASIF) classifications compared with standard radiographs. Bernstein et al[37] found that the addition of CT scans resulted in a slight increase in reliability but did not improve interobserver reliability when using the Neer classification. More importantly, they found that experts were still unable to agree which fragments were fractured with the addition of CT scans.

Magnetic resonance imaging is rarely used in the evaluation and management of proximal humerus fractures; however, it may be helpful in identifying associated soft tissue injury and early posttraumatic osteonecrosis. Its cost-effectiveness in the setting of proximal humeral fractures has not yet been determined. In general, it should be reserved for specific fracture patterns to address specific concerns.

■ Classification

The purpose of a fracture classification system is to provide a method for describing fractures, which in turn should provide guidelines for treatment and prognosis. The system must be comprehensive and ideally should encompass all possible factors and variations. The complex anatomy of the proximal humerus and glenohumeral articulation necessitates a large number of fracture types; however, a classification system should rely on specific, clearly identifiable factors.[38,39] It is also essential for the classification system to have acceptable inter- and intraobserver reliability. Most importantly, this reliability should be based on routine radiographs that are easily and reproducibly obtained in a standard clinical setting.[29,39]

History of Proximal Humerus Classifications

The early classification systems for proximal humerus fractures were simplistic and often based on the mechanism of injury. They had relatively no correlation with treatment or prognosis. Kocher's original classification was based on the different anatomic levels of the fracture. He divided the fractures into four groups: supertubercular, per tubercular, infratubercular, and subtubercular. The classification did not address fracture displacement, dislocation, or mechanisms of injury. Watson-Jones later proposed a classification system that was based on the mechanism injury. He divided the fractures into three groups: contusion crack fractures (Fig. **3–12A**), impacted adduction fractures (Fig. **3–12B**), and impacted abducted fractures (Fig. **3–12C**). This

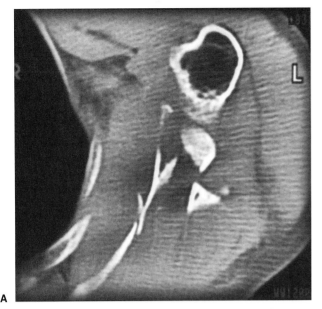

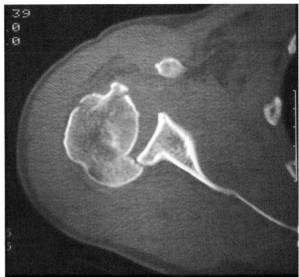

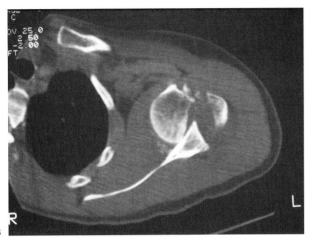

FIGURE 3–10 Computed tomography (CT) scans are very useful in the evaluation of glenoid fractures **(A)**, proximal humerus fracture-dislocations **(B)**, and dislocations associated with impression fractures **(C)**.

system was limited by the fact that humeral rotation significantly altered the radiographic appearance and, thereby, altered the classification.[6]

In 1934 Codman recognized that fractures of the proximal humerus tended to occur along the old epiphyseal lines that separated the articular surface, greater and lesser tuberosities, and shaft into four distinct segments (Fig. **3–13**). Codman's recognition of these four segments was the basis of the Neer classification system described in 1970.[14,24]

The Neer Classification

Neer based his classification system on the study of 300 displaced proximal humerus fractures (Fig. **3–14**). The purpose of the classification system was to identify all possible types of proximal humerus fractures, document the anatomic findings, and provide a standard

terminology that would represent the specific injury pattern. Neer based his classification on Codman's four fragment patterns, noting that all fractures differed in which segments were involved and in how displaced they were. The Neer classification did not address the level of the fracture, number of fracture lines, or the mechanism of injury. Neer intended his classification to be based on a "concept" or mental picture of the pathomechanics of the fracture, not a numerical classification.[38]

The four segment classification is based on the displacement of one or more of the segments. For a segment to be considered displaced, it must be either greater than 1 cm. displaced, or angulated more than 45°. If none of these criteria is met, the fracture is considered nondisplaced or minimally displaced; that is, a "one-part" fracture. Two-part fractures are named by the segment that is displaced. Three-part fractures all have a displaced

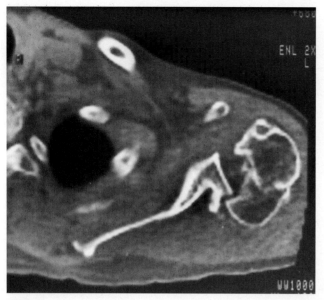

FIGURE 3–11 The CT scan can assist in determining the chronicity of dislocations as shown here. Reactive bone along the posterior glenoid neck is evident.

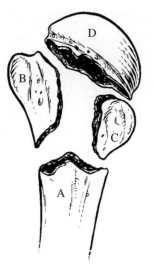

FIGURE 3–13 Codman's classification is based on the location of the epiphyseal lines in the proximal humerus and identified four specific fragments. A, humeral shaft; B, greater tuberosity; C, lesson tuberosity; D, articular segment.

surgical neck component and are named by the displaced tuberosity. Four-part fractures have all four segments displaced.[38]

One-Part Fractures

One-part fractures or minimally displaced fractures include all fractures in which no segment is displaced more than 1 cm or angulated/rotated more than 45°. This group represents 80 to 85% of all proximal humerus fractures.[24] Fracture stability is maintained by the soft tissues that remain intact, allowing the fracture to move as a single unit.

Two-Part Fractures

There are four types of two-part fractures. Two-part anatomic neck fractures represent a rare fracture type in which there is isolated displacement of the articular segment at the level of the anatomic neck without

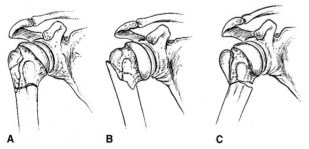

A   B   C

FIGURE 3–12 (A–C) The Watson-Jones classification is based on the mechanism of injury, particularly the role of abduction and adduction forces.

displacement or involvement of the tuberosities. A high incidence of osteonecrosis is anticipated with this fracture type because of its separation from the metaphyseal portion of the proximal humerus.

Two-part surgical neck fractures occur at the surgical neck distal to the tuberosities (Fig. 3–15). The pectoralis major is the major deforming force, resulting in medial displacement of the humeral shaft. Rotator cuff attachments remain intact, holding the proximal fragment in a relatively neutral position. Neer described three subtypes of two-part surgical neck fractures: impacted, unimpacted, and comminuted. The impacted type is angulated greater than 45° and usually has an apex anterior alignment. In the unimpacted type, the shaft is displaced medially and there is complete loss of contact between the two fragments. The comminuted type consists of a segment of comminution at the surgical neck level that extends to the proximal shaft, resulting in an unstable pattern.

Two-part greater tuberosity fractures are common and frequently occur in association with anterior glenohumeral dislocations (Fig. 3–16). Some authors have questioned whether the definition of displacement (i.e., measuring 1 cm) is appropriate for the greater tuberosity segment and believe that a lower threshold should apply to the greater tuberosity, particularly for displacement superiorly into the subacromion space. A threshold of 5 mm has been suggested because greater amounts of displacement would lead to mechanical interference with the gliding mechanism in the subacromial space.[40] Two-part lesser tuberosity fractures are relatively uncommon. They can occur as isolated injuries but more commonly occur in association with posterior glenohumeral dislocations (Fig. 3–17). Significant medial displacement of the fragment may block internal rotation.

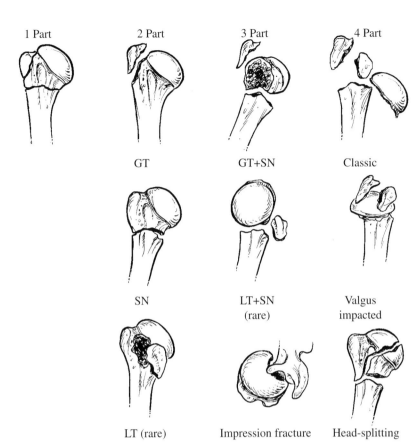

1 Part   2 Part   3 Part   4 Part

GT   GT+SN   Classic

SN   LT+SN   Valgus
       (rare)   impacted

LT (rare)   Impression fracture   Head-splitting

FIGURE 3–14 The Neer classification is based on the four segments described by Codman and adds fracture-dislocations, impression fractures, and head-splitting fractures.

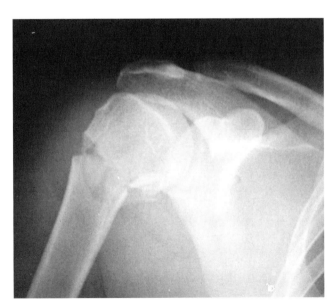

FIGURE 3–15 Two-part surgical neck fracture.

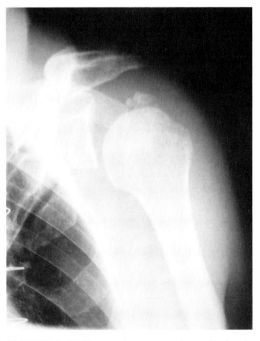

FIGURE 3–16 Two-part greater tuberosity fracture.

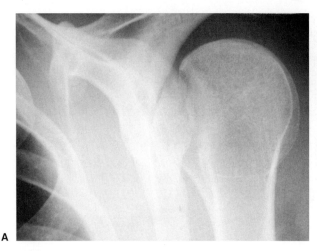
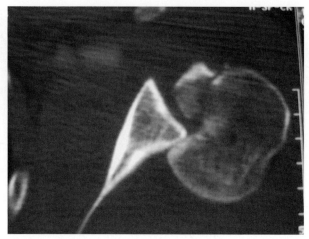

FIGURE 3–17 Scapular lateral **(A)** and CT scan **(B)** of two-part lesser tuberosity posterior fracture-dislocation.

Three-Part Fractures

The two types of three-part fractures both have a displaced surgical neck component with one tuberosity that is displaced and one tuberosity that remains in continuity with the head. If the greater tuberosity is displaced (a three-part greater tuberosity fracture), the head assumes a position of internal rotation due to the unopposed pole of the subscapularis muscle on the intact lesser tuberosity. This is the more commonly encountered fracture pattern (Fig. **3–18**). If the lesser tuberosity is displaced (a three-part lesser tuberosity fracture), the head is externally rotated due to the unopposed pull of the supraspinatus/infraspinatus/terres minor on the greater tuberosity.

Four-Part Fractures

In a classic four-part fracture, both tuberosities are detached from the articular segment (Fig. **3–19**). Typically, the articular segment is laterally displaced and is not in contact with the glenoid. These fractures have the highest risk for osteonecrosis due to the complete disruption of the blood supply to the humeral head. The valgus impacted four-part fracture is a subtype of the "classic" four-part fracture (Fig. **3–20**). In this pattern, the articular segment is impacted into the shaft in a valgus orientation. Both tuberosities displace away from the shaft as a result of the inferior impaction of the articular surface.[38] This fracture has a relatively reduced risk of osteonecrosis most probably because of preservation of some of the blood supply entering the humeral head through intact capsular attachments.[10,41]

The Neer classification also included fracture dislocations that could occur with two-part, three-part, and four-part fractures in which the humeral head could be dislocated either anteriorly or posteriorly. Six specific subtypes of fracture dislocations are described.

The Neer classification also describes two types of articular surface fractures: impression fractures and head-splitting fractures. Impression fractures are most commonly associated with chronic dislocations. Posterolateral impression fractures are primarily associated with chronic anterior dislocations (Fig. **3–21**) and anterior-medial impression fractures are associated with chronic posterior dislocations (Fig. **3–22**). Head-splitting fractures are a result of a central impacting force or associated with other displaced segments[24,38] (Fig. **3–23**).

Reliability of the Neer Classification

Fracture classifications have been described as a "tool" that not only should help the surgeon choose an appropriate

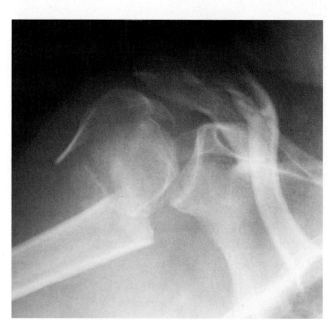

FIGURE 3–18 Three-part fracture involving the greater tuberosity and surgical neck.

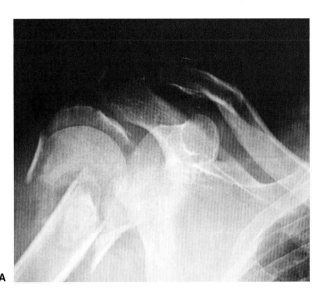

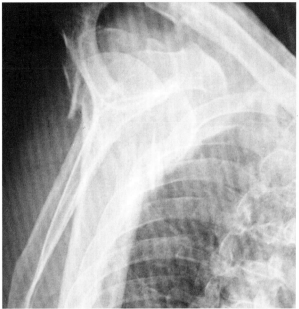

FIGURE 3–19 Four-part fractures. The "classic" pattern with lateral extrusion of the articular surface is evident on AP **(A)** and lateral **(B)** radiographs.

treatment method but also should predict outcomes.[39] A large number of studies addressed the reliability of the Neer classification system, focusing specifically on the intra- and interobserver reliability. Intraobserver reliability assesses whether the classification produces the same result when repeated by the same observer. If the observer assesses a proximal humerus fracture on two occasions or in two patients, the same classification should be

chosen. Interobserver reliability assesses whether the test produces the same result when applied by different observers. If different observers assess a proximal humeral fracture using the same set of x-rays, the same classification should be chosen.[38,42]

Sidor et al[42] conducted a study to assess the degree of intraobserver and interobserver reliability of the Neer classification system using the standard trauma series

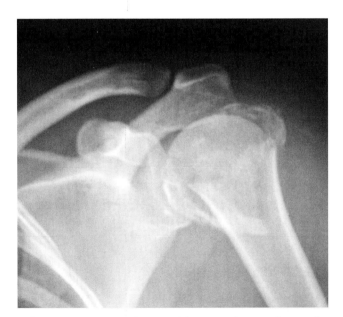

FIGURE 3–20 Valgus-impacted four-part fracture has a characteristic appearance with a valgus-impacted position of the articular segment, resulting in outward displacement of the tuberosities.

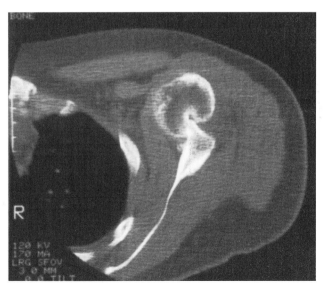

FIGURE 3–21 CT scan of chronic anterior dislocation showing the presence of a large posterolateral humeral head impression fracture.

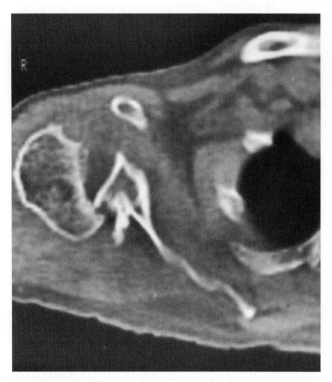

FIGURE 3–22 CT scan of chronic posterior dislocation with an anteromedial humeral head impression fracture.

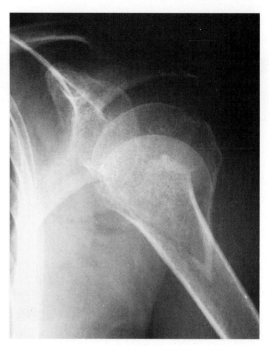

FIGURE 3–23 Head-splitting fracture with the double subchondral density consistent with a split in the articular surface.

for 50 proximal humerus fractures. Radiographs were reviewed, on two separate occasions (6 months apart), by an orthopaedic shoulder specialist, an orthopaedic traumatologist, a skeletal radiologist, and two orthopaedic residents. Inter- and intraobserver reliability were determined and kappa reliability coefficients were calculated. Kappa coefficients ranged from 1.0 (complete agreement) to 0 (chance agreement). A kappa value of 0.61 to 0.8 was considered as substantial agreement. The authors found a moderate level of interobserver reliability with both experienced and inexperience surgeons. The kappa reliability coefficient ranged from 0.37 to 0.62. A kappa value of >0.81 (excellent agreement) was not obtained for any paired evaluation. Intraobserver reliability was found to be slightly higher, with kappa values ranging from 0.5 to 0.68. The shoulder specialist was the only observer to score a kappa value >0.8.[42] Brien et al[43] and Siebenrock and Gerber[44] both found poor to moderate interobserver and intraobserver reliability for the Neer classification system. Kappa values ranged from 0.35 to 0.45 and 0.4 to 0.6, respectively, for the two studies. A study by Bernstein et al[37] found that the disagreement of the Neer classification did not relate to observers determining if a fragment was displaced, based on angulation or displacement, but instead the disagreement stemmed from determining if fragment separation occurred at all. In close to half of their cases, the observers could not agree on which segments were even involved.

Kristiansen and Christensen[45] found the Neer classification system to have a low level of reliability but also found fragment criteria to have prognostic significance. Minimally displaced one-part fractures essentially all had excellent outcomes, whereas 50% of displaced fractures had unsatisfactory outcomes. They concluded that the classification system had great prognostic value despite the problems with reliability.

The problems with the reliability of the Neer classification system are an important factor, but, at the same time, it is only one measure of a classification. Classifications that are less reliable may in fact be more clinically useful and have greater prognostic capability.[38] Neer's system has simplified proximal humerus fractures and decreased confusion in the treatment of this injury. In a recent review article, Neer[38] stated that his classification "is not a radiographic system but is a pathoanatomic classification of fracture displacement and accurate assessment of fracture displacement may require special roentgen studies and even operative assessment."

AO/ASIF Classification

The AO/ASIF classification system (Fig. **3–24**) of proximal humerus fractures focuses on the blood supply of two articular segments. This more complex classification system with 27 subgroups attempts to provide detailed therapeutic and prognostic guidelines. Proximal humerus

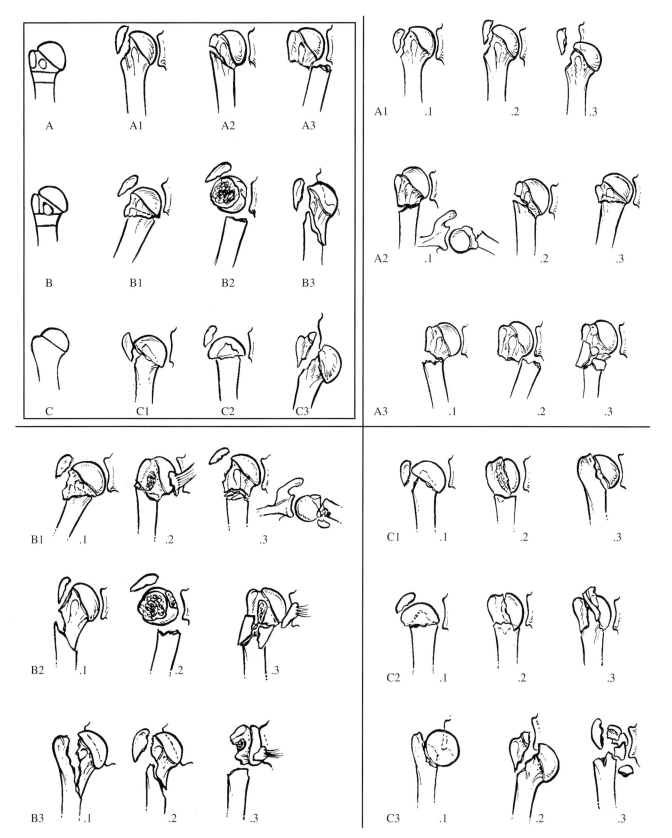

FIGURE 3–24 The AO/ASIF classification of proximal humerus fractures focuses on the extra- versus intraarticular location of the fracture and the potential for the development of osteonecrosis.

fractures are divided into three types: extraarticular unifocal, extraarticular bifocal, and articular fractures. These are then further divided into groups, based on degree and direction of displacement, presence of impaction, and associated dislocation.[29]

Type A fractures are extraarticular and involve one tuberosity. These fractures are extracapsular and do not compromise the blood supply of the articular surface, and thereby have little or no risk of osteonecrosis. Type B fractures are also extraarticular but involve both tuberosities with a concomitant metaphyseal fracture or glenohumeral dislocation. In spite of the number of fragments and associated displacement, this fracture group also has a low risk of osteonecrosis. Type C fractures involve the articular surface with disruption of the blood supply to the humeral head. These fractures are the most severe and are at high risk for osteonecrosis. Each of these groups is then subdivided into three numerical groups in which higher numbers reflect increased severity.[10,29,46]

In general, the complexity of this classification system has precluded its widespread utilization in the United States. It is used more commonly in Europe. Assessment of intra- and interobserver reliability has not shown it to be significantly better than the Neer classification when these patients are evaluated. Siebenrock and Gerber[44] studied the reliability of both the Neer and AO/ASIF classification systems. Kappa reliability values were found to be moderate for both systems (Neer, 0.4 to 0.6; AO, 0.53 to 0.58).[44]

■ Conclusion

Proximal humerus fractures are common injuries encountered by orthopaedic surgeons. Although up to 85% of these fractures are minimally displaced, it is the other 15 to 20% that present the most significant challenge, beginning with the proper classification. Clinical evaluation is required, including a detailed history and physical examination. By integrating the radiographic characteristics and specific attributes of the exam, fracture stability can be determined. The trauma series is the most commonly used radiographic method of assessing these fractures. The Neer classification system, based on Codman's description of the four fragments of the proximal humerus, is currently the most widely accepted classification for proximal humerus fractures. It is based on displacement of one or more of the four described segments: articular surface, greater tuberosity, lesser tuberosity, and humeral shaft. Numerous studies have addressed the Neer classification system and have demonstrated varying levels of reliability. Imaging techniques, as well as our understanding of the pathoanatomy, continue to improve. It is hoped that these two factors will lead us

to more reliable classifications that will ultimately guide treatment and predict prognosis in proximal humerus fractures.

REFERENCES

1. Rose SH, Melton LJ III, Morrey BF, Ilstrup DM, Riggs BL. Epidemiologic features of humeral fractures. Clin Orthop 1982;168:24–30
2. Horak J, Nillson BE. Epidemiology of fracture of the upper end of the humerus. Clin Orthop 1975;112:250–253
3. Court-Brown CM, Garg A, McQueen MM. The epidemiology of proximal humeral fractures. Acta Orthop Scand 2001;72:365–371
4. Lind T, Kroner K, Jensen J. The epidemiology of fractures of the proximal humerus. Arch Orthop Trauma Surg 1989;108:285–287
5. Bengner U, Johnell O, Redlund-Johnell I. Changes in the incidence of fracture of the upper end of the humerus during a thirty-year period. Clin Orthop 1988;231:179–182
6. Bigliani LU, Flatow EL, Pollock RG. Fracture of the proximal humerus. In: Rockwood CA, Matsen FA, eds. The Shoulder. Philadelphia: WB Saunders, 1990:337–389
7. Cornell CN, Schneider K. Proximal humerus. In: Koval KJ, Zuckerman JD, eds. Fractures in the Elderly. Philadelphia: Lippincott-Raven, 1998:85–92
8. Cofield RH. Comminuted fractures of the proximal humerus. Clin Orthop 1988;230:49–57
9. Norris TR, Green A. Proximal humerus fractures and glenohumeral dislocations. In: Browner BD, Jupiter JB, Levine AM, Trafton PG, eds. Skeletal Trauma. Philadelphia: WB Saunders, 1998:1549–1656
10. Flatow EL. Fractures of the proximal humerus. In: Bucholz RW, Heckman JD, eds. Rockwood and Green's Fractures in Adults. Philadelphia: Lippincott Williams & Wilkins, 2002:997–1040
11. Hawkins RJ, Neer CS II, Pianta RM, Mendoza FX. Locked posterior dislocation of the shoulder. J. Bone Joint Surg Am. 1987;69:9–18
12. Glessner JR. Intrathoracic dislocation of the humeral head. J Bone Joint Surg 1961;43-A:428–430
13. Patel MR, Pardee ML, Singerman RC. Intrathoracic dislocation of the head of the humerus. J Bone Joint Surg Am 1963;45:1712–1714
14. Neer CS III. Displaced proximal humeral fractures. II. Treatment of three-part and four-part displacement. J Bone Joint Surg Am 1970;52:1090–1103
15. Zuckerman JD, Flugstad DL, Teitz CC, King HA. Axillary artery injury as a complication of proximal humeral fractures. Two case reports and a review of the literature. Clin Orthop 1984;189:234–237
16. Smyth EH. Major arterial injury in closed fracture of the neck of the humerus. Report of a case. J Bone Joint Surg Br 1969;51:508–510
17. Visser CPJ, Coene LN, Brand R, Tavy DLJ. Nerve lesions in proximal humeral fractures. J Shoulder Elbow Surg 2001;10:421–427
18. Fairbank TJ. Fracture-subluxations of the shoulder. J Bone Joint Surg Br 1948;30:454–460
19. Hawkins RJ, Angelo RL. Displaced proximal humeral fractures: selecting treatment, avoiding pitfalls. Orthop Clin North Am 1987;18:421–431
20. Shaw JL. Bilateral posterior fracture-dislocation of the shoulder and other trauma caused by convulsive seizures. J Bone Joint Surg Am 1971;53:1437–1440
21. Kelly JP. Fractures complicating electro-convulsive therapy and chronic epilepsy. J Bone Joint Surg Br 1954;36-B:70–79

22. McLaughlin HL. Posterior dislocation of the shoulder. J Bone Joint Surg Am 1952;24-A:584–590

23. Richardson JB, Ramsay A, Davidson JK, Kelly IG. Radiographs in shoulder trauma. J Bone Joint Surg Br 1988;70:457–460

24. Neer CS II. Displaced proximal humeral fractures. I. Classification and evaluation. J Bone Joint Surg Am 1970;52:1077–1089

25. Sidor ML, Zuckerman JD, Lyon T, Koval K, Schoenberg N. Classification of proximal humeral fractures. The contribution of the scapular lateral and axillary radiographs. J Shoulder Elbow Surg 1994;3:24–27

26. Rockwood CA, Jensen KL. X-ray evaluation of shoulder problems. In: Rockwood CA, Matsen FA, eds. The Shoulder. Philadelphia: WB Saunders, 1990:199–203

27. Neviaser RJ. Radiologic assessment of the shoulder. Plain and arthrographic. Orthop Clin North Am 1987;18:343–349

28. Silfverskiold JP, Straehley DJ, Jones WW. Roentgenographic evaluation of suspected shoulder dislocation: a prospective study comparing the axillary view and the scapular 'Y' view. Orthopedics 1990;13:63–69

29. Sidor ML, Koval KJ, Zuckerman JD. The radiographic evaluation and classification of proximal humerus fractures. In: Flatow E, Ulrich C, eds. Musculoskeletal Trauma. Oxford: Butterworth-Heinemann, 1996

30. Bloom MH, Obata WG. Diagnosis of posterior dislocation of the shoulder with use of Velpeau axillary and angle-up roentgenographic views. J. Bone Joint Surg 1967;49:943–949

31. Horsefield D, Jones SN. A useful projection in radiography of the shoulder. J Bone Joint Surg 1987;69-B:338

32. Kuhlman JE, Fishman EK, Ney DR, Magid D. Complex shoulder trauma: three-dimensional CT imaging. Orthopedics 1998;11:1561–1563

33. Castagno AA, Shuman WP, Kilcoyne RF, Haynor DR, Morris ME, Matsen FA. Complex fractures of the proximal humerus: role of CT in treatment. Radiology 1987;165:759–762

34. Sallay PI, Pedowitz RA, Mallon WJ, Vandemark RM, Dalton JD, Speer KP. Reliability and reproducibility of radiographic interpretation of proximal humeral fracture pathoanatomy. J Shoulder Elbow Surg 1997;6:60–69

35. Sjoden GOJ, Movin T, Guntener P, et al. Poor reproducibility of proximal humeral fracture: additional CT of minor value. Acta Orthop Scand 1997;68:239–242

36. Sjoden GOJ, Movin T, Asplin P, Guntener P, Shalabi A. 3D-Radiographic analysis does not improve the Neer and AO classifications of proximal humeral fractures. Acta Orthop Scand 1999;70:325–328

37. Bernstein J, Adler LM, Blank JE, Dalsey RM, Williams GR, Iannotti JP. Evaluation of the Neer system of classification of proximal humeral fractures with computerized tomographic scans and plain radiographs. J Bone Joint Surg Am 1996;78:1371–1375

38. Neer CS II. Four-segment classification of proximal humeral fractures: purpose and reliable use. J Shoulder Elbow Surg 2002;11:389–400

39. Burstein AH. Fracture classification systems: do they work and are they useful? J Bone Joint Surg Am 1993;75:1743–1744

40. Park TS, Choi IY, Kim YH, Park MR, Shon JH, Kim SI. A new suggestion for the treatment of minimally displaced fractures of the greater tuberosity of the proximal humerus. Bull Hosp Jt Dis 1997;56:171–176

41. Resch H, Beck E, Bayley I. Reconstruction of valgus-impacted humeral head fracture. J Shoulder Elbow Surg 1995;4:73–80

42. Sidor ML, Zuckerman JD, Lyon T, Koval K, Cuomo F, Schoenberg N. The Neer classification system for proximal humeral fractures: an assessment of interobserver reliability and intraobserver reproducibility. J Bone Joint Surg Am 1993;75:1745–1750

43. Brien H, Noftall F, MacMaster S, Cummings T, Landells C, Rockwood P. Neer's classification system: a critical appraisal. J Trauma 1995;38:257–260

44. Siebenrock KA, Gerber C. The reproducibility of classification of fractures of the proximal end of the humerus. J Bone Joint Surg Am 1993;75:1751–1755

45. Kristiansen B, Christensen SW. Proximal humeral fractures: late results in relation to classification and treatment. Acta Orthop Scand 1987;58:124–127

46. Jakob RP, Kristiansen T, Mayo K, Ganz R, Muller ME. Classification and aspects of treatment of fractures of the proximal humerus. In: Bateman JE, Welsh RP, eds. Surgery of the Shoulder. Philadelphia: BC Decker, 1984:330–343

4

One-Part Fractures

STEVEN S. SHIN AND JOSEPH D. ZUCKERMAN

Fractures about the shoulder make up 5% of all fractures.[1] Among patients aged 15 to 64, proximal humerus fractures make up almost 2% of all fractures, whereas among those older than 65, proximal humerus fractures make up 4% of all fractures.[2,2a] Of all proximal humerus fractures, up to 85% are minimally displaced or nondisplaced, whereas 15% are displaced.[1,3–13] These minimally displaced or nondisplaced fractures have received little attention in the orthopaedic literature, however. Only a few studies have reported the results of treatment of these fractures.[2,3,14,15]

■ Description

A one-part fracture of the proximal humerus, as defined by Neer, is a fracture with less than 1 cm of displacement and less than 45° of angulation between fracture fragments, regardless of the number of fracture lines.[9,16] The AO/Association for the Study of Internal Fixation (ASIF) North America classification of proximal humerus fractures is: type A (extraarticular unifocal fracture), type B (extraarticular bifocal fracture), and type C (articular fracture). Each category is then further subdivided to give a complex system that according to its authors "does not apply as uniformly...as it does in diaphyseal fractures."[17,17a] Using the AO/ASIF system, minimally displaced fractures can be classified as either type A or B, depending on whether one or multiple fractures lines are present. In a study by Koval et al,[18] one-part fractures were most commonly found to be fractures of the surgical neck (42%) and greater tuberosity (30%) (Figs. **4–1** and **4–2**). Multiple fracture lines in the proximal humerus accounted for the remainder of minimally displaced fractures (28%) (Fig. **4–3**). Proper classification of one-part fractures is important because it will determine the treatment plan. Minimally displaced fractures are primarily treated nonoperatively; however, if more significant displacement is identified (i.e., greater than 1 cm displacement or more significant angulation), the fracture is no longer a one-part fracture, and operative management should be considered. This emphasizes the importance of proper radiographic imaging of the fracture.

Fractures of the greater tuberosity (Fig. **4–4**) warrant special mention because some authors believe that less than 5 mm of displacement should be accepted.[19–21] Santee[20] reported that healing of a fracture of the greater tuberosity in slight displacement might result in disability. McLaughlin[21] reported that patients who had 5 to 10 mm of displacement of the fragment often had a prolonged convalescence, with some having permanent pain and disability and with 20% needing a reconstructive procedure. Miller,[22] however, maintained that incomplete reduction was compatible with a good functional result providing the greater tuberosity was not left in an elevated position under the acromion. Jakob and co-workers[6] recommended nonoperative treatment for displacement of 5 to 10 mm because the tuberosity usually remains in an acceptable position. At present, the issue of greater tuberosity fractures with borderline (greater than 5 mm and less than 10 mm) displacement remains uncertain, with both nonoperative and operative treatment recommendations. This type is discussed in Chapter 5.

Most one-part fractures result from a fall onto the outstretched upper extremity or onto the shoulder from a standing height. They occur most commonly in elderly, osteoporotic patients, with the prevalence twice as common in women as in men.[1,6,8] In younger patients, proximal humerus fractures are usually caused by higher energy trauma, such as a motor vehicle accident.

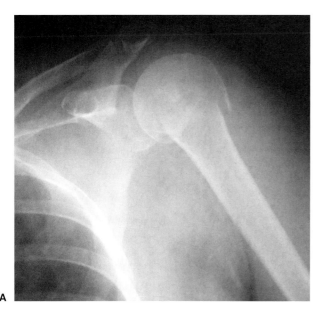

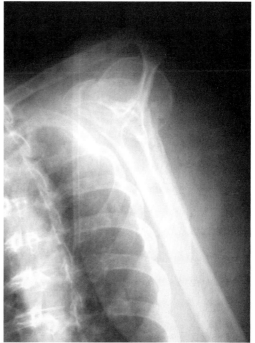

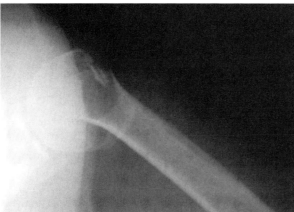

FIGURE 4–1 Trauma series of a one-part surgical neck fracture. The scapular anteroposterior (AP) **(A)**, lateral **(B)**, and axillary **(C)** views show preservation of the alignment of the proximal humerus. There is a nondisplaced greater tuberosity fracture line.

■ Clinical Evaluation

For patients who sustain a proximal humerus fracture, a thorough history should be taken, including the age of the patient, associated medical conditions, work requirements, handedness, recreational activities, and expectations. It should be accompanied by a complete clinical evaluation of the involved shoulder and the ipsilateral upper extremity. In higher energy injuries, the neck and chest should be evaluated. Ipsilateral fractures of the humeral shaft, elbow, forearm, or wrist can occur. The patient with a one-part fracture may have pain, tenderness, and swelling about the shoulder, but to a lesser degree than with more displaced fractures. There will most likely be no appreciable crepitus or deformity about the shoulder. Ecchymosis may be present (Fig. **4–5**), but lacerations and open fractures are rare. The patient may also be unable or unwilling to raise the arm. A thorough neurovascular exam must be performed and documented carefully. Because the axillary nerve is the most frequently injured nerve in proximal humerus fractures, an exam of the sensation over the lateral deltoid and motor function of the three parts of the deltoid is required if pain allows. In a prospective follow-up study by Visser et al,[23] nerve lesions were identified by electromyogram (EMG) in 59% of nondisplaced fractures, with the axillary and suprascapular nerves being the most commonly affected.

The examiner should determine if the proximal humerus moves as one unit or not, to gain assurance that the motion is occurring at the glenohumeral joint and not at the fracture site.[18] With one hand supporting the patient's forearm and elbow and the other placed at the proximal humerus, the examiner carefully rotates the patient's shoulder and determines if the proximal humerus

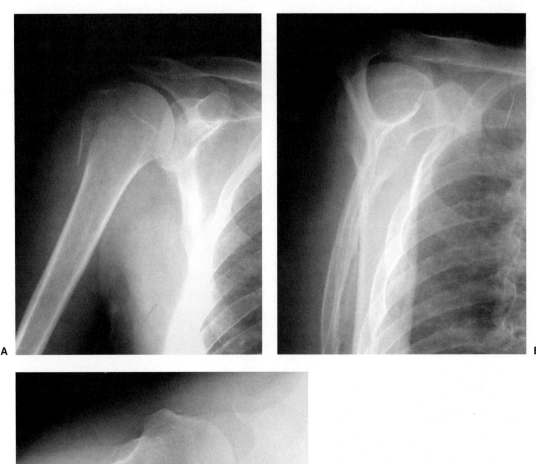

FIGURE 4–2 Scapular AP **(A)**, lateral **(B)**, and axillary **(C)** views of a one-part greater tuberosity fracture. The fragment is less than 1 cm displaced.

moves as "one part" (Fig. **4–6**). Only if the fracture moves as a unit can the patient proceed with early passive shoulder exercises. Nonunion or malunion may result if early motion is implemented in fractures that are unstable.[16]

Radiographs/Imaging Studies

The standard trauma series of shoulder radiographs (scapular anteroposterior [AP], scapular lateral, and axillary lateral views) are necessary for the evaluation of any proximal humerus fracture and are the next step in evaluation. Correct classification of the fracture depends on being able to visualize the degree of displacement or angulation of the fracture fragments. The axillary lateral view is useful for determining displacement of the humeral head on the glenoid and posterior displacement

of the greater tuberosity fragment. For stable fractures, carefully obtained internal and external rotation views may help visualize the proximal humerus. The external rotation view is useful for seeing the anatomic neck and the greater tuberosity. Computed tomography (CT), although potentially helpful in displaced fractures, is generally not necessary for one-part fractures; however, if the amount of posterior displacement of a greater tuberosity fracture is in question, a CT scan should be obtained.

■ Treatment

Nonoperative treatment is the primary treatment for one-part proximal humerus fractures. Healing occurs largely due to the substantial soft tissue envelope

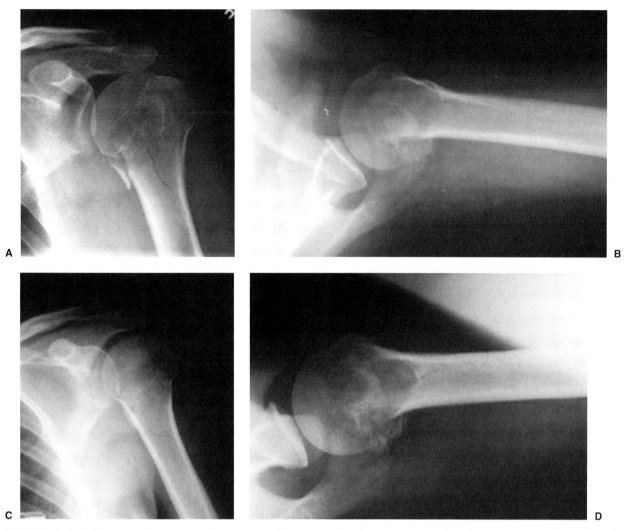

FIGURE 4–3 A 57-year-old woman with a one-part fracture characterized by multiple fracture lines. Nonoperative management consisting of sling immobilization resulted in fracture healing and an excellent functional result (American Shoulder and Elbow Surgeons [ASES] score 94).

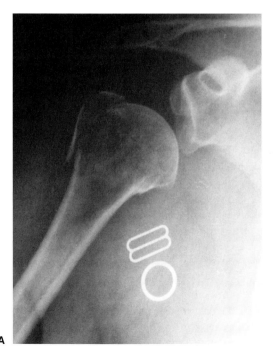

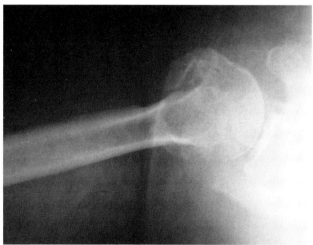

FIGURE 4–4 A 66-year-old with a proximal humerus fracture with surgical neck and greater tuberosity components. The AP view (A) shows borderline displacement of the greater tuberosity, as does the scapula lateral (B) view. The displacement is between 5 and 10 mm. Note the "pseudosubluxation" on the AP view (A).

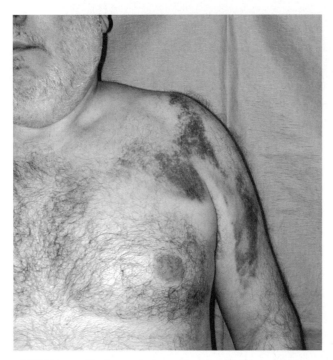

FIGURE 4–5 Ecchymosis is evident in this 63-year-old man 4 days following one-part fracture. The ecchymosis can extend from the shoulder down to the elbow and along the anterior and lateral chest wall.

surrounding the proximal humerus that remains intact.[8,16] Satisfactory, good, or excellent results have been reported in 80 to 97% of patients treated nonoperatively for one-part proximal humerus fractures.[3,10,14,18]

The goal of treatment in one-part fractures is to prevent the development of stiffness while maintaining or improving the range of motion of the affected shoulder. Therefore, progressive mobilization of the shoulder

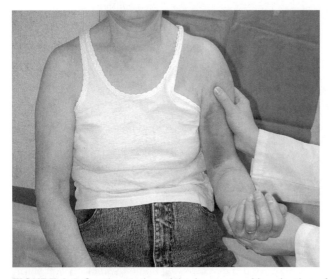

FIGURE 4–6 Gentle rotation of the humerus with palpation of the proximal portion provides an assessment of fracture stability.

should follow a very brief period of immobilization in a sling for pain relief. In a prospective controlled trial, Kristiansen et al[15] reported the functional results following 1 and 3 weeks of immobilization, and found that 1 week of immobilization resulted in a better outcome than 3 weeks of immobilization primarily because of diminished pain; however, no difference in pain, function, or mobility was found after 6 months and no further recovery of shoulder function was seen after 12 and 24 months.

Preferred Technique

We prefer to treat all one-part proximal humerus fractures nonoperatively and have seen good clinical results after early mobilization of these fractures. The goals of treatment are healing of the fracture and functional recovery. The patient should be reevaluated within 1 week of injury (and sling application) to make certain that displacement of the fracture has not occurred. This is especially important for fractures of the greater tuberosity, where even less displacement is tolerated. If the fracture is deemed stable on exam, the patient is referred to a physical therapist to begin immediate, supervised active range-of-motion (ROM) exercises of the elbow, wrist, and hand as well as assisted ROM for the affected shoulder. If there are concerns about the stability of the fracture, the patient should continue using the sling for 2 more weeks before starting therapy. The patient should also be instructed in home exercises that can be performed without the therapist. The sling should be worn until the fracture is united clinically (usually 3 to 6 weeks) and removed for the exercise sessions. The shoulder exercises should be performed in the supine position for forward elevation, external rotation, and internal rotation (to the chest wall). The patient should participate in one to three weekly supervised therapy sessions and perform three to four daily therapy sessions at home. When the sling is discontinued, the patient can perform active ROM exercises, initially in the supine position and then gradually progressing to the sitting position. Isometric strengthening exercises for the deltoid and rotator cuff muscles can be added at the same time. Isotonic resistive (Theraband) exercises for these muscles can be performed when good active shoulder ROM is achieved. Gentle stretching exercises are also added at this time. At about 12 weeks after the time of injury, a more vigorous stretching program can be implemented.

In a prospective study of functional outcomes after early mobilization of one-part proximal humerus fractures, we found that patients regained 87% of forward elevation, 79% of external rotation, and 89% of internal rotation, compared with the opposite side.[18] Unlike previous studies, we found a high incidence of residual

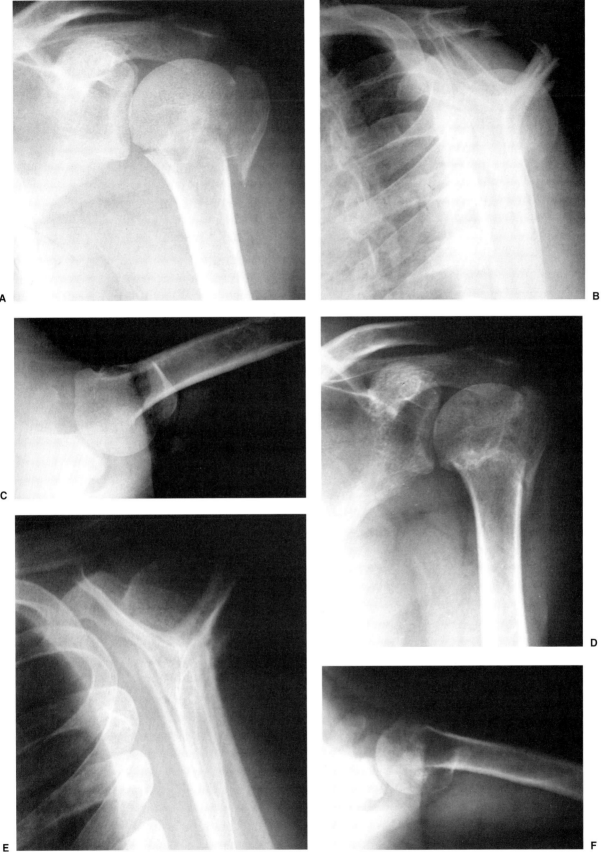

FIGURE 4–7 A 55-year-old man with proximal humerus fracture following a fall. Trauma series **(A–C)** shows multiple fracture lines without significant displacement of any "part." Six months following the surgery the fracture has healed **(D–F)**, and the patient has achieved an excellent functional result.

shoulder pain (67%) with a significant number (27%) of patients describing the pain as moderate to severe. Moreover, almost 30% of patients required some form of medication for pain relief. Nearly two thirds (65%) of patients reported some limitation of function, with 42% reporting a significant restriction of overall function. The most affected activities of daily living were inability to sleep on the affected side (40%), inability to carry a package at the side (46%), and inability to use the hand overhead (51%).

These results differ from previously reported series of proximal humerus fractures. It may be that there are different subtypes of minimally displaced proximal humerus fractures that may benefit from a different treatment protocol. The physical therapy program described above is a rough guideline that is individualized to each of our patients with a one-part fracture. Next we describe the case of a patient with a one-part fracture of the proximal humerus who received our treatment protocol.

■ Case Study

The patient is a 55-year-old, right-hand-dominant man who works as a banker. He fell onto his right shoulder while playing basketball and now complains of right shoulder pain. He has pain with attempted shoulder movement and has noted some swelling around the shoulder. He has no other complaints. His past medical history is unremarkable, and he takes no medications. He denies smoking and drug use and drinks alcohol socially.

On physical examination, mild swelling was noted about the right shoulder. There was no ecchymosis present at the shoulder or chest wall. Both shoulders appeared symmetric. Mild tenderness to palpation was noted at the anterolateral aspect of the shoulder. Examination of the neck revealed full range of motion and no tenderness to palpation. Spurling's test was negative. Sensation over the deltoid was intact to light touch and active contraction was seen in all three parts of the deltoid. The distal neurovascular exam was normal in the right upper extremity. Careful passive range of motion of the right shoulder demonstrated that the proximal humerus moved as one unit. He had passive forward elevation to 60°, external rotation to 50°, and internal rotation to the ilium with all motions limited by pain. Active range of motion was limited by pain. Deltoid contraction was present but painful.

AP, scapular lateral, and axillary lateral radiographs of the right shoulder revealed multiple fracture lines of the proximal humerus, including fractures of the greater tuberosity and surgical neck (Fig. **4–7**). There was no

angulation and no more than 5 mm of displacement at any fracture.

Because each fracture fragment did not satisfy the Neer classification criterion of being a separate "part," the patient was diagnosed with a one-part fracture of the proximal humerus. Nonoperative treatment was indicated for this patient in the form of a sling for comfort and physical therapy. The sling was discontinued after 1 month of use. He began physical therapy 6 days after the injury and completed the program as described earlier. At 6-month follow-up, the patient had no pain, full strength in all of his muscle groups, and excellent range of motion (active forward elevation to 170°, active external rotation to 60°, and internal rotation to T10). He returned to his preinjury activities, including basketball, which he plays three times per week.

■ Conclusion

Proximal humerus fractures are commonly encountered by the orthopaedic surgeon, and minimally displaced fractures account for the vast majority of these fractures. Proper clinical evaluation, along with the appropriate radiographs, is necessary for accurate diagnosis and treatment of one-part fractures, whether they are a borderline isolated greater tuberosity fracture or a proximal humerus fracture with multiple fracture lines. Nonoperative management of these fractures is the primary treatment modality. If displacement of the fracture occurs, operative management may be necessary. Few studies have reported the functional outcomes of nonoperative management of one-part proximal humerus fractures. In our experience, short-term immobilization with early ROM exercises of the involved shoulder and extremity can give acceptable results.[18]

REFERENCES

1. Rose SH, Melton LJ, Morrey BF, et al. Epidemiologic features of humeral fractures. Clin Orthop 1982;168:24–30
2. Nordquist A, Petersson CJ. Incidence and causes of shoulder girdle injuries in an urban population. J Shoulder Elbow Surg 1995;4:107–112
2a. Nordquist A, Petersson CJ. Incidence and causes of shoulder girdle injuries in an urban population. J Shoulder Elbow Surg 4:107–112, 1995.
3. Clifford PC. Fractures of the neck of the humerus: a review of the late results. Injury 1980;12:91–95
4. Hall MC, Rosser M. The structure of the upper end of the humerus with reference to accompanying small fractures. Can Med Assoc J 1963;88:290
5. Horak J, Nilsson B. Epidemiology of fractures of the upper end of the humerus. Clin Orthop 1975;112:250–253
6. Jakob RP, Kristiansen T, Mayo K, Ganz R, Muller ME. Classification and aspects of treatment of fractures of the proximal humerus. In:

Bateman JE, Welsh RP, eds. Surgery of the Shoulder. Philadelphia: BC Decker, 1984

7. Lind T, Kroner K, Jensen J. The epidemiology of fractures of the proximal humerus. Arch Orthop Trauma Surg 1989;108: 285–287

8. Neer CS II. Displaced proximal humeral fractures. I. Classification and evaluation. J Bone Joint Surg Am 1970;52:1077–1089

9. Neer CS II. Displaced proximal humeral fractures. II. Treatment of three-part and four-part displacement. J Bone Joint Surg Am 1970;52:1090–1103

10. Young TB, Wallace WA. Conservative treatment of fractures and fracture-dislocations of the upper end of the humerus. J Bone Joint Surg Br 1985;67:373–377

11. DePalma AF. Surgery of the Shoulder, 3rd ed. Philadelphia: JB Lippincott, 1983:372–406

12. Hawkins RJ, Bell RH, Gurr K. The three-part fracture of the proximal part of the humerus: operative treatment. J Bone Joint Surg Am 1986;68:1410–1414

13. Moriber LA, Patterson RL Jr. Fractures of the proximal end of the humerus. J Bone Joint Surg Am 1967;49:1018

14. Kristiansen B, Christensen SW. Proximal humeral fractures. Late results in relation to classification and treatment. Acta Orthop Scand 1987;58:124–127

15. Kristiansen B, Angermann P, Larsen TK. Functional results following fractures of the proximal humerus. A controlled clinical study comparing two periods of immobilization. Arch Orthop Trauma Surg 1989;108:339–341

16. Norris TR. Fractures of the proximal humerus and dislocations of the shoulder. In: Browner BD, Jupiter JB, Levine AM, Trafton PG, eds. Skeletal Trauma. Fractures, Dislocations, Ligamentous Injuries, vol 2. Philadelphia: WB Saunders, 1992:1201–1290

17. Muller ME, Allgower M, Willeneger H. The Technique of Internal Fixation of Fractures, Segmuller G, trans. New York: Springer-Verlag, 1965

17a. Muller ME, Allgower M, Willeneger H. The Technique of Internal Fixation of Fractures. Segmuller G, trans. New York, Springer-Verlag, 1965.

18. Koval KJ, Gallagher MA, Marsicano JG, Cuomo F, McShinawy A, Zuckerman JD. Functional outcome after minimally displaced fractures of the proximal part of the humerus. J Bone Joint Surg Am 1997;79:203–207

19. Park TS, Choi IY, Kim YH, Park MR, Shon JH, Kim SI. A new suggestion for the treatment of minimally displaced fractures of the greater tuberosity of the proximal humerus. Bull Hosp Jt Dis 1997;56:171–176

20. Santee HE. Fractures about the upper end of the humerus. Ann Surg 1924;80:103–114

21. McLaughlin HL. Dislocation of the shoulder with tuberosity fracture. Surg Clin North Am 1963;43:1615–1620

22. Miller SR. Practical points in the diagnosis and treatment of fractures of the upper fourth of the humerus. Ind Med 1940;9: 458–460

23. Visser C, Coene L, Brand R, Tavy D. Nerve lesions in proximal humerus fractures. J Shoulder Elbow Surg 2001;10:421–427

5

Two-Part Fractures and Fracture-Dislocations

FRANK A. LIPORACE AND KENNETH J. KOVAL

Proximal humerus fractures are most commonly classified according to the number of parts.[1,2] According to Neer, a part is defined as a fracture fragment that is at least 45° angulated or 1 cm displaced. Fragments include the humeral shaft, humeral head, greater tuberosity, and lesser tuberosity (Fig. 5–1).[1–3] Two-part fractures occur when one of the four fragments fulfills the displacement criteria. All two-part fractures may be accompanied by a concomitant dislocation.

Displacement of fragments is influenced by the muscular attachments.[1,4] The most commonly displaced two-part fractures are those of the surgical neck.[1,5] With a surgical neck fracture, the humeral shaft is displaced anteriorly and medially secondary to the influence of the pectoralis major. The humeral head (with its attached tuberosities) remains in neutral position due to the balanced pull of the rotator cuff. When there is a greater tuberosity fracture, the attached supraspinatus, infraspinatus, and teres minor retract the greater tuberosity posteriorly and superiorly. In a two-part lesser tuberosity fracture, displacement of the lesser tuberosity occurs medially due to the influence of the subscapularis.

The majority of patients who sustain two-part fractures are in the older age group.[1,6–8] Osteoporosis and sedentary lifestyle frequently play a role by increasing the susceptibility of the proximal humerus to relatively minor trauma. Fractures in the younger age groups are more often a result of higher energy trauma.[8–11] The majority of two-part fractures are primarily surgical neck fractures occurring in patients older than 65 years.[12–14] Isolated greater tuberosity fractures are responsible for less than 2% of all proximal humerus fractures,[12] although this incidence may be underreported.[15] Two-part anatomic neck fractures and two-part lesser tuberosity fractures account for less than 1% of two-part fractures. Greater tuberosity fractures have been cited as occurring 5 to 33% of the time in association with anterior dislocations.[16–18] Lesser tuberosity fractures also occur in association with posterior dislocations.[12] This chapter focuses on the clinical and radiographic evaluations and treatment of two-part fractures and fracture dislocations.

■ Clinical Evaluation

After determining the patient's chief complaint, clinical evaluation should proceed with an account of the events leading to injury. The mechanism can be either direct (i.e., a lateral blow to the shoulder) or indirect (i.e., fall on an outstretched hand, electroconvulsive therapy, seizure, etc.). The indirect mechanism often results in greater fracture displacement than the direct mechanisms.[19] Indirect mechanisms are also responsible for fracture-dislocations, often in the younger population.[19] A loss of consciousness or other constitutional symptoms should alert the clinician to a possible underlying medical condition, especially in the elderly.[19]

Patients usually complain of shoulder pain with tenderness to palpation and limited range of shoulder motion. Crepitus may be appreciated when attempting to actively or passively range the shoulder. Ecchymosis may be present and can extend distally. A detailed neurovascular examination is essential, as with all orthopaedic injuries. A careful, sensory examination is necessary to delineate the location of potential nerve injury.[20] With proximal humerus fractures, up to a 45% incidence of nerve injury has been reported. This most commonly occurs with surgical neck fractures and fracture-dislocations.[21] Older patients and those with clinical evidence of hematoma have an increased risk of nerve

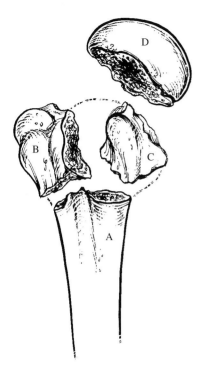

FIGURE 5–1 The four parts of the proximal humerus. A, humeral shaft; B, greater tuberosity; C, lesser tuberosity; D, articular segment.

injury. The axillary nerve is most commonly involved, followed by the suprascapular, radial, and musculocutaneous nerves. Fortunately, the majority of nerve injuries are neuropraxias from low-energy trauma and resolve within 4 months.[22]

Although the axillary artery lies just anteromedial to the proximal humerus,[23] the incidence of vascular injury in association with two-part fractures is very small. In two studies reporting a total of more than 300 patients, there were no cases of vascular complications in association with proximal humeral fractures.[2,24] The proximity of vascular structures and risk of injury is greater with high-energy fractures and fracture-dislocations, particularly with significant medial displacement. With a pure anterior dislocation, damage can occur at the thoracoacromial, subscapular, or circumflex humeral trunks.[25] Suspicion of injury should be high in the presence of an expanding hematoma, absent distal pulses, a cold extremity, and a pulsatile painful mass with a bruit.[26] Because there is extensive collateral flow in the shoulder, pulses may be palpable in up to 27% of cases with an axillary artery injury.[27] A Doppler exam and arteriogram should therefore be performed whenever an arterial injury is suspected.[28,29] When a vascular injury is present, the sequence of bone and arterial repair is controversial and is usually based on the degree of ischemia present.[28,30]

Careful assessment of fracture stability is required. Motion through the distal fragment should be evaluated

to determine if the fracture moves as a unit. Also, any abnormal contours, such as a fullness or concavity, either anteriorly or posteriorly, should increase the suspicion for an associated glenohumeral dislocation.

Radiographic/Imaging Studies

Radiographic evaluation of the injury requires the trauma series: anteroposterior (AP) and lateral shoulder views in the plane of the scapula and an axillary view. Classification and treatment is often influenced by the findings in each of these views. The scapula AP can delineate fracture fragment angulation, alignment, and displacement.[21,31–34] The scapula lateral is particularly helpful in evaluating shaft displacement and glenohumeral joint orientation, and in visualizing posteriorly displaced fragments. An axillary view provides information about displacement of the tuberosities, associated dislocations, and humeral head impression fractures often seen with fracture-dislocations.[27,35–39]

When patients are in too much pain to be removed from a sling, the Velpeau axillary view can be obtained by having the patient lean backward 30° over the x-ray table. An x-ray cassette is placed beneath the shoulder and the beam is directed from superiorly to inferiorly, through the glenohumeral joint.[32]

Computed tomography (CT) scans may be of assistance if the trauma series radiographs are indeterminate and with fracture-dislocations.[21,39,40] Fragment rotation, tuberosity displacement, head impression fractures, and head-splitting components can be further delineated with CT scans.[21] Although CT scans may clarify certain injuries, their effect on intraobserver reliability and interobserver reproducibility for classification of injuries has been questioned.[41] Bernstein et al[41] found that the addition of CT scans to plain radiography increased the kappa coefficient for intraobserver reliability from 0.64 (plain radiographs) to 0.72 (plain radiographs and CT scan) but had no effect on interobserver reliability. Additionally, magnetic resonance imaging (MRI) can aid with defining associated soft tissue injuries of the rotator cuff, biceps tendon, and glenoid labrum, although it is uncommon for this information to have a significant impact on the treatment plan selected.

■ Treatment

The decision to proceed with operative management is based on a careful consideration of patient and fracture factors, including the patient's physiologic age, arm dominance, associated injuries, fracture pattern, degree of displacement, and bone quality; the decision is also based on the surgeon's experience.[27] Specific guidelines are discussed in the following sections for each fracture.

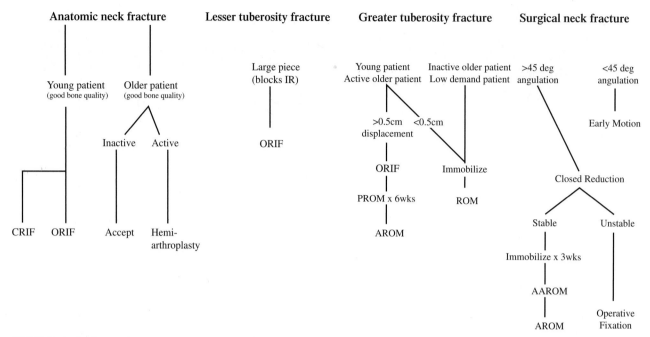

FIGURE 5–2 General algorithm for treatment of two part proximal humerus fractures. AAROM, active-assisted range of motion; AROM, active range of motion; CRIF, closed reduction and internal fixation; IR, internal fixation; ORIF, open reduction and internal fixation; PROM, passive range of motion.

An outline of the principles of treatment is described in the algorithm in Fig. 5–2.

■ Two-Part Surgical Neck Fractures

With this fracture pattern, the tuberosities and humeral head are one fragment that remains neutral or slightly abducted while the humeral shaft displaces medially and anteriorly as a result of the pull of the pectoralis major. Approximately 22% of proximal humerus fractures are two-part surgical neck patterns.[12] Patient age and functional status are important factors in determining treatment.

Closed Treatment without Reduction

Impacted surgical neck fractures with angulation that approaches or even exceeds 45° can be considered for nonoperative management with institution of an early range-of-motion program. If the examination confirms the fracture is stable, it may be reasonable to accept the angulation in patients whose activities will not be adversely affected. These will usually be older, more sedentary individuals who do not require frequent overhead use of the involved extremity. Although it is true that significant angulation limits forward elevation, there are patients in whom the potential limitations will not have a significant impact on function. Selecting these patients requires a careful assessment of functional needs and treatment expectations. For these selected patients, treatment consists of sling immobilization for approximately 4 to 5 weeks until fracture healing has progressed. Range-of-motion exercises should be initiated as early as patient comfort allows. It is important for the exercises to be structured and supervised to avoid an aggressive approach that could displace the fracture site and interfere with healing.

Active range of motion of the elbow, wrist, and hand, with the arm at the side, may begin immediately. Assisted range of motion of the shoulder can be started when the acute discomfort subsides, as can isometric deltoid exercises. Throughout the course of therapy, the patient is instructed to perform a home exercise program four times per day.

To perform assisted flexion, the patient is instructed to lie supine and grasp the wrist of the injured extremity with the contralateral hand. Using the unaffected extremity, the injured arm is pulled up and overhead; that is, forward elevation (Figs. 5–3A–C). For assisted external rotation, the patient lies supine with arms at the side and elbows flexed 90°. The patient places a stick or similar object into both hands and uses the uninvolved side to push the injured extremity into external rotation. It is then used in the opposite direction for internal rotation back to the chest (Fig. 5–3D,E).

Isometric exercises promote muscle tone of the anterior, middle, and posterior portions of the deltoid, and can be performed as comfort allows. Isometric

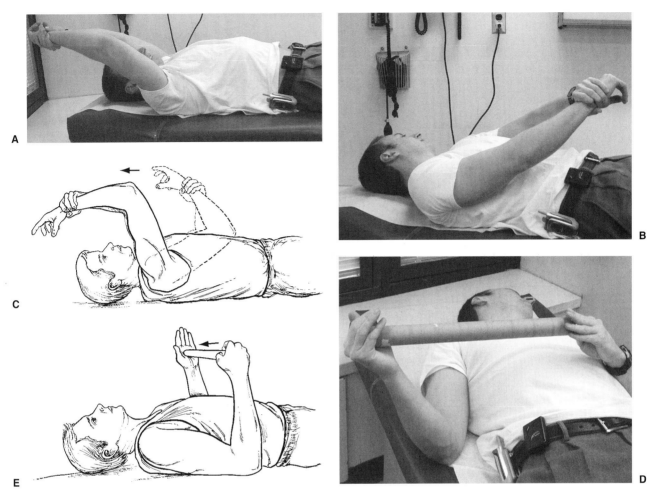

FIGURE 5–3 Clinical photographs **(A,B)** and schematic **(C)** of assisted flexion exercise; and a clinical photograph **(D)** and schematic **(E)** of assisted external rotation exercise.

internal and external rotation exercises can be performed after 2 to 3 weeks as fracture healing progresses.

At 4 to 6 weeks, therapy can progress to active range of motion, including forward elevation, external rotation out to the side, and internal rotation behind the back. More vigorous stretching can be initiated 8 to 10 weeks after fracture and resistive strengthening at about 12 weeks postinjury.

Closed Treatment with Reduction

Fractures with more than 45° of angulation or greater than 1 cm may require fracture reduction. The typical pattern of these fractures consists of varus and apex anterior angulation that could potentially limit forward elevation. Active patients with a high level of functional demands should undergo closed reduction to improve alignment.

Closed reduction is most easily performed under regional or general anesthesia with the aid of fluoroscopy.

Adduction of the distal fragment relaxes the pectoralis major. Gentle traction should be applied (to correct the angulation) combined with lateral displacement of the humeral shaft (to correct medial translation) as the humerus is flexed to 90°. In this position a gentle impacting force should be applied to the humerus to engage the two fragments into a stable position (Fig. **5–4**). The fracture is then visualized using fluoroscopy, and stability is assessed. Posterior angulation is better tolerated than anterior or varus angulation, so an overcorrection of this nature may be acceptable.[27] If the alignment is acceptable, Velpeau immobilization should be used for 2 to 3 weeks. At that time, if follow-up radiographs confirm the alignment, assisted range of motion can be instituted along with a sling. At 6 weeks the sling can be discontinued and active range of motion is started as described previously. Radiographs should be done weekly for the first 2 to 3 weeks to ensure maintenance of reduction. Eighty percent of the stable, reduced two-part fractures will

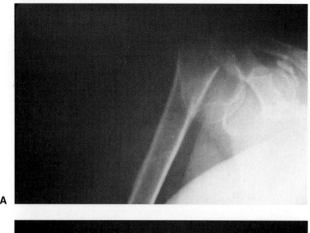
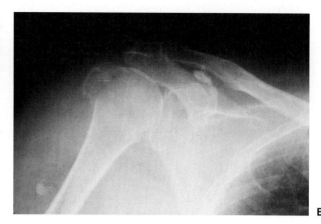
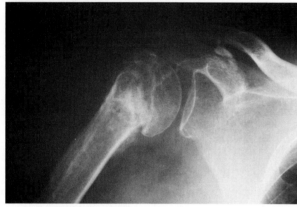

FIGURE 5–4 (A) Angulated surgical neck fracture underwent closed reduction **(B)**. At 6-month follow-up, the fracture is healed in acceptable position **(C)**.

heal by 6 weeks.[42] At 12 weeks, strengthening exercises can begin. Closed treatment has yielded a high level of satisfactory or excellent results when reduction can be achieved and maintained. In a study of 80 patients, 81% had good or excellent results overall when treated by closed means.[43]

If reduction cannot be obtained or maintained, operative management should be considered. Treatment options include closed reduction with percutaneous pinning and open reduction and internal fixation (plate and screws, tension-band wiring, suturing, and/or intramedullary fixation).[7,44–48]

Surgical Reduction and Fixation

Closed Reduction and Percutaneous Pinning
This approach is best utilized in patients with good bone stock and minimal comminution in which the fracture can be adequately reduced by closed manipulation.[49] Up to 70% good or excellent results have been obtained when using this technique[7]; however, biomechanically pin fixation is less rigid than other fixation methods.[50,51]

The equipment necessary for this technique includes fluoroscopy, terminally threaded 2.5-mm pins, and a tissue protector for pin placement. The patient is placed

on the operating table with the injured shoulder off the lateral aspect of the table. Prior to prepping and draping, fluoroscopy is positioned to confirm that adequate AP and axillary images can be obtained by moving the image around the patient. Closed reduction is attempted with longitudinal traction on the arm and laterally directed traction of the shaft (Fig. **5–5**). Anterior angulation is corrected with traction and flexion of the humerus.[7]

While an assistant manually maintains the fracture reduction, the operating surgeon inserts the pins with either a retrograde (lateral, anterior, or anterolateral) or antegrade (superolateral) technique. It has been shown that multiplanar pin constructs in the proximal humerus optimize torsional stiffness, and placement of an antegrade greater tuberosity pin optimizes bending stiffness.[51] Placing percutaneous pins superior to the deltoid insertion may help avoid injury to the radial nerve in the spiral groove. Retrograde pin placement requires the use of a soft tissue protector to avoid axillary nerve injury. When pinning retrograde, it is also important to avoid the biceps tendon while ensuring pin placement in both fracture fragments (the anteriorly located shaft and the posteromedially located head). Both goals can be accomplished by aiming pins from anterolateral to posteromedial.

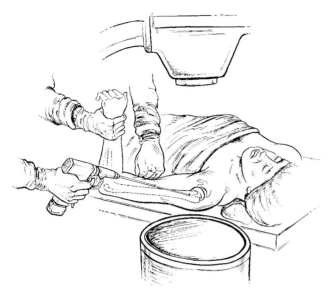

FIGURE 5–5 Patient positioning for percutaneous pinning procedure including fluoroscopy setup and reduction maneuver for closed percutaneous pinning.

An initial retrograde anterolateral pin can be placed through a small puncture wound in the lateral aspect of the humeral shaft. Due to the humerus's natural retroversion and posteromedial location of the head relative to the shaft, proper retrograde pin placement is performed from anterolateral to posteromedial directed toward the center of the humeral head. The initial pin is angled 45° to the shaft in the coronal plane and 30° to the shaft in the sagittal plane. Under fluoroscopic guidance, the pin is placed just beneath the subchondral bone without penetrating the articular surface. A second pin can be placed parallel (either superior or inferior) to the first. If adequate space exists, a third retrograde pin may begin more anteriorly to allow for wide pin placement within the head. Care must be taken to avoid the biceps tendon when placing this pin. Finally an antegrade superolateral to inferomedial pin may be placed. Other pins may be added for further stability if necessary (Fig. **5–6**). All pins should be shortened to a subcutaneous position just under the skin. Multiplanar fluoroscopy should then be instituted, while moving the shoulder through a range of motion, to ensure that the fracture is adequately stabilized and that there are no pins violating the articular surface. A Velpeau dressing is applied and the arm is immobilized for 3 weeks. Patients are followed with weekly radiographs, to ensure that pin migration has not occurred. Formal therapy should not be started until the proximal pin(s) is removed. With clinical and radiographic evidence of healing, assisted range of motion is begun. The pins are usually removed 4 to 6 weeks after surgery.

Care must be taken to avoid the axillary nerve, cephalic vein, biceps tendon, and the posterior humeral circumflex artery when performing this procedure. A cadaveric study has shown that all of these structures are located between 2 and 11 mm from the placement of the pins as described (Fig. **5–7**).[52] These authors recommended that lateral pins should be placed distal enough to avoid the axillary nerve, and the greater tuberosity pins should be placed with the arm in external rotation and directed to a point 20 mm from the inferior aspect of the humeral head.[52]

Closed Reduction and Percutaneous Fixation with Cannulated Screws

An alternative method of percutaneous fixation utilizes cannulated screws (Fig. **5–8**). Patient positioning and fracture reduction are performed in a similar fashion to that described earlier; however, instead of placing a larger diameter pin, guidewires for 4.5-mm partially threaded cannulated screws are inserted to the level of the subchondral bone. Screw length can be determined in two ways. The depth gauge for the guidewire can be seated to the bone and confirmed under fluoroscopic visualization, or an equal-length guidewire can be placed alongside the protruding guidewire to the level of the bone. The area that does not overlap is then measured as the appropriate screw length. A 3.2-mm cannulated drill bit is inserted over the guidewire using a dull guide to protect the soft tissues. A partially threaded 4.5-mm cannulated screw is then inserted over the guidewire and the guidewire is removed. This is repeated for the other guidewires. After all screws have been placed, the shoulder is placed through a range of motion and visualized under fluoroscopic guidance to confirm appropriate hardware placement, fracture alignment, and stability of the construct (Fig. **5–8**).[53]

This technique has the potential for earlier passive range of motion without waiting for selective pin removal as when percutaneous pins are used. A report on 19 patients treated with percutaneous cannulated screws for displaced proximal humerus fractures yielded 84% good or excellent results with a 93% union rate.[53]

Open Reduction and Internal Fixation

When closed reduction is unsuccessful, open reduction with internal fixation should be considered. Success with plate and screw fixation has been reported.[54–56] A series of 98 patient with either two- or three-part proximal humerus fractures yielded 76% good to excellent results when fixed with a T-plate.[57] In a biomechanical study comparing 10 modes of internal fixation, the plate and screw fixation was shown to be the strongest construct for patients with or without osteopenic bone.[58] Plate fixation, however, carries the risk of devascularizing the proximal fragment thereby increasing the risk of

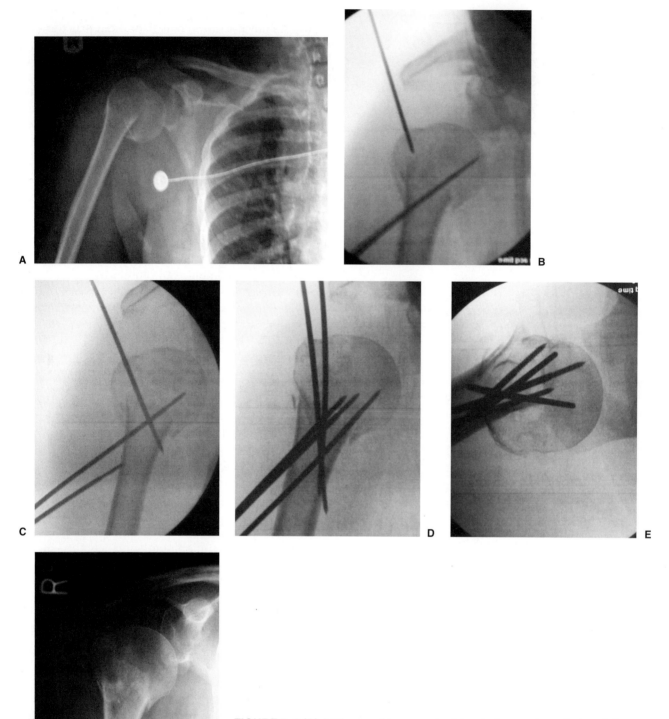

FIGURE 5–6 (A) A 62-year-old woman sustained a two-part surgical neck fracture as a result of a fall. **(B–E)** Closed reduction was performed followed by pin placement. A retrograde pin is placed first to secure the head to the shaft followed by a second pin inserted from a superolateral to an inferomedial position to fix the nondisplaced greater tuberosity fragment. Additional threaded 2.5-mm Schantz pins are placed sequentially to enhance fixation. **(F)** Four months following pin removal, radiographs demonstrate a healed fracture with acceptable alignment.

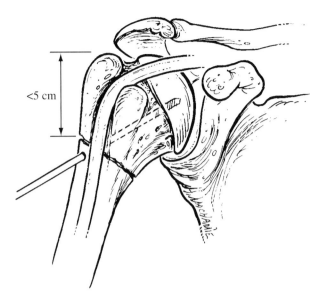

FIGURE 5–7 Pin placement should avoid neurovascular structures based on the described "safe zone."

osteonecrosis.[59,60] Osteonecrosis has been reported up to 3.5 years after injury in the proximal humerus.[61,62] The most common complications after open reduction and plating include prominent hardware, loss of fixation, and osteonecrosis.[62–65]

Biomechanically, interfragmentary suture has been shown to be least effective in stabilizing proximal humeral fractures.[58] The addition of intramedullary rods to a figure-of-eight interfragmentary construct significantly improved maximum resistance to load.[58,66] This augmented fixation becomes even more important when there is existing comminution.[67] Clinically, up to 71% good or excellent results with an average of 145° of elevation, 43° of external rotation, and internal rotation to T11 have been reported with the use of intramedullary rods combined with figure-of-eight tension band.[67]

Locked intramedullary fixation has been used for the treatment of proximal humerus fractures. A biomechanical study comparing tension band wiring supplemented

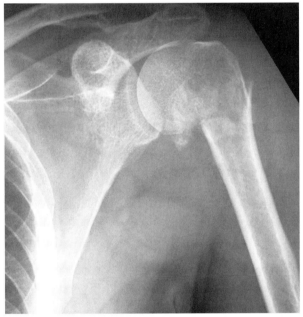

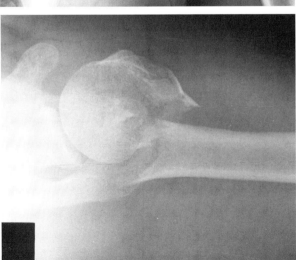

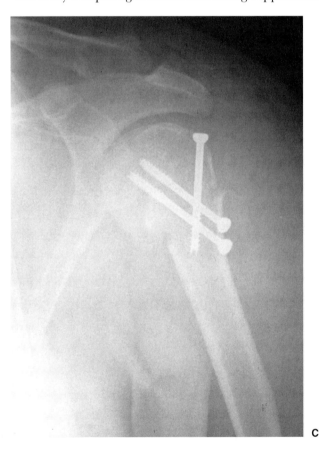

FIGURE 5–8 Preoperative **(A,B)** and postoperative **(C)** radiographs of a displaced surgical neck fracture treated by closed percutaneous cannulated screw fixation.

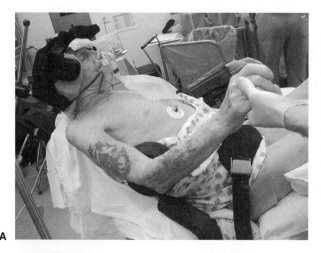

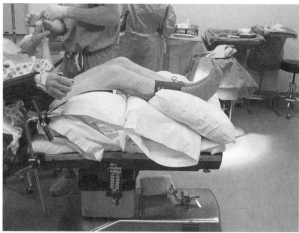

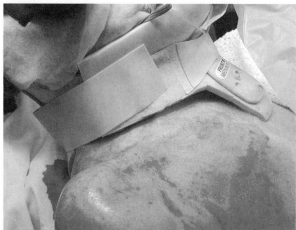

FIGURE 5–9 Patient positioning for open reduction and internal fixation of the proximal humerus includes the beach chair position **(A)**, pillows under the knees with the heels padded **(B)**, and a modified cervical collar **(C)**.

with Enders nails, plate and screws, and a locked intramedullary nail showed that the plate/screw construct and the locked intramedullary nail were superior to the tension band/Enders nail construct. There was no statistically significant difference in the stability provided by the locked intramedullary nail compared with the plate/screw construct.[68]

Open reduction with internal fixation is performed using a deltopectoral approach. The patient is placed in the beach chair position on the operating room table with the head elevated ~30° (Fig. **5–9A**). Care is taken to pad all bony prominences. The patient's operative side should be moved off the operating table to allow unimpeded range of motion during the procedure. Two pillows are placed under the thighs and one under the calves to allow the heels to be free of excessive pressure and to help maintain the beach chair position (Fig. **5–9B**). To control the patient's neck safely in the beach chair position, a cervical spine collar is applied to the neck with a cutout modification made to allow complete access to the operative side (Fig. **5–9C**). The entire shoulder girdle with

upper extremity should be prepped and draped in the operative field.

An incision is made from a point just lateral to the coracoid, obliquely toward the insertion of the deltoid tuberosity, laterally on the humerus (Fig. **5–10**). Skin and subcutaneous tissues are dissected to the level of the muscle layer, and flaps are elevated medially and laterally. The deltopectoral interval is identified at the junction of the deltoid and pectoralis major muscle fibers. The fat stripe covering the cephalic vein is a helpful landmark in this interval. Most branches of the cephalic vein enter from the lateral side, and frequently the surgeon mobilizes this vein laterally, but the direction of mobilization is a matter of surgeon preference. Once the vein is retracted, the deltopectoral interval can be bluntly developed. At times, release of the superior 1 cm of the pectoralis major insertion can make this easier. A self-retaining retractor should be placed in the interval, exposing the coracoid process, conjoined tendon, coracoacromial ligament, lesser tuberosity/subscapularis insertion, and bicipital groove. The clavipectoral

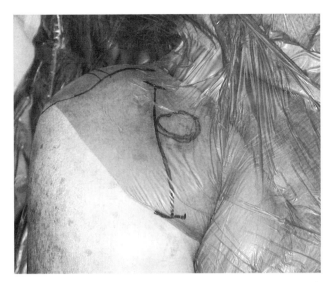

FIGURE 5–10 Skin incision for deltopectoral approach to the proximal humerus (circular mark indicates the coracoid process).

fascia, confluent with the coracoacromial ligament proximally, should be incised along the lateral edge of the short head of the biceps tendon up to the coracoacromial ligament. This allows a retractor to be placed beneath the conjoined tendon. Next, a Darrach retractor can be used to develop the subacromial and subdeltoid spaces.

The biceps tendon is identified and tagged with a suture or vessel loop. The biceps tendon provides an orientation to the greater and lesser tuberosities. The lesser tuberosity is located medial to the biceps tendon, and the greater tuberosity is located superiorly and laterally. Once located, the biceps tendon is followed to the bicipital groove to the rotator interval.

There are several important anatomic structures in this area that should be avoided. Throughout exposure, care should be taken to preserve the deltoid attachment. The cephalic vein should remain to limit postoperative swelling of the extremity. The "three sisters" (anterior humeral circumflex artery and two accompanying veins) are located on the inferior one third of the subscapularis tendon. This is part of the vascular supply to the humeral head and should be preserved. Also, the musculocutaneous and axillary nerves are in close proximity to surgical dissection and retraction. The musculocutaneous nerve's entry point into the conjoined tendon is variable, though frequently it is only 5 cm distal to the tip of the coracoid. The axillary nerve can be palpated by sweeping a finger along the anteroinferior border of the subscapularis tendon, near the 6 o'clock position on the glenoid.

Adequate exposure of fracture fragments includes removal of fracture hematoma and interposed soft tissue. Control of the proximal fragment can be performed with sutures placed at the tuberosity–tendon interface. Fracture reduction and fixation can then be performed using a variety of techniques.

Modified Intramedullary Nails with Tension Band

After exposure of the surgical neck fracture, the humeral shaft and head fragments are mobilized. A No. 2 nonabsorbable suture is placed into the posterior aspect of the rotator cuff to enhance manipulation of the proximal fragment. Drill holes are placed in the humeral shaft fragment, 1 or 2 cm distal to the fracture site, on either side of the bicipital groove. Number 5 nonabsorbable sutures are passed through these drill holes; they will be used as the tension band after nail insertion. Eighteen-gauge wire may be substituted for nonabsorbable suture; although it provides greater immediate stability, it is more difficult to handle and carries the risk of breakage and migration, making it a less desirable option.

The humeral head is reduced onto the shaft. Fracture reduction is obtained by forward elevation of the humeral shaft with gentle traction on the sutures to control the proximal fragment. The fracture is impacted and the arm is extended while maintaining tension on the sutures to prevent loss of reduction. Tension on the rotator cuff sutures extends the proximal fragment while the arm is extended and prevents apex anterior angulation.

Once adequate reduction is achieved, fixation is accomplished using a combination of tension band suture and flexible intramedullary nails (Fig. **5–11**). Enders nails (3.5 mm) are superior to straight rods/pins such as Rush rods in that they provide three-point fixation, which enhances rotational stability. Furthermore, with use of Enders nails, a figure-of-eight suture or wire can be placed through the eyelet to prevent proximal migration and impingement that often occurs with non-fenestrated straight rods. The slot of the Enders nail is long, however, and a significant amount of metal may still protrude proximally. Therefore, the nail can be modified with placement of an additional hole above the slot (Fig. **5–12**). This allows for deeper insertion of the nail into the humeral head, placing the proximal end below the rotator cuff tendon. The addition of the tension band configuration with intramedullary nails has been found to add greater longitudinal and rotational stability over either tension banding or intramedullary nailing alone.

While maintaining reduction, small longitudinal incisions are made at the insertion of the rotator cuff fibers into the greater tuberosity. The two Enders nails are inserted through the anterior and posterior aspect of the greater tuberosity. An awl or drill bit is used to

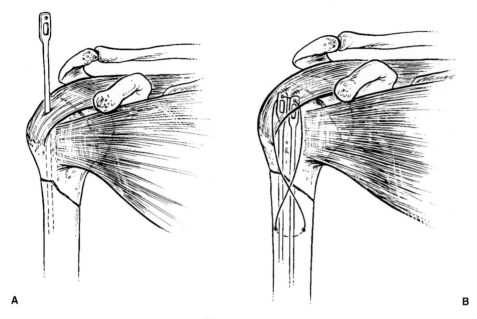

A

B

FIGURE 5–11 (A,B) Graphic representation of modified Enders nail and tension band suture fixation of a surgical neck fracture.

enter the bone. It is better to place the posterior nail first because levering on this partially inserted nail will aid in holding the reduction and preventing the humeral head from angulating. The second nail is then inserted 1.0 to 1.5 cm anterior to the first nail. It is best to use nails of different lengths to prevent the possibility of a distal stress riser.[67,69] Nails between 22 and 27 cm in length are generally adequate. Before completely burying the nails, the previously placed suture is placed through the eyelet of one nail, then deep to the rotator cuff between the two nails, and then through the second nail. The nails are impacted below the rotator cuff and the suture tied in a figure-of-eight manner, which helps to prevent proximal nail migration.[67] Prior to tying the suture, fracture reduction should be confirmed fluoroscopically (Fig. **5–13**).

Once the figure of eight is secured, the stability of the fixation is assessed through a range of motion. The findings will determine the postoperative rehabilitation parameters to avoid stress on the repair. The rotator cuff incisions should be closed and a suction drain used if necessary. A standard closure is performed and the upper extremity is placed in a sling.

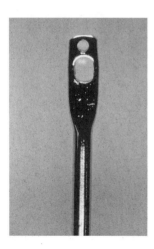

FIGURE 5–12 Enders nail modified with a drill hole placed proximal to the standard slot.

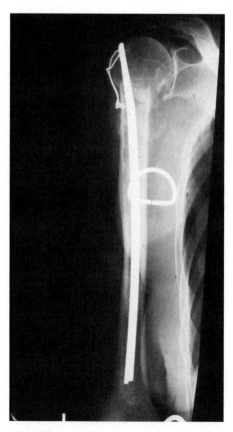

FIGURE 5–13 Postoperative radiograph of surgical neck fracture fixation with Enders nails.

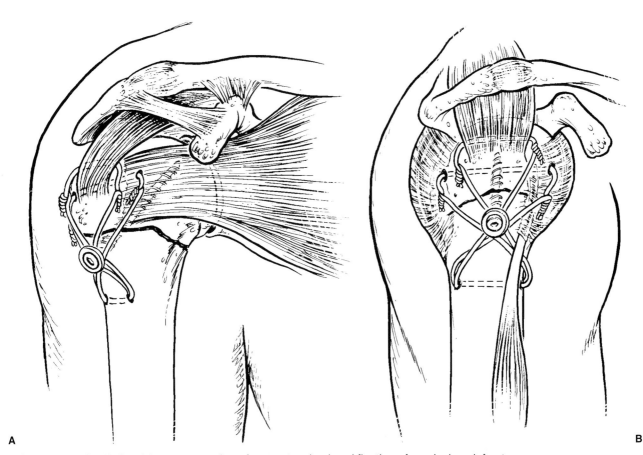

A   B

FIGURE 5–14 (A,B) Graphic representation of screw-tension band fixation of surgical neck fractures.

Lag Screw Fixation with Tension Band

This technique also utilizes a standard deltopectoral approach as described. The fracture site is identified and fracture hematoma removed. Provisional reduction and impaction of the humeral shaft and head is performed under direct visualization with confirmed fluoroscopy. A 6.5-mm lag screw (32-mm thread) is inserted from the lateral humeral shaft cortex, about 1 to 2 cm distal to the fracture site and angled superiorly, into the central portion of the humeral head. Countersinking the screw avoids the need for use of a washer and prevents the screw from propagating a fracture of the lateral humeral cortex. Two tension band wires of 18-gauge stainless steel or No. 5 nonabsorbable suture can be used. Two drill holes are placed through the lateral cortex just distal to the screw. The wires or sutures are passed through the holes in an "in-and-out" fashion. One wire/suture is then passed under the supraspinatus tendon and the second is passed through a drill hole in the greater and lesser tuberosities or through the subscapularis tendon and across the rotator interval into the anterior portion of the supraspinatus insertion (Fig. 5–14).[70]

Clinically, this construct has provided adequate fixation to allow initiation of early postoperative passive range of motion.[70,71] Thirteen patients with proximal humerus fractures, fixed with this technique, were evaluated with a mean follow-up of 20 months. Average forward flexion was 160°, external rotation was 46°, and internal rotation was to T10. Ten of the 13 patients achieved a good result.[70]

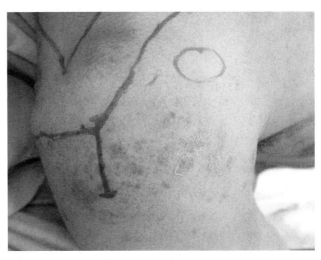

FIGURE 5–15 Lateral deltoid splitting incision for insertion of locked intramedullary nail.

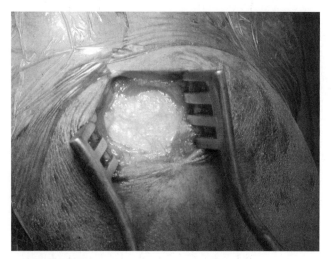

FIGURE 5–16 Deltoid split provides visualization of the subacromial bursae.

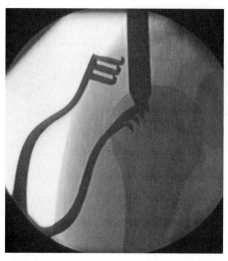

FIGURE 5–18 After an awl is used to prepare the starting point, a ball-tipped guidewire is inserted and passed across the fracture site.

A deltopectoral approach may be utilized when open reduction is needed to obtain proper reduction with alignment of the fracture. If a closed reduction can be performed, however, a much more limited exposure is needed for nail insertion. A lateral incision can be made extending from the anterolateral corner of the acromion up to 5 cm distally (Fig. **5–15**). The deltoid fibers are split to visualize the subacromial space. Bursal excision provides exposure or the rotator cuff (Fig. **5–16**).

With either approach, an incision in line with the fibers of the supraspinatus is made ~1.5 cm posterior to the anterior edge of the greater tuberosity just adjacent to the articular surface (Fig. **5–17**). A starting hole is made with an awl or cannulated drill bit (Fig. **5–18**). As fracture reduction is maintained, the ball-tipped guidewire is passed across the fracture site under fluoroscopic guidance. Proximal reaming is performed to allow passage and seating of the nail 5 mm below the

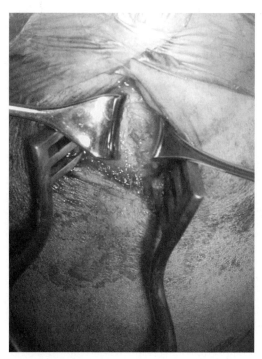

FIGURE 5–17 In-line incision is made between the supraspinatus fibers.

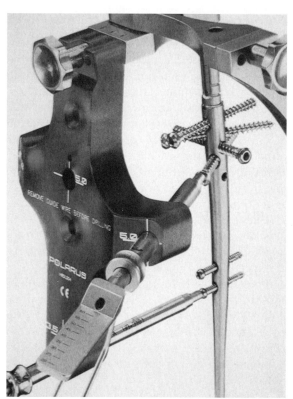

FIGURE 5–19 Intramedullary nail attached to the jig for locking screw insertion.

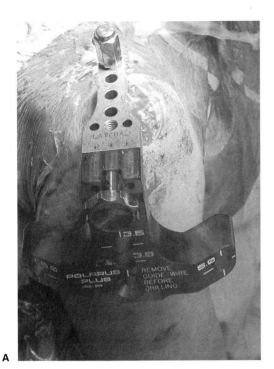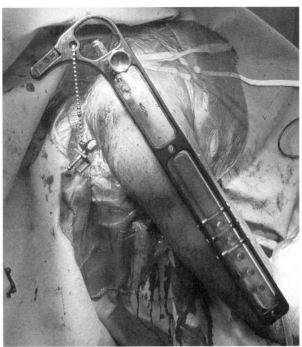

FIGURE 5–20 Intraoperative view of the jig for insertion of proximal **(A)** and distal **(B)** screw insertion.

surface of the bone. Exchange of the initial ball-tipped guidewire for a smooth guidewire is then performed. The nail is prepared for insertion by attaching the jig for locking screw insertion (Fig. **5–19**). The nail is placed over the guidewire and seated to the appropriate level. Proximal locking of the nail is performed using the prefabricated jig (Fig. **5–20**). A soft tissue protector, inserted to the bone, should be used during drilling and

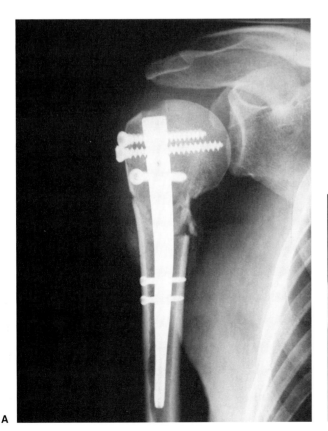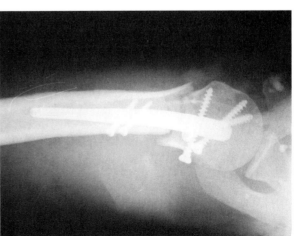

FIGURE 5–21 (A,B) Postoperative radiographs of short intramedullary locked nails.

placing locking screws to prevent deltoid and axillary nerve injury. Avoiding use of the anterior locking holes proximally will decrease the chance of biceps tendon injury. If a short nail is used, a distal locking screw can be placed using the proximal jig (Fig. **5–21**). If a full-length intramedullary nail is being used with anterior to posterior locking screws, a formal anterior incision should be made with careful dissection down to bone for protection of the brachial artery, median nerve, and biceps tendon. Standard free-hand techniques with fluoroscopic guidance should be used for placement of distal locking bolts. It is always necessary to use soft tissue protectors throughout drilling and screw placement to avoid complications. Some systems also allow for the use of a distal locking bolt-targeting guide.

In one study, 16 of 20 patients treated with a locked intramedullary nail for displaced proximal humerus fractures had satisfactory to excellent results.[72] Another series of 21 patients with displaced surgical neck fractures treated with a locked humeral nail yielded 86% satisfactory to excellent results.[73]

Blade Plate Fixation

Using a fixed-angle device such as a blade plate provides more stable proximal fixation, especially for patients with osteoporotic bone. When use of a blade plate is planned, it is important to ensure that the proximal fragment is large enough to allow proper placement of the blade and that the bone quality of the shaft is adequate for bicortical fixation. A blade plate may be fashioned from a semitubular plate[48] or can be prefabricated with a 90° bend (Synthes, Paoli, Pennsylvania).

With the patient in the beach chair position, an extended deltopectoral incision is made. If necessary, provisional fracture fixation can be obtained with Kirschner wires (K-wires) or terminally threaded pins. Fluoroscopic confirmation of fracture reduction should be performed. Sutures should be placed through the individual fracture fragments as previously described. When using the prefabricated 90° blade plate, a 2.0-mm threaded guidewire is placed through the drill guide perpendicular to the humeral shaft and 0.5 to 1.0 cm posterior to the bicipital groove at a level 1 to 2 cm distal to the top of the greater tuberosity. The guidewire is inserted, passing through the center of the humeral head and into the subchondral bone (Fig. **5–22**).[74] The length of the blade plate is determined using the measuring guide. In general, a blade 5 mm shorter than this measurement should be used to minimize the risk of penetrating the subchondral bone. With the drill guide in place, a 4.5-mm drill is passed through each of the large holes in the guide, on either side of the guidewire (Fig. **5–23**). A 3.2-mm drill is passed through the angled holes in the drill guide and the 4.5-mm cannulated drill is passed over the guidewire. The

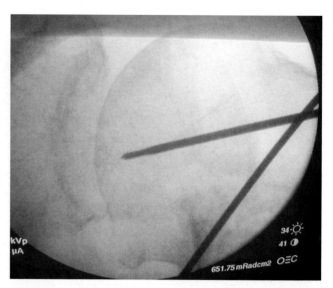

FIGURE 5–22 Insertion of guidewire for blade plate fixation of proximal humerus.

4.5-mm, 90° cannulated blade plate is inserted over the guidewire until the side plate lies flush against the lateral cortex of the humeral shaft (Fig. **5–24**). If the fracture pattern allows, the most proximal screw in the plate should be inserted obliquely toward the tip of the blade in the head of the humerus. If this is not possible, the sutures that have been passed through the anterior, superior, and posterior portions of the rotator cuff can be passed through this hole to augment stability.[74] The screws are then placed through the plate to complete the fixation (Fig. **5–25**).

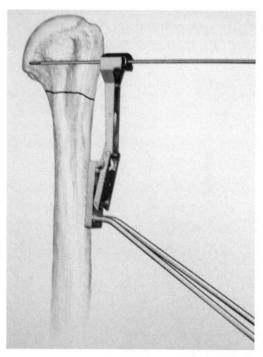

FIGURE 5–23 Drill guide placed over guidewire for drilling to prepare path for the blade.

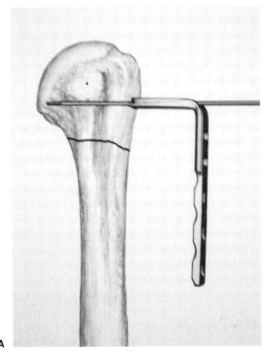
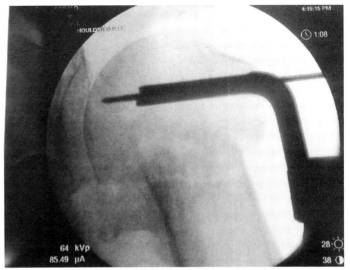

FIGURE 5–24 (A,B) The blade plate is inserted over the guidewire.

A study of 42 elderly patients treated with blade plate fixation for proximal humerus fractures yielded a 100% union rate and greater than 70% good to excellent results at an average 3.4-year follow-up.[55] All patients were allowed to begin rehabilitation immediately after surgery. The authors suggested that rigid fixation of displaced fractures of the proximal humerus with a blade plate in the elderly patient provides sufficient primary stability to allow early rehabilitation.[55]

Locked Humeral Plating

The 3.5 mm locking compression plate (LCP) proximal humerus locking plate (Synthes) is a relatively new alternative for proximal humerus fixation that offers the benefits of a fixed-angle device with multiple points of fixation. This may be particularly helpful in patients with osteoporotic bone. Because this implant has been available for a relatively short period of time, mid- and

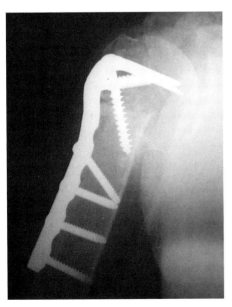
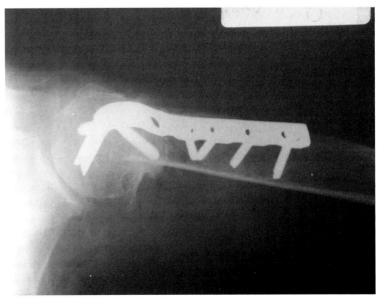

FIGURE 5–25 (A,B) Postoperative radiographs of blade plate fixation of surgical neck fracture.

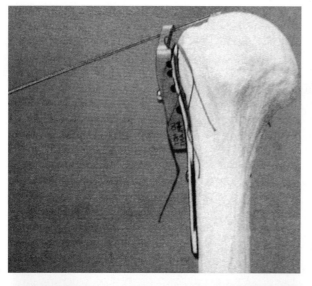

A

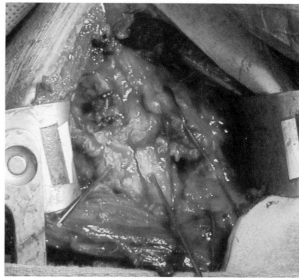

B

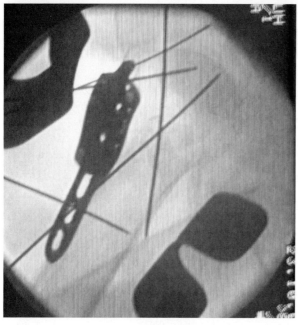

C

FIGURE 5–26 Sawbone model showing placement of the plate and superior guidewire **(A)**; intraoperative photograph **(B)** and fluoroscopy **(C)** of provisional Kirschner wire (K-wire) fixation and plate placement.

long-term outcomes have not been documented, but early results have been promising.

With the patient in the beach chair position, a standard deltopectoral approach is performed. Provisional fracture reduction and fixation is obtained with K-wires and is confirmed with orthogonal fluoroscopic views. After the plate is locked to the insertion guide, the plate should be placed approximately 8 mm distal to the rotator cuff attachment on the greater tuberosity. If the plate is placed too proximally it can interfere with gliding of the subacromial space. Excessive distal placement will compromise proper placement of the locked screws into the humeral head. To confirm proper plate placement, a 1.6-mm K-wire can be placed through the proximal hole in the insertion

guide. This wire should just engage the proximal portion of the humeral head. A second K-wire should be placed through the distal hole of the insertion guide (Fig. **5–26**). This wire should be located about 5 mm proximal to the calcar, if the plate is appropriately positioned. Additionally, the plate should be centered against the lateral aspect of the greater tuberosity, posterior to the biceps tendon (Fig. **5–27**).

The plate can be definitively fixed to the humerus by either inserting the proximal humeral head locking screws, which provides the option to insert the distal humeral shaft screws in compression mode, or by inserting the distal humeral shaft screws first. To insert the proximal locking screws, the triple sleeve (3.5-mm locking sleeve, 2.8-mm drill sleeve, and 1.6-mm wire

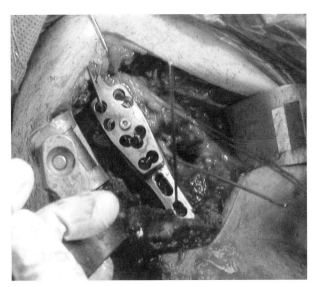

FIGURE 5–27 Provisional plate placement on lateral humeral cortex posterior to biceps tendon.

sleeve) is placed into the insertion guide. A 1.6-mm K-wire is inserted through the sleeve assembly to the level of the subchondral bone (Fig. **5–28A**). The measuring device is placed over the K-wire and pushed against the sleeve assembly (Fig. **5–28B**). The K-wire and its sleeve are then removed and the near cortex is drilled with the 2.8-mm drill bit through the remaining drill sleeve (Fig. **5–28C**). The drill sleeve is removed and the appropriate-length 3.5-mm locking screws are inserted through the remaining sleeve (Fig. **5–28D**).

Distal humeral shaft screws may be inserted in standard or compression mode, or they can be locked to the plate. If using locking screws, the threaded drill guide must be used. Once the 2.8-mm drill hole is made, the drill guide is removed and the depth gauge is used to determine the appropriate length screw. The screw is then inserted in the same orientation as the drill sleeve (Fig. **5–28E**). When the fixation of the plate is completed, the insertion guide should be removed and orthogonal fluoroscopic views obtained to confirm fracture alignment and placement of the fixation device (Fig. **5–29**).

■ Two-Part Anatomic Neck Fractures

In an anatomic neck fracture, the fracture line is medial to the rotator cuff insertion, resulting in an articular surface fragment devoid of bone and soft tissue attachments. As a result, there is theoretically a high risk of osteonecrosis. This is a rare fracture, and as a result there are no large series documenting treatment outcomes. Closed reduction can be expected to result in malunion. Operative management of this

fracture consisting of open reduction and stabilization should be considered, especially in younger active patients. Prosthetic replacement should be considered when this fracture is encountered in elderly patients. If reduction and fixation is considered the appropriate treatment, closed reduction and percutaneous pinning can be considered. Longitudinal traction on the arm may reduce the articular segment into an acceptable position. Internal or external rotation may further allow manipulation of the fragment into a reduced position by contact with the glenoid. If the position is confirmed fluoroscopically, two or three threaded 2.5-mm Schantz pins can be inserted directly into the fragment through the lateral humeral cortex. Follow-up radiographs should be obtained after 10 to 14 days to confirm fixation. The shoulder should be immobilized for 6 weeks when the pins are removed. We do not begin range-of-motion exercises until the fracture appears healed and the pins have been removed. In general, the fixation of the articular segment is limited by the amount of purchase of the pins. Because the fragment can be relatively small, we prefer a cautious approach to mobilization.

If closed reduction is not possible, an open reduction can be performed. A standard deltopectoral approach, with the patient in the beach chair position, is utilized. It may be possible to reduce this fracture by entering the joint through the rotator interval. If this is not successful, the subscapularis tendon should be divided 1 cm medial to its insertion. This allows visualization of the anatomic neck and glenohumeral joint. Once anatomic reduction is obtained, screws or terminally threaded pins can be inserted through the tuberosities, into the subchondral bone of the head. Screws remain permanently,[71] but if pins are used, they should be removed 6 weeks postoperatively if there is clinical and radiographic evidence of healing. The previously described rehabilitative approach is utilized. In older patients, primary prosthetic replacement should be considered. This is also performed using the deltopectoral approach with division of the subscapularis tendon as described to enter the glenohumeral joint. The fragment should be removed. When the tuberosities remain intact, the humeral head replacement component can be inserted without the need for tuberosity fixation. The advantage of prosthetic replacement is the ability to initiate an early range-of-motion program without concern about the stability of fixation. Assisted range of motion is initiated on the first postoperative day with external rotation limited by the subscapularis repair. A sling is worn for 3 to 4 weeks when an active range-of-motion program is begun combined with isometric strengthening. Stretching and resistive strengthening are begun 8 to 10 weeks following surgery.

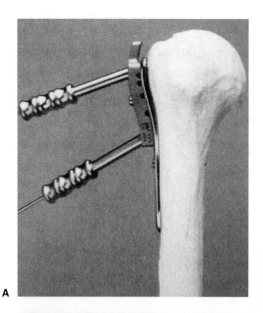

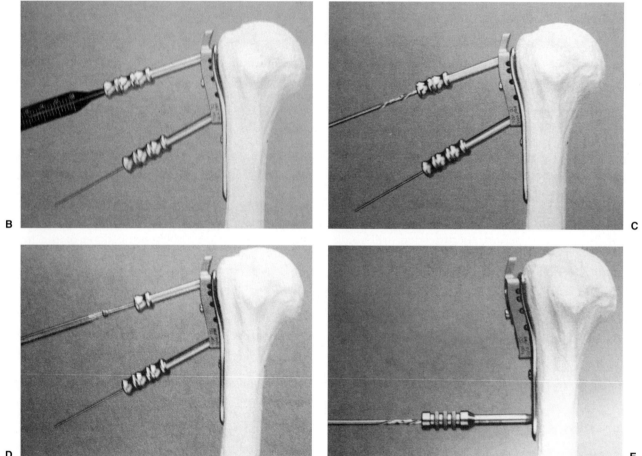

FIGURE 5–28 (A) Sawbone model shows the triple sleeve with guide pin inserted. **(B)** Measuring device for screw length. **(C)** Insertion of drill through locked sleeve. **(D)** Insertion of locking screw. **(E)** Procedure for insertion of locked shaft screws through locked sleeve.

■ Two-Part Greater Tuberosity Fractures

Although Neer[1] defined a part as 1 cm displaced or 45° angulated, for two-part greater tuberosity fractures 5 mm of superior displacement is probably sufficient to inter-fere with subacromial gliding and compromise overhead elevation.[75,76] Anatomically, displacement is determined by the pull of the attached supraspinatus, infraspinatus, and teres minor, which often results in some combination of superior and posterior displacement. With greater than 5 mm of superior displacement, operative management

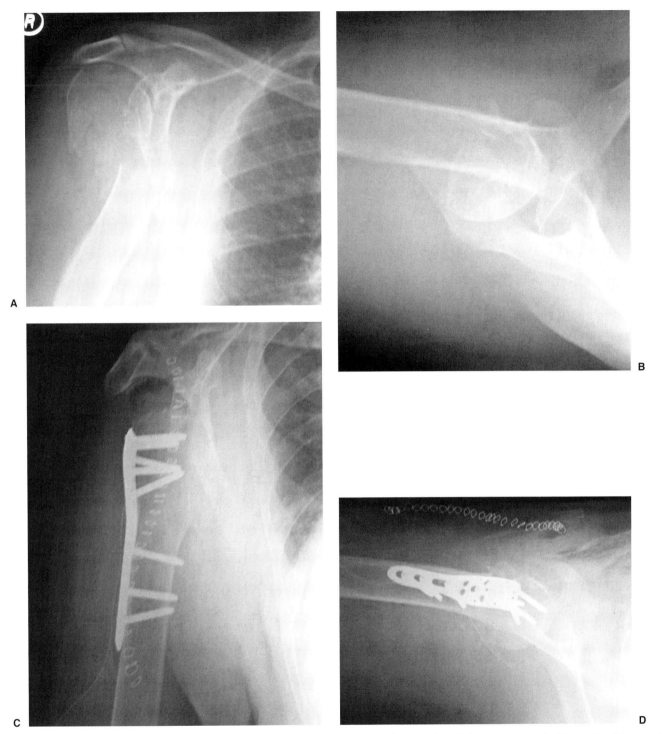

FIGURE 5–29 Preoperative **(A,B)** and postoperative **(C,D)** radiographs of surgical neck fracture treated with proximal humeral locking plate.

is generally indicated. Clifford[43] reported only 50% good results when treating these fractures closed.

The patient is positioned as previously described in the beach chair position. A 5- to 6-cm incision is made in Langer's lines over the anterolateral corner of the acromion. The placement of the incision is dictated by the relative anterior or posterior position of the

fragment.[45] The deltoid is split in line with its fibers less than 5 cm distal to the lateral aspect of the acromion to avoid injury to the axillary nerve.[23]

Subacromial adhesions are released with the aid of a Darrach elevator. The ability to rotate the humerus combined with flexion and extension provides necessary visualization of the fracture fragment and its bed.

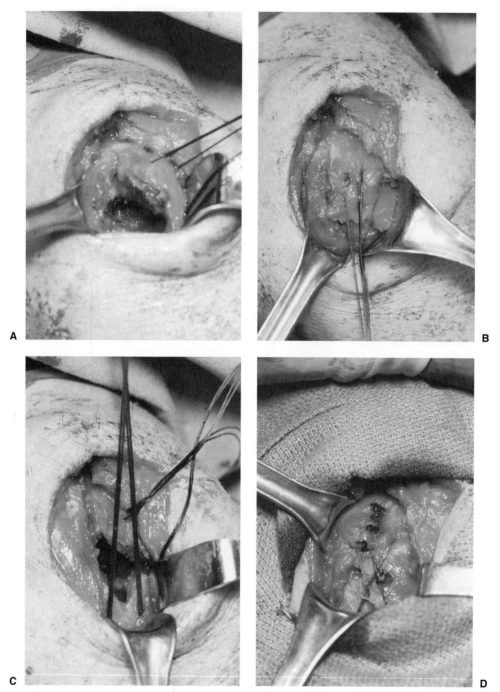

FIGURE 5–30 Technique of open reduction and internal fixation (ORIF) of two-part greater tuberosity fracture. Sutures are placed in the mobilized greater tuberosity fragment **(A,B)** and through the lateral humeral cortex distal to the fracture bed **(C)**. The sutures are tied in a figure-of-eight fashion with closure of the longitudinal tear of the rotator cuff **(D)**.

The greater tuberosity fragment and its bed are exposed and debrided of fracture hematoma. To gain control of the fragment, No. 2 nonabsorbable sutures are placed at the rotator cuff insertion into the fragment. One, two, or three sutures can be used depending on the size of the fragment (Fig. **5–30A,B**). Before reduction, two drill holes are placed into the lateral humeral cortex 1 to 1.5 cm distal to the fracture bed.

Two No. 5 nonabsorbable sutures are passed through the drill holes in an "in-and-out" fashion (Fig. **5–30C**). The fracture fragment is secured to the fracture bed with these sutures in a figure-of-eight fashion, passed through the rotator cuff insertion, and tied over the bony portion of the fragment. Any rotator cuff defects in either the rotator interval or the area between the rotator cuff tendons should be repaired with No. 1 or 2

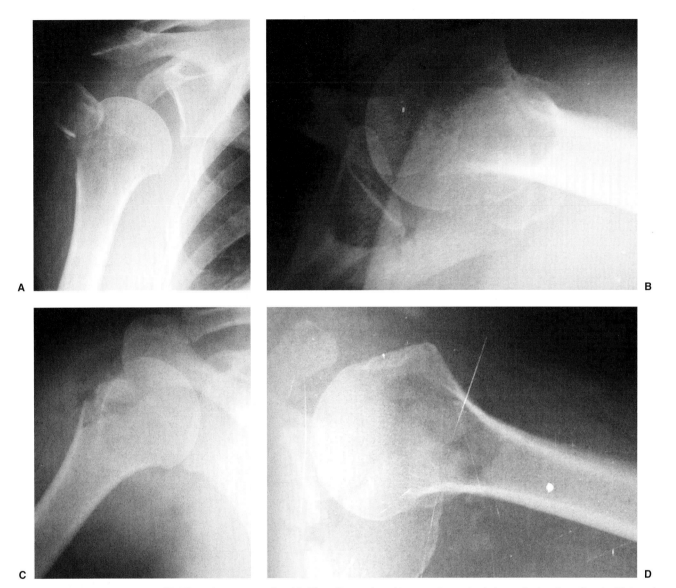

FIGURE 5–31 Preoperative **(A,B)** and postoperative **(C,D)** radiographs of two-part greater tuberosity fracture fixed with tension bend suture technique.

nonabsorbable sutures (Fig. **5–30D**). Postoperative radiographs should be obtained to confirm the fragment is reduced (Fig. **5–31**).

Alternatively, large fracture fragments can be fixed with two partially threaded cancellous screws with washers that are placed perpendicular to the fracture bed (Fig. **5–32**). This technique should be reserved for large fragments in good-quality bone where secure fixation can be obtained. Screw fixation has to be utilized judiciously because of the potential for and the risk of intraarticular penetration.[77]

Before closure, the shoulder is placed through a range of motion to determine the parameters for postoperative passive range of motion that can begin immediately after surgery. The deltoid split should also be closed. Active range of motion can be

started 6 weeks postoperatively using the program described previously. In one study of 12 patients, this technique resulted in 100% good or excellent results.[45]

■ Two-Part Lesser Tuberosity Fractures

Isolated two-part lesser tuberosity fractures in the absence of an associated posterior dislocation are quite uncommon. The fragment is displaced medially by the pull of the subscapularis. It may be of limited significance unless it is large and thereby causing a block to motion or it includes a significant portion of the articular surface.[76] If a large fragment is displaced, open reduction

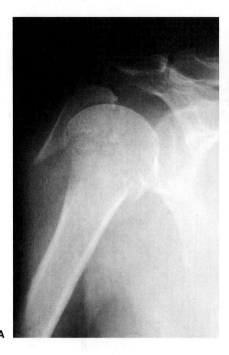

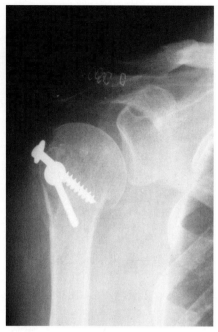

A

B

FIGURE 5–32 Preoperative **(A)** and postoperative **(B)** radiographs of two-part greater tuberosity fracture fixed with cancellous screws.

and internal fixation is indicated using a deltopectoral approach (Fig. **5–33**). Fixation can utilize either wire or heavy suture with the figure-of-eight tension band technique or screw fixation in patients with good bone quality. Assisted range of motion should be initiated within the limits identified intraoperatively. Due to the uncommon nature of these fractures, there have been no large series reported with long-term results.

■ Two-Part Surgical Neck Fracture with Glenohumeral Dislocation

Although uncommon, displaced surgical neck fractures can occur in association with anterior dislocation and less commonly with posterior dislocation (Fig. **5–34**). In addition, some apparent anterior or posterior glenoid dislocation may occur in association with nondisplaced and frequently unrecognized surgical neck fractures, which further reinforces the need for gentle manipulation of these injuries in an effort to reduce the dislocated fragment. We prefer to reduce the injuries under regional or general anesthesia in the operating room, rather than with sedation in the emergency room. By achieving complete muscular relaxation, this approach minimizes the potential for excessive force to be used. Once reduced the alignment should be evaluated to determine the treatment required based on the guidelines discussed earlier in this chapter. If a closed reduction cannot be performed, then open reduction is necessary using a deltopectoral approach. The proximal

fragment can usually be reduced with manipulation. If it cannot be reduced easily, the rotator interval should be opened for more direct manipulation of the head. In rare situations, subscapularis tenotomy may be necessary to expose the articular surface and the glenohumeral joint and to reduce the head. After reduction, internal fixation should be performed using one of the techniques described previously (Fig. **5–34**) with the appropriate postoperative rehabilitation program.

■ Two-Part Greater Tuberosity Fractures with Dislocation

Up to one third of anterior shoulder dislocations are associated with greater tuberosity fractures (Fig. **5–35A,B**). This is the most common type of shoulder fracture-dislocation, especially in a patient under 40 years of age.[16] After gentle closed reduction under sedation, the position should be confirmed with a full set of radiographs (Fig. **5–35C,D**). Sling immobilization should be used for 4 weeks. Active range of motion of the elbow, wrist, and hand can be performed immediately. After 2 weeks, we allow passive forward elevation to 90°, external rotation, and internal rotation to the chest. After the immobilization is discontinued, an active range of motion program is started including internal rotation behind the back.

If superior displacement is more than 5 mm following closed reduction or is identified on early follow-up radiographs, operative management is indicated with the

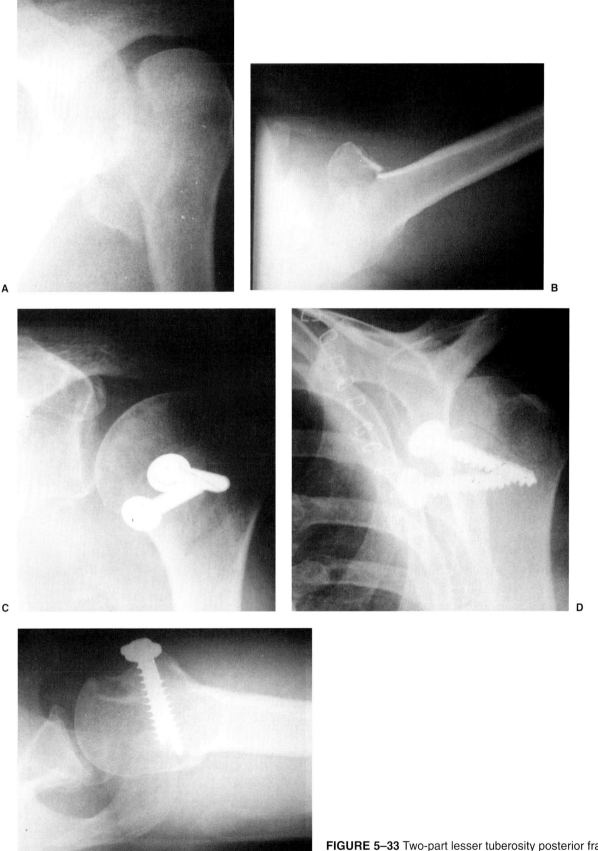

FIGURE 5–33 Two-part lesser tuberosity posterior fracture dislocation **(A,B)** treated with ORIF with cancellous screws **(C–E)**.

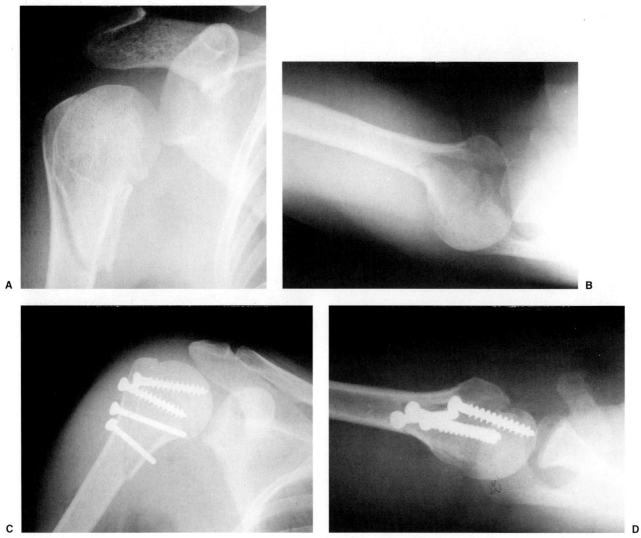

FIGURE 5–34 Two-part surgical neck fracture-dislocation **(A,B)** treated by open reduction and fixation with multiple screws **(C,D)**.

techniques previously described.[76] Any rotator cuff or interval tear should be repaired at the time of surgery.

■ Two-Part Lesser Tuberosity Fractures with Dislocation

Lesser tuberosity fracture-dislocations usually represent an avulsion fracture in association with a posterior dislocation (Fig. **5–33**). Closed reduction should be performed with sedation, using gentle traction and slight adduction of the forward flexed arm. Manipulation of the humeral head can aid the reduction. If the fracture displacement is less than 1 cm after reduction, the arm can be immobilized in a "gun-slinger"–type orthosis (10 to 15° of external rotation, 10° extension, and 10 to 15° abduction). If the fragment is large and significant displacement exists, operative management consisting

of open reduction through a deltopectoral approach should be performed as described. Based on the stability and security of fixation as assessed intraoperatively, either a sling or "gun-slinger"–type orthosis can be used. Passive range of motion is indicated immediately after surgery. When fracture union has occurred (i.e., after 6 weeks), the sling or orthosis is removed and active range of motion is begun, progressing to a strengthening program after 6 more weeks.

■ Conclusion

When treating two-part fractures of the proximal humerus, it is important to obtain a complete history, perform a comprehensive physical exam, and obtain a complete radiographic series for proper and complete assessment of the injury. The patient's medical condition, physiologic age,

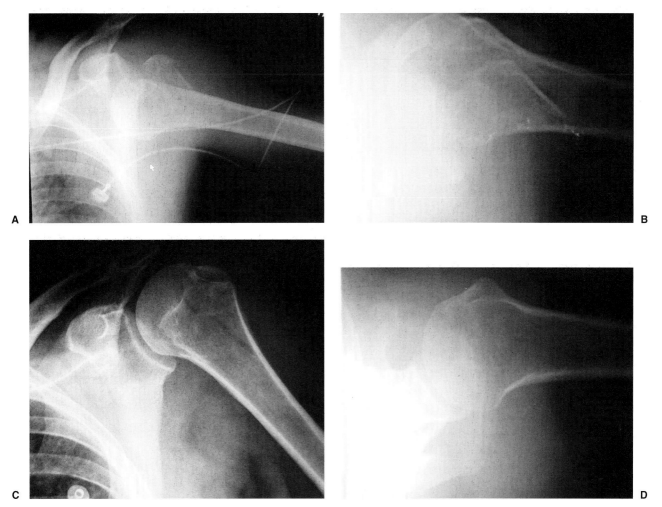

FIGURE 5–35 (A,B) Two-part greater tuberosity fracture-dislocation. **(C,D)** Following closed reduction the greater tuberosity fragment is reduced.

and ability to perform activities of daily living are important in determining treatment. If operative treatment is indicated, the fracture pattern, patient factors, and surgeon experience are also important considerations.

REFERENCES

1. Neer CS II. Displaced proximal humeral fractures. I. Classification and evaluation. J Bone Joint Surg Am 1970;52:1077–1089
2. Neer CS II. Displaced proximal humeral fractures. II. treatment of three-part and four-part displacement. J Bone Joint Surg Am 1970;52:1090–1103
3. Codman EA. Rupture of the Supraspinatus Tendon and Other Lesions in or About the Subacromial Bursa. Boston: Thomas Todd, 1934
4. Neer CS II. Four-segment classification of displaced proximal humeral fractures. AAOS: Instr Course Lect 1975;24:160–168
5. Chun JM, Groh GI, Rockwood CA Jr. Two-part fractures of the proximal humerus. J Shoulder Elbow Surg 1994;3:273–287
6. Hawkins RJ, Bell RH, Gurr K. The three-part fracture of the proximal part of the humerus: operative treatment. J Bone Joint Surg Am 1986;68:1410–1414
7. Jaberg H, Warner JJP, Jakob RP. Percutaneous stabilization of unstable fractures of the humerus. J Bone Joint Surg Am 1992;74:508–515
8. Kristiansen B, Barfod G, Bredesen J, et al. Epidemiology of proximal humeral fractures. Acta Orthop Scand 1987;58:75–77
9. Horak J, Nilsson BE. Epidemiology of fracture of the upper end of the humerus. Clin Orthop 1975;112:250–253
10. Hall MC, Rosser M. The structure of the upper end of the humerus with reference to osteoporotic changes in senescence leading to fractures. Can Med Assoc J 1963;8:290–294
11. Rose SH, Melton LJ, Morrey BF, et al. Epidemiologic features of humeral fractures. Clin Orthop 1982;168:24–30
12. Jakob RP, Kristiansen T, Mayo K, et al. Classification and aspects of treatment of fractures of the proximal humerus. In: Bateman JE, Welsh RP, eds. Surgery of the Shoulder. Philadelphia: BC Decker, 1984
13. Wentworth ET. Fractures involving the shoulder. NY J Med 1940;40:1282
14. Lind T, Kroner K, Jensen J. The epidemiology of fractures of the proximal humerus. Arch Orthop Trauma Surg 1989;108:285–287
15. Cowell HR. Patient care and scientific freedom. J Bone Joint Surg Am 1994;76:640–641
16. Schweiger G, Ludolph E. Fractures of the shoulder joint. Unfallchirurg 1980;6:225–232

17. Greeley PW, Magnuson PB. Dislocation of the shoulder accompanied by fracture of the greater tuberosity and complicated by spinatus tendon injury. JAMA 1934;102:1835–1838

18. Rowe CR. Prognosis in dislocations of the shoulder. J Bone Joint Surg Am 1956;38-A:957–977

19. Kristiansen B, Christensen SW. Fractures of the proximal end of the humerus caused by convulsive seizures. Injury 1984;16:108–109

20. Bloom S, Dahlback LO. Nerve injuries in dislocations of the shoulder joint and fractures of the neck of the humerus: a clinical and electromyographical study. Acta Chir Scand 1970;136:461-466

21. Bigliani LU. Fractures of the shoulder. Part I. Fractures of the proximal humerus. In: Rockwood CA, Green DP, Bucholz RW, eds. Fracture in Adults, 3rd ed. Philadelphia: JB Lippincott, 1991:871–927

22. DeLatt EAT, Visser CPJ, Coene LNJEM, Pahlplatz PVM, Tavy DLJ. Nerve lesions in primary shoulder dislocations and hmeral neck fractures. J Bone Joint Surg Br 1994;76:381–383

23. Netter FH. Upper limb. In: The CIBA Collection of Medical Illustrations, vol 8. Summit, NJ: CIBA-GEIGY, 1987:20–74

24. Morris GC Jr, Beall AC Jr, Roof WR, et al. Surgical experience with 220 acute arterial injuries in civilian practice. Am J Surg 1960;99:775

25. Milton GW. The circumflex nerve and dislocation of the shoulder. Br J Phys Med 1954;17:136–138

26. White EM, Kattapuram SV, Jupiter JB. Case report 241. Skeletal Radiol 1983;10:178–182

27. Cuomo F. Proximal humerus fractures in the elderly: instructional course lecture #247. American Academy of Orthopaedic Surgeons, annual meeting, San Francisco, February 14, 1997

28. Zuckerman JD, Flugstad DL, Teitz CC, King HA. Axillary artery injury as a complication of proximal humeral fractures. Clin Orthop 1984;189:234–237

29. Barra JA, LeSaout J, Gaultier Y. Manifestations tardives des complications vasculaires des trauma tismes fermes de l'epaule. J Chir (Paris) 1978;115:151–157

30. Stromqvist B, Lidgren L, Norgren L, Odenbring S. Neurovascular injury complicating displaced proximal fractures of the humerus. Injury 1987;18:423–425

31. McLaughlin HL. Posterior dislocation of the shoulder. J Bone Joint Surg Am 1952;24-A:584–590

32. Bloom MH, Obata WG. Diagnosis of posterior dislocation of the shoulder with use of Velpeau axillary and angle-up roentgenographic views. J Bone Joint Surg Am 1967;49:943–949

33. Brems-Dalgaard E, Davidsen E, Sloth C. Radiographic examination of the acute shoulder. Eur J Radiol 1990;11:10–14

34. Zuckerman JD, Buchalter JS. Shoulder injuries. In: Zuckerman JD, ed. Comprehensive Care of Orthopaedic Injuries in the Elderly. Baltimore: Urban & Schwarzenberg, 1990:307

35. Hawkins RJ, Angelo RL. Displaced proximal humeral fractures: selecting treatment, avoiding pitfalls. Orthop Clin North Am 1987;18:421–431

36. Rockwood CA, Szaleay EA, Curtis RJ, Young DC, Kay SP. X-ray evaluation of shoulder problems. In: Rockwood CA, Matsen FA, eds. The Shoulder, vol 1. Philadelphia: WB Saunders, 1990:178–184

37. Neviaser RJ. Radiologic assessment of the shoulder: plain and arthrographic. Orthop Clin North Am 1987;18:343–349

38. Whiston TB. Fractures of the surgical neck of the humerus: a study in reduction. J Bone Joint Surg Br 1954;36:423–427

39. Sidor ML, Zuckerman JD, Lyon T, Koval K, Cuomo F, Schoenberg N. The Neer classification of proximal humeral fractures: an assessment of inter-observer reliability and intraobserver reproducibility. J Bone Joint Surg Am 1993;75:1745–1750

40. Castagno AA, Shuman WP, Kilcoyne RF, Haynor DR, Morris ME, Matsen FA. Complex fractures of the proximal humerus: role of CT in treatment. Radiology 1987;165:759–762

41. Bernstein J, Adler LM, Blank JE, et al. Evaluation of the Neer system of classification of proximal humeral fractures with computerized tomographic scans and plain radiographs. J Bone Joint Surg Am 1996;78:1371–1375

42. Jones AR, Brashear HR, Dameron TB. Surgical neck fracture of the humerus with severe displacement: factors related to union. Orthop Trans 1987;11:457

43. Clifford PC. Fractures of the neck of the humerus: a review of the late results. Injury 1980;12:91–95

44. Bosworth DM. Blade plate fixation: technic suitable for fractures of the surgical neck of the humerus and similar lesions. JAMA 1949;141:1111–1113

45. Flatow EL, Cuomo F, Maday MG, et al. Open reduction and internal fixation of two-part displaced surgical neck fractures of the proximal humerus. J Bone Joint Surg Am 1991;73:1213–1218

46. Instrum KA, Fennell CW, Shrive N, et al. Semitubular blade plate fixation in proximal humeral fractures. J Shoulder Elbow Surg 1998;7:462–466

47. Jupiter JB, Mullaji AB. Blade plate fixation of proximal humeral non-unions. Injury 1994;25:301–303

48. Sehr JR, Szabo RM. Semitubular blade plate for fixation in the proximal humerus. J Orthop Trauma 1988;2:327–332

49. Dahners LE. Internal fixation of proximal humeral fractures. J South Orthop Assoc 1995;4:3–8

50. Naidu SH, Bixler B, Capo JT, Moulton MJ, Raidn A. Percutaneous pinning of proximal humerus fractures: a biomechanical study. Orthopedics 1997;20:1073–1077

51. Wheeler DL, Colville MR. Biomechanical comparison of intramedullary and percutaneous pin fixation for proximal humeral fracture fixation. J Orthop Trauma 1997;11:363–367

52. Rowles DJ, McGrory JE. Percutaneous pinning of the proximal part of the humerus. An anatomic study. J Bone Joint Surg Am 2001;11:1695–1699

53. Chen CY, Chao EK, Tu YK, Ueng SW, Shih CH. Closed management and percutaneous fixation of unstable proximal humerus fractures. J Trauma 1998;45:1039–1045

54. Wijgman AJ, Roolker W, Patt TW, Raaymakers EL, Marti RK. Open reduction and internal fixation of three and four-part fractures of the proximal part of the humerus. J Bone Joint Surg Am 2002;84:1919–1925

55. Hintermann B, Trouillier HH, Schafer D. Rigid internal fixation of fractures of the proximal humerus in older patients. J Bone Joint Surg Br 2000;82:1107–1112

56. Moda SK, Chadha NS, Sangwan SS, et al. Open reduction and fixation of proximal humeral fractures and fracture-dislocations. J Bone Joint Surg Br 1990;72:1050–1052

57. Hessmann M, Baumgaertel F, Gehling H, Klingelhoeffer I, Gotzen L. Plate fixation of proximal humerus fractures with indirect reduction: surgical technique and results utilizing three shoulder scores. Injury 1999;30:453–462

58. Koval KJ, Blair B, Takei R, Kummer FJ, Zuckerman JD. Surgical neck fractures of the proximal humerus: a laboratory evaluation of ten fixation techniques. J Trauma 1996;40:778–783

59. Laing PG. The arterial supply to the adult humerus. J Bone Joint Surg Am 1956;38:1105–1116

60. Gerber C, Schneeberger AG, Vinh T. The arterial vascularization of the humeral head. J Bone Joint Surg Am 1990;72:1486–1494

61. Lee CK, Hansen HR. Post-traumatic avascular necrosis of the humeral head in displaced proximal humeral fractures. J Trauma 1981;21:788–791

62. Kuner EH, Siebler G. Fracture-dislocations of the proximal humerus. Unfallchirugie 1987;13:64–71

63. Paavolainen P, Bjorkenheim JM, Slatis P, et al. Operative treatment of severe proximal humeral fractures. Acta Orthop Scand 1983;54:374–379

64. Sturzenegger M, Fornaro E, Jacob RP. Results of surgical treatment of multifragmented fractures of the humeral head. Arch Orthop Trauma Surg 1982;100:249–259

65. Kristiansen B, Christiensen SW. Plate fixation of proximal humeral fractures. Acta Orthop Scand 1986;57:320–323

66. Williams GR Jr, Copley LA, Iannotti JP, Lisser SP. The influence of intramedullary fixation on figure-of-eight wiring for surgical neck fractures of the proximal humerus: a biomechanical study. J Shoulder Elbow Surg 1997;6:423–428

67. Flatow EL, Cuomo F, Maday MG, et al. Open reduction and internal fixation of two-part displaced fractures of the greater tuberosity of the proximal part of the humerus. J Bone Joint Surg Am 1991; 73:1213–1218

68. Ruch DS, Glisson RR, Marr AW, Russell GB, Nunley JA. Fixation of three-part proximal humeral fractures: a biomechanical evaluation. J Orthop Trauma 2000;14:36–40

69. Contreras D, Day L, Bovill D, Appleton A. Combined Enders rods and tension banding for humeral neck fractures. Presented at the 57th annual meeting, American Academy of Orthopaedic Surgeons, New Orleans, February 9, 1990

70. Cornell CN, Levine D, Pagnani MJ. Internal fixation of proximal humerus fractures using the screw-tension band technique. J Orthop Trauma 1994;8:23–27

71. Cornell CN. Tension-band wiring supplemented by lag-screw fixation of proximal humerus fractures: a modified technique. Orthop Rev 1994;suppl:19–23

72. Rajasekhar C, Ray PS, Bhamra MS. Fixation of proximal humeral fractures with the Polarus nail. J Shoulder Elbow Surg 2001;10:7–10

73. Lin J, Hou SM, Hang YS. Locked nailing for displaced surgical neck fractures of the humerus. J Trauma 1998;45: 1051–1057

74. Williams GR Jr, Wong KL. Two-part and three-part fractures: open reduction and internal fixation versus closed reduction and percutaneous pinning. Orthop Clin North Am 2000;31:1–21

75. McLaughlin H. Common shoulder injuries. Am J Surg 1947;3: 282–295

76. Warren R. Management of displaced fractures of the proximal humerus. Contemp Orthop 1987;15:61–93

77. Zuckerman JD, Matsen FA. Complications about the glenohumeral joint related to the use of screws and staples. J Bone Joint Surg Am 1984;66:175–180

6

Three-Part Fractures and Fracture-Dislocations

KENNETH A. EGOL AND KENNETH J. KOVAL

Proximal humerus fractures are common fractures and account for 10% of fractures in patients over age 65.[1] Understanding the anatomy about the proximal humerus is paramount to developing a proper treatment plan for displaced three-part fractures. This chapter addresses three-part fractures and fracture-dislocations. Three-part fractures include more commonly surgical neck and greater tuberosity fractures, and less commonly surgical neck and lesser tuberosity fractures. The three-part greater tuberosity pattern can be associated with anterior dislocations, whereas the lesser tuberosity pattern can be associated with posterior dislocations.

■ Clinical Evaluation

A detailed history should include handedness, and an assessment of activities of daily living and occupational as well as recreational activities. Chronicity of the injury should be documented, as it impacts the treatment options. Conditions predisposing to seizure such as medications, recent trauma, or stroke should be identified and treated in concert with the management of the fracture. On physical examination, one should expect swelling and tenderness about the shoulder girdle. If anterior dislocation is present, the head of the humerus may be palpable. Crepitation may be elicited with passive range of shoulder motion. Ecchymosis about the proximal humerus is usually present at 24 to 48 hours after injury and may track down the affected extremity or down the axilla.

A careful neurologic examination is essential, as many patients with complex fracture patterns with or without dislocation may have an axillary or musculocutaneous nerve neuropraxia. Neurologic injury may be present in

up to 45% of these injuries.[2] Vascular examination must be performed. The presence of distal pulses, however, does not rule out a more proximal vascular injury, due to the rich collateral circulation about the shoulder. Penetrating injuries, a palpable thrill, or a bruit about the shoulder girdle necessitate vascular surgery consultation.

Radiographic/Imaging Studies

As with all fractures about the shoulder, a standard shoulder trauma series should be obtained including anteroposterior, scapular lateral, and axillary views. The axillary view is critical to evaluate reduction of the glenohumeral joint (Fig. 6–1).[3] If the patient cannot tolerate the positioning for the axillary, a Velpeau axillary view can be obtained. Computed tomography (CT) scan may provide additional useful information about involvement of the head (Hill-Sachs or head-splitting component) and tuberosity displacement. Although not required routinely, reformatted reconstruction views can be obtained to provide additional information about fracture anatomy.

■ Treatment

Nonoperative

Most displaced three-part proximal humerus fractures require operative treatment. Exceptions to this are elderly patients with minimal functional ability and patients in whom surgery would be considered high risk. In these cases, a period of 7 to 10 days of immobilization (either for patient comfort or when the fracture moves as a unit) is followed by a structured and supervised

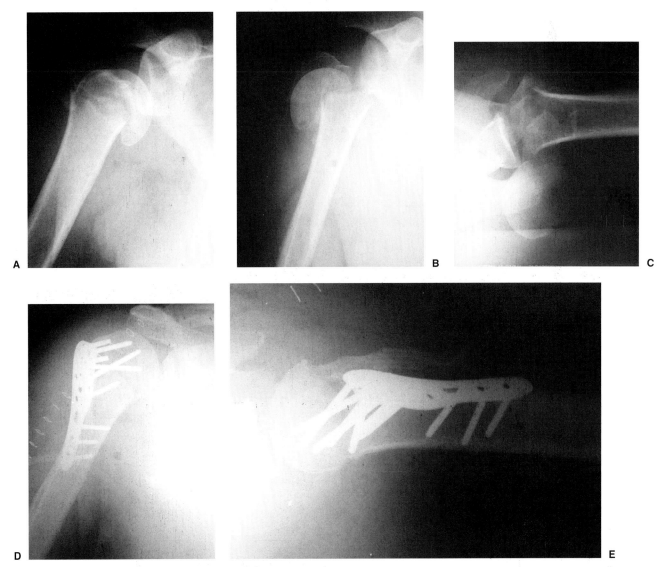

FIGURE 6–1 A 48-year-old, right-hand-dominant man was injured while skiing and sustained this three-part fracture-dislocation. The anteroposterior (AP) radiographs **(A,B)** do not show the posterior dislocation that is evident on the axillary view **(C)**. Open reduction and internal fixation (ORIF) was performed with a locking plate **(D,E)**. The postoperative axillary view **(E)** shows a concentric reduction.

rehabilitation program (Fig. **6–2**). This program should include pendulum exercises as well as gentle passive range-of-motion exercises.[4,5] Once there is radiographic evidence of healing, active range-of-motion exercises can be started. In one retrospective small series, two trauma centers compared their results for three- and four-part fractures. Sixteen patients (seven three-part fractures) treated nonoperatively were compared with 18 patients (eight three-part fractures) who underwent operative treatment. At follow-up no significant differences were found with regard to pain, function, and motion. As would be expected, there were no complications in the nonoperatively treated group.[6]

Other studies have reported good functional results with nonoperative treatment of comminuted proximal humerus fractures. In a long-term follow-up study of 17 patients with three- and four-part fractures, mean Constant shoulder scores averaged 59 for three-part and 47 for four-part fractures at 10 years.[7] These numbers compared favorably with a second series of operatively treated three- and four-part fractures at 3 years. Mean Constant scores were 51 for three-part and 46 for four-part fractures.[8]

Operative

A three-part fracture consists of a surgical neck fracture with either a greater or lesser tuberosity fracture. Most three-part fractures are treated with reduction and fixation. In some cases, when bone stock is poor,

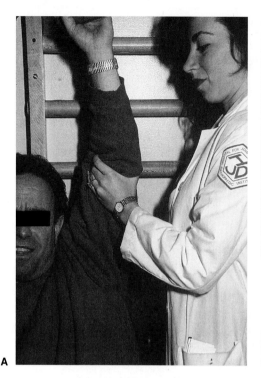

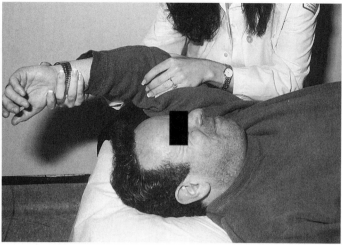

FIGURE 6–2 (A,B) A structured, supervised rehabilitation program relies on the interactions between the patient, the therapist, and the orthopaedic surgeon.

prosthetic replacement may be chosen. The technique for prosthetic replacement is described in Chapter 7. Operative treatment options include closed reduction and percutaneously placed pins or cannulated screws if closed reduction is chosen. If open treatment is chosen, internal fixation options vary and include plate and screws, Enders rod and tension band fixation, tension band fixation alone, and locked intramedullary nailing.

Percutaneous Pinning

Percutaneous pinning of three-part proximal humerus fractures is an attractive option when a closed reduction can be obtained. The advantages of this technique include minimal soft tissue dissection, decreased bleeding, and generally reduced morbidity.[9] In addition, the minimized scarring and adhesions with early range of shoulder motion can be beneficial with respect to final shoulder range of motion.

The operative technique is demanding and requires proper radiographic image intensification. Closed manipulation of the fracture fragments should correct the adducted position of the humeral shaft (secondary to the medial pull of the pectoralis muscle) combined with varying degrees of internal and external rotation to bring the proximal fragment in opposition to the tuberosity. Longitudinal traction, with adduction and internal rotation helps to reduce the humeral head to the shaft (Fig. 6–3).[10,11] With the reduction confirmed fluoroscopically, terminally threaded Schantz pins or

threaded Kirschner wires (K-wires) are inserted lateral to medial and anteriorly to posteriorly. Pin insertion should be done with careful consideration of the anatomic structures at risk. In particular are the long head of the biceps and cephalic vein. Based on one anatomic study, a relative safe zone for lateral pin placement is from a point approximately two head diameters distal to the top of the humeral head to the deltoid tuberosity.[9] At least one pin is directed from superolateral to inferomedial to capture the greater tuberosity fragment. This pin should be placed while the patient's shoulder is held in external rotation to minimize risk to the axillary nerve and directed to exit medially 2 cm distal to the inferior medial articular surface.[9] The use of terminally threaded 2.5-mm Schantz pins should prevent pin migration, which has been reported as a complication of this technique.[12] This technique is most suitable for younger patients with good-quality bone. Fixation is likely to be less secure in older patients, although the technique can be utilized successfully in these patients with proper attention to detail and close postoperative follow-up.

Jaberg et al[13] reported on their experience with 48 patients treated with percutaneous wire fixation. Their cohort included two-, three-, and four-part fractures. Of the eight patients in their series with three-part fractures, all had a good or excellent result. Complications included pin tract infections in four and symptomatic osteonecrosis in two patients with anatomic neck fractures. In an attempt to avoid the two largest complications with this technique, pin tract infection

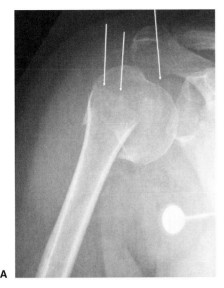

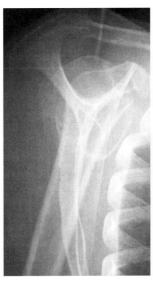

FIGURE 6–3 A 76-year-old man with displaced three-part fracture involving the surgical neck and the greater tuberosity **(A–C)**. Closed reduction and percutaneous pinning was performed **(D,E)**. Follow-up radiographs 6 months later show the fracture to be healed with excellent alignment **(F,G)**.

A

B

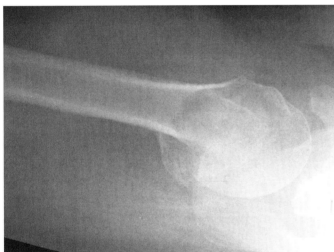

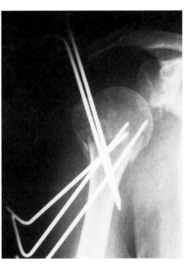

C

D

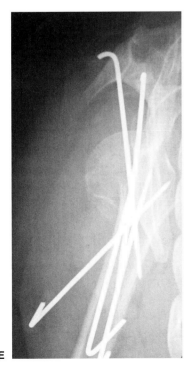

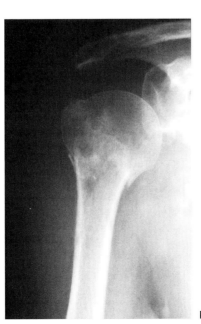

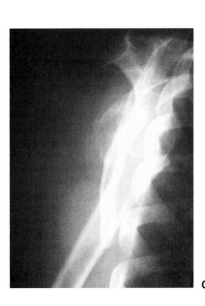

E

F

G

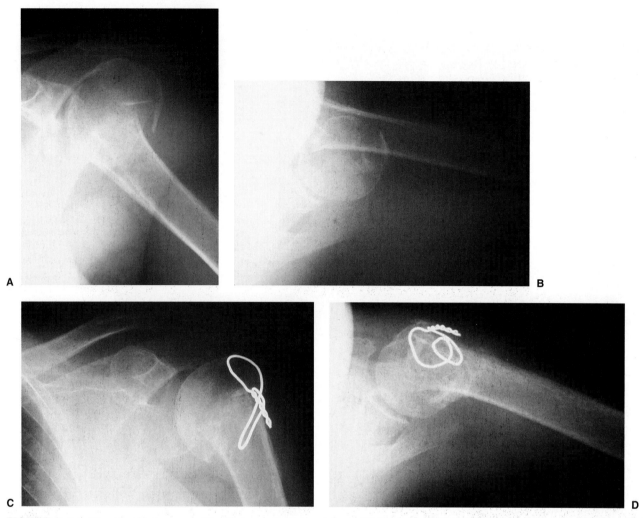

FIGURE 6–4 A 69-year-old woman with a three-part greater tuberosity fracture **(A,B)** treated by the open tension band wire technique **(C,D)**.

and stiffness from the period of immobilization required secondary to a prominent superolateral pin, some authors have advocated the use of cannulated screws. Chen et al[11] reported on 18 patients who were treated with percutaneous pinning or cannulated screw fixation of two- and three-part fractures including six three-part fractures in their series. All but one of the fractures united and all of the three-part fractures had satisfactory clinical outcomes. One patient who was pinned with K-wires had a skin problem that resolved after wire removal.

In another series of three- and four-part proximal humerus fractures, 27 patients (including nine with three-part fractures) were treated with percutaneous screw fixation.[10] At 2-year follow-up, the three-part group had an average constant score of 91 and no cases of osteonecrosis. The small numbers and mixture of fracture patterns in all of these series make it difficult to draw meaningful conclusions.

Tension Band Technique

The tension band technique described by Hawkins et al[14] is an open procedure (Fig. **6–4**). We utilize the tension band techniques in elderly patients with poor-quality bone. Because all of these techniques depend more on the rotator cuff–tendon bone interface than on the often thin and osteoporotic tuberosity fragments, hardware failure is less likely. The patient is placed in the beach chair position with the head secured. A deltopectoral incision is made with the arm in abduction to facilitate mobilization of the deltoid muscle. Once the fracture fragments are identified, the tuberosity fragment is reduced to the articular segment, which is then reduced to the shaft. The technique was originally described with the use of wire, but we prefer the use of No. 5 nonabsorbable braided suture. Two drill holes are placed in the shaft in an in-and-out technique. These sutures are then passed in a figure-of-eight fashion through the supraspinatus tendon insertion across the rotator interval. Additional sutures (two or three) are passed in a similar fashion, including one encompassing the infraspinatus tendon insertion and another encompassing the subscapularis. These sutures are tied securely to achieve the desired fixation. The rotator interval is then repaired and the shoulder tested to assess stability and determine parameters for the postoperative rehabilitation plan.

The Hawkins technique utilized wire passed through the bone of the tuberosity and the articular segment. They reported their results on 15 patients with three-part fractures using this technique. All 15 fractures united by 6 weeks. The active forward elevation averaged 126°. There was one poor functional result in a patient who had sustained an axillary nerve injury. There was one early failure of the tension band and two cases of osteonecrosis. One patient required revision to hemiarthroplasty.[14]

An alternate to this technique is the modification of adding a supplemental cancellous lag screw to enhance fixation.[15,16] The screw is placed from the lateral humeral cortex and angled toward the articular surface. The tension band fixation is placed around the head of the screw. In a series of 13 patients Cornell et al[15] used this technique to treat two- and three-part fractures. At final follow-up at an average of 20 months, all fractures had united. Four of the five patients with three-part fractures had good functional shoulder scores and one had a fair result. There were no complications in this series.

Enders and Suture Tension Band

This technique combines intramedullary fixation using modified Enders rods with a suture tension band technique for secure head and tuberosity fixation (Fig. **6–5**). This technique is preferable when there is medial neck comminution and the surgical neck is tipped into a varus position. A deltopectoral approach is utilized. The incision starts just lateral to the coracoid process and curves distal and lateral toward the deltoid tuberosity. The cephalic vein is identified and retracted laterally to protect its branches. Next the clavipectoral fascia is incised, and the conjoined tendon of the coracobrachialis and biceps is retracted medially. Partial release of the pectoralis major may facilitate shaft reduction by removing a deforming force. The displaced tuberosity, whether it is the greater or lesser tuberosity, is identified and mobilized. Tag sutures are placed into the rotator cuff to help mobilize the fracture fragments. The tuberosity is reduced and repaired to the head fragment first. This can be done with wire as described by Hawkins et al,[14] or, as we prefer, heavy nonabsorbable suture. Flexible rods such as Enders are placed through the head down the humeral shaft. Rotational

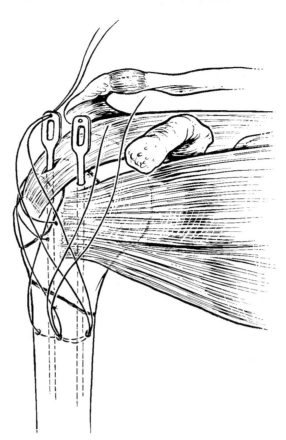

FIGURE 6–5 Graphic representation of the modified Enders rod-tension band technique.

stability is obtained by the three-point bend on the rods.[17] Some implant manufacturers (Smith and Nephew Richards, Memphis, Tennessee) have modified the Enders rod by adding a hole superior to the eyelet in the rod (Fig. **6–5**). This enables the Enders to be buried deeper within the bone and minimizes the risk of encroachment on the subacromial space. The tension band is then passed through the rotator cuff and the superior eyelets of the Enders and tied in a figure-of-eight fashion through drill holes in the shaft (Fig. **6–6**). Passing the suture through the humeral head and tuberosities prior to passage of the rods will limit the superior migration of the rods as long as the tension band is intact. The shoulder is then placed through a range of motion to assess stability. A passive range of shoulder motion program is begun immediately. Active motion is started 6 weeks after surgery when fracture healing has occurred (Fig. **6–6**).

In one series of 22 patients with two- and three-part fractures (nine were three-part) utilizing this technique, all of the three-part fractures achieved good or excellent results. The average range of motion was 153° of forward elevation, 46° of external rotation, and internal rotation to T12 for the three-part group. All fractures united, and two patients required removal of hardware.

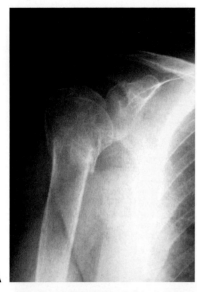
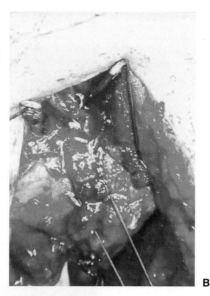
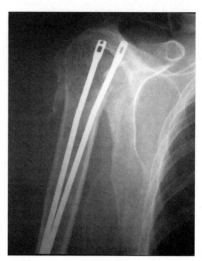

A

B

C

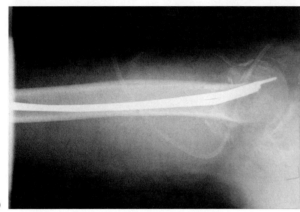

D

FIGURE 6–6 (A) A 57-year-old man with a three-part greater tuberosity fracture treated by the modified Enders rod-tension band technique. **(B)** The intraoperative photograph shows passage of the Enders rods through the tuberosities with nonabsorbable sutures in place. **(C,D)** Postoperative radiographs show excellent fracture reduction.

One patient fell and sustained a periprosthetic fracture at the tip of the Enders nails.[17]

Open Reduction: Plates and Screws

Open reduction and internal fixation is best suited for younger patients with good bone stock. Osteopenic bone may lead to loss of screw purchase and thus fixation failure.[18] If plates and screws are to be used, the deltopectoral approach is utilized once again. Care is taken to avoid stripping the fracture fragments of their soft tissue attachments. K-wires can be utilized to provide provisional stabilization. Plate and screw fixation can be achieved using several different implants including large-fragment T-buttress plates, small fragment cloverleaf plates, and distal tibial periarticular plates rotated 180° (Fig. **6–7**). If the three-part fracture includes the surgical neck and greater tuberosity, placement of the plate over the greater tuberosity fragment with screws through the plate will secure the greater tuberosity. If the fracture involves the lesser tuberosity (less frequent), a screw needs to be placed across the lesser tuberosity fragment in an

anterior to posterior direction. If screws are to be used in the head of the humerus, they should be cancellous screws to maximize purchase in the soft metaphyseal bone.

Esser[19] reported on 36 patients who had sustained three- and four-part fractures, all treated with open reduction and internal fixation using a modified cloverleaf or T-buttress plate. There were 21 patients with a three-part fracture or fracture-dislocations. In this series at a mean follow-up of 6.7 years, 15 patients had an excellent result, four had fair result, and two had a poor result. Three of the patients who were treated with a T-plate needed hardware removal for subacromial impingement. Hardware loosening was noted in five patients. There were no cases of osteonecrosis in this series.

In another small series, Moda et al[20] reported on 25 patients with various displaced fractures treated by open reduction and internal fixation with a T-plate or a blade plate. The five three-part fractures in the series were all fixed with a T-plate. According to Neer's criteria, four of the three-part patients had a satisfactory result and

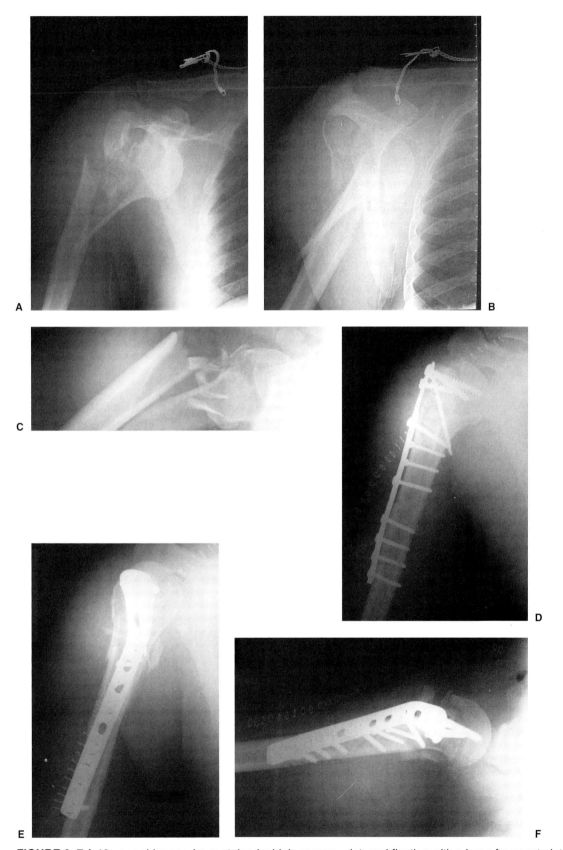

FIGURE 6–7 A 46-year-old man who sustained a high-energy three-part fracture involving the surgical neck and greater tuberosity **(A–C)**. The patient underwent open reduction and internal fixation with a large fragment plate and screws. Postoperative radiographs **(D–F)** reveal an anatomic reduction.

one had a poor result. Once again there were no cases of osteonecrosis in this series and only two patients developed significant stiffness.

In a large series of 98 patients treated with plate and screw fixation of two-, three-, and four-part fractures, 37 patients in the study population had sustained a three-part fracture. The authors utilized three separate outcome measures: the Constant score, the Neer score, and the UCLA score. Nonunion and osteonecrosis were identified in two of the three-part fractures in the series. Overall results were favorable, with 76% of patients having a good to excellent result according to the UCLA score, 69% according to the Neer score, and 59% according to the Constant score. Secondary varus deformity was identified in 12% of cases and malrotation in 8% of cases. The authors concluded that this was a very good treatment option for displaced two-, three-, and four-part fractures as long as technical errors such as malreduction and improper plate placement were avoided.[21]

A recent study evaluated longer term (average follow-up 10 years) results of open reduction and internal fixation of three- and four-part fractures and fracture-dislocations. The authors used both the wire tension band technique and T-plate and screw fixation. Twelve of the 22 patients with three-part fractures had an excellent result, nine a good result, and one a poor result based on the Constant score.[22] Two of the patient with good or excellent results developed asymptomatic osteonecrosis of the humeral head. There were 18 patients with three-part fracture-dislocations in the series: three had an excellent result, 11 a good result, and four a poor result. Five of the 11 patients with a good result in this group developed osteonecrosis, as did two of the patients with a poor result. The importance of these findings is that a good clinical result is possible even when humeral head osteonecrosis develops.

Other plate and screw implants can be utilized including the 90° cannulated blade plate or newly designed pre-contoured locking plates (Synthes, Paoli, Pennsylvania) These implants may have an advantage in osteoporotic bone. The fixed-angle nature of the implants may be beneficial in cases where there is concern about conventional plate and screw constructs. Both of these plates require access to the lateral humeral cortex for application (Figs. **6–1** and **6–8**).

Intramedullary Nail

Newly designed intramedullary (IM) nails with the ability to place a cancellous screw through the nail have added to the orthopaedic surgeon's armamentarium for the treatment of two- and three-part fractures. These implants are potentially helpful when the surgical neck fracture extends distally into the proximal humeral shaft or if the tuberosity fracture is nondisplaced; an IM nail can be placed with screws to fix the greater or lesser tuberosity fragments. With this technique, the patient is placed in the beach chair position with adequate image intensification for two views of the proximal humerus oriented 90° to each other. A 2-cm incision is made off the lateral edge of the acromion (Fig. **6–9A**). The deltoid is split between the anterior and middle thirds, with care taken to avoid splitting the deltoid too distally (4 cm distal to the acromial tip), which could injure the axillary nerve. The supraspinatus is incised longitudinally, and an awl is used to prepare a starting hole just lateral to the articular surface (Fig. **6–9B**). A reduction tool can be used to reduce the head to the shaft. The tuberosity is reduced with direct manipulation and rotation. If the tuberosity fragment is not reduced, a percutaneously placed joystick can aid in the reduction. The rod is placed over a guidewire to fix the head and shaft (Fig. **6–9C**). Large cancellous screws are placed via a targeting jig through the tuberosities for fixation (Fig. **6–10**).

Although there are no clinical series published in the literature that utilize IM nails, a biomechanical comparison of three modes of fixation used for the treatment of three-part proximal humerus fractures showed intramedullary fixation to be as stable a construct as plate and screw fixation. Ruch et al used a cadaveric three-part fracture model with Enders tension band, a cloverleaf plate, a screw construct, and an intramedullary device (Polaris nail, Accumed, Beaverton, Oregon). Specimens were potted and tested in cantilever bending and torsion. Both the plate and screw construct and IM nail construct were superior to the stability of the tension band construct. One problem with this study is that the cadaveric specimens were stripped of soft tissue. The intact rotator cuff is important in adding to the stability of the tension band construct.[23]

Prosthetic Replacement

In younger patients we generally attempt to fix all three-part fractures and fracture-dislocations. In selected older patients, in whom there is poor bone quality and extensive comminution, fixation may not be an option. In these patients, hemiarthroplasty with tuberosity and rotator cuff reconstruction would be preferred.

To do a humeral head replacement for three-part fractures, the patient is placed in the beach chair position with the head firmly secured in the head rest. A deltopectoral approach is utilized. Proximal humeral replacement should be cemented for fixation. There are several pitfalls that must be avoided when performing a shoulder hemiarthroplasty, including compromised tuberosity fixation, component malposition, and improper tension in the myofascial sleeve.[24] The details

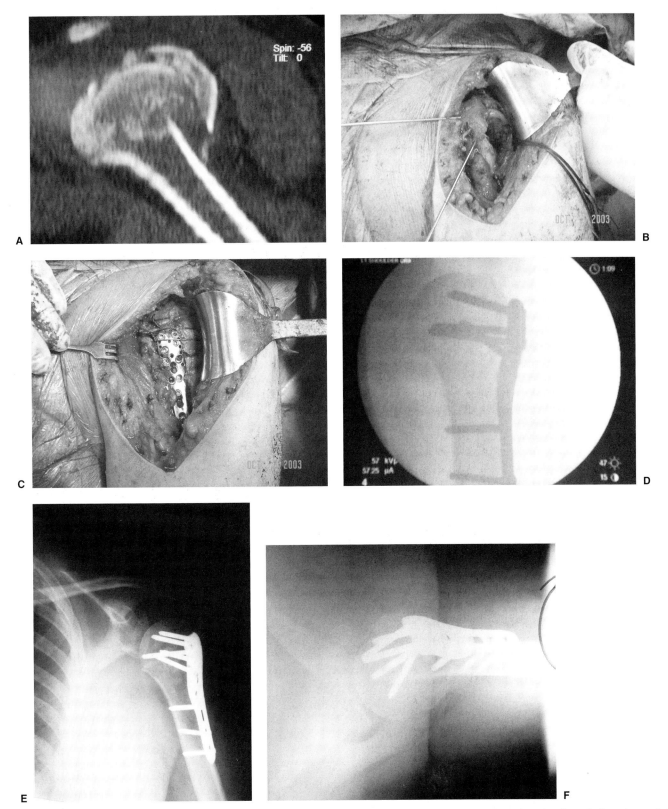

FIGURE 6–8 (A) A 38-year-old woman sustained an impacted valgus fracture visualized on computed tomography (CT) scan reconstruction. **(B)** During open reduction, elevation of the humeral head segment results in a void that is filled with cancellous allograft. **(C)** The greater tuberosity is reduced and a lateral humeral locking plate is placed. Supplemental suture fixation of the greater tuberosity is added to enhance fixation. **(D)** Intraoperative fluoroscopy is used to confirm the reduction. **(E,F)** Postoperative radiographs demonstrate excellent reduction and alignment.

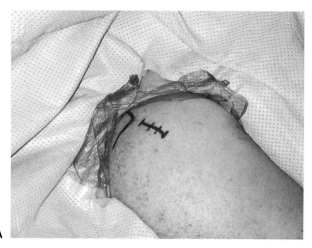

A

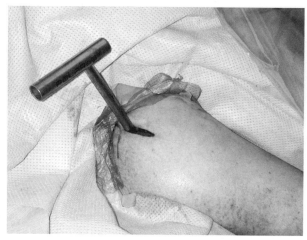

B

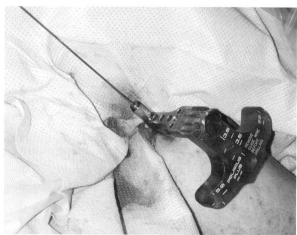

C

FIGURE 6–9 **(A)** Operative sequence for intramedullary nailing of a proximal humerus fracture includes identification of the lateral border of the acromion as the starting point for the incision. Care must be taken to limit extension of the deltoid split to avoid axillary nerve injury. **(B)** An awl is utilized to open the entry portal in the proximal humerus. **(C)** The nail is passed over a guidewire with the targeting jig attached.

of this operative technique is described in Chapter 7. The primary difference in performing this technique for three- and four-part fractures is the need to osteotomize the intact tuberosity from the articular segment. Frequently, nondisplaced fractures are present, which facilitates this step. It is important for the tuberosity to have sufficient bone to enhance reattachment and healing.

The greater and lesser tuberosities are repaired to one another and to the humeral shaft with heavy nonabsorbable braided sutures. The surgeon must be careful to bring the greater tuberosity below the prosthetic articular surface to avoid subacromial impingement. Loss of tuberosity fixation can lead to weakness or instability. Component malpositioning can also lead to instability. The recommendations are to place the humeral head in 20° to 40° of retroversion. Acceptable guidelines for testing intraoperative stability include anterior translation of the head upon the glenoid of 25% and posterior translation of 50%. Finally, seating the implant too low will decrease tension in the myofascial sleeve and thus potentially lead to weakness, instability, and decreased range of shoulder motion. Careful assessment of prosthetic height and humeral head size is integral to maintaining the proper length/tension relationship.

Most studies with regard to outcome following hemiarthroplasty for comminuted proximal humerus fracture show similar results. The operation is reliable for producing a comfortable shoulder; however, motion and function are limited. In a study of 18 patients who had undergone acute hemiarthroplasty for three- and four-part fractures, 11 of 18 were pain free, but range of motion was significantly limited compared with the opposite side.[25]

One study showed better functional outcomes in a small patient group. Skutek et al[23] looked at 13 consecutive active elderly patients (mean age 62) who underwent hemiarthroplasty for three- and four-part fractures. The authors' specific aim was to assess shoulder hemiarthroplasty's effect on recreational activities. Only three of the 13 patients had three-part fractures in this series. At a mean follow-up of 50 months, eight patients had a good or excellent result according to the Hospital for Special Surgery (HSS) score. Ten of the 13 patients returned to their preinjury activities, which included cycling, swimming, and dancing.

We reported a series of 26 patients who underwent humeral head replacement for acute three- and four-part proximal humerus fractures. Postoperative pain,

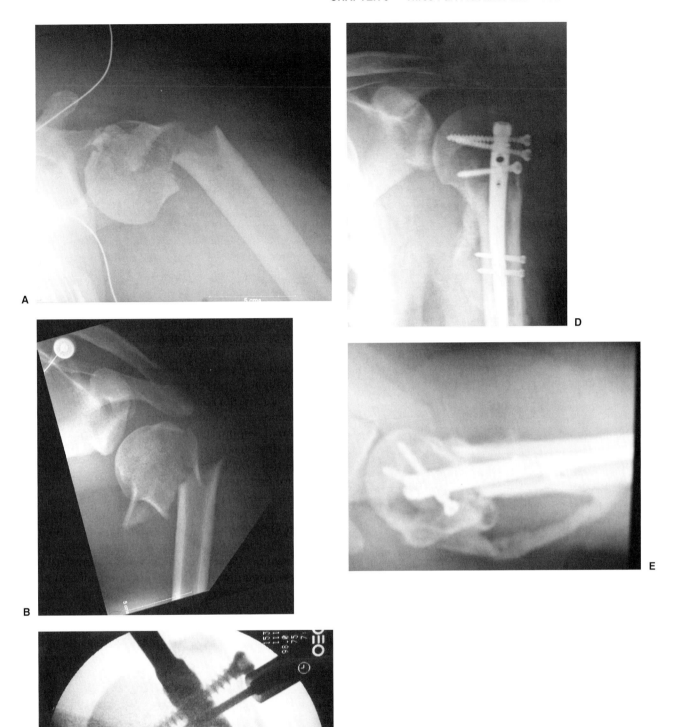

FIGURE 6–10 (A,B) A 32-year-old man involved in a motor vehicle accident sustained a left proximal humerus fracture as well as bilateral lower extremity fractures. Intramedullary fixation was selected to allow for earlier weightbearing. (C) Intraoperative fluoroscopy demonstrating fixation of the greater tuberosity fragment with an oblique locking bolt. (D,E) Radiographs obtained 6 months postoperatively, demonstrating healing of the fracture. Heterotopic ossification is evident anteriorly, but it did not inhibit motion.

active range of motion, and function were evaluated in 22 patients at a mean follow-up of 30 months (range 12 to 66 months) with the American Shoulder and Elbow Surgeons evaluation form. Seventy-three percent of patients reported only slight or no pain. Active forward elevation averaged 107°, external rotation averaged 31°, and the average internal rotation was to the second lumbar vertebra. Seventy-three percent of patients reported difficulty with at least three of 15 functional tasks tested. Lifting, carrying a weight, and using the hand at or above shoulder level were the most common limitations. When we compared the outcomes of the 12 three-part and 14 four-part fractures, frequently better active range of motion was recovered in the three-part group.

■ Conclusion

Fractures involving the proximal humerus are diverse injuries. The three-part fracture or fracture dislocation is a severe injury to the upper extremity. Nondisplaced or minimally displaced fractures as well as displaced fractures in frail elderly patients or poor surgical candidates may be treated nonoperatively. Nonoperative treatment, however, is not benign neglect. All nonoperatively treated patients should be started on an early therapy program. Most displaced three-part fractures are treated operatively. Good outcomes have been seen with various modes of fixation from closed reduction and percutaneous fixation to formal open reduction and internal fixation. The choice of implant is surgeon and fracture dependent. For selected cases, hemiarthroplasty is the treatment of choice. It is a particularly excellent option for low-demand elderly patients with regard to pain relief. All operative treatment of proximal humerus fractures requires meticulous attention to the surgical principles of minimal soft tissue stripping, utilization of appropriately selected implants, and good intraoperative and postoperative radiographic assessment. Avoiding pitfalls and use of a structured and supervised postoperative rehabilitation protocol with respect to passive followed by active motion and progressive strengthening will maximize functional outcomes in patients who have sustained these significant injuries.

REFERENCES

1. Baron JA, Karagas M, Barrett J, et al. Basic epidemiology of fractures of the upper and lower limb among Americans over 65 years of age. Epidemiology 1996;7:612–618
2. Stableforth PG. Four-part fractures of the neck of the humerus. J Bone Joint Surg Br 1984;66:104–108
3. Simon J, Puopolo SM, Egol KA, Zuckerman JD, Koval KJ. Accuracy of the Axillary Projection to Determine Fracture Angulation of the Proximal Humerus. San Francisco: American Academy of Orthopaedic Surgeons, 2000
4. Koval KJ, Gallagher MA, Marsicano JG. Functional outcome after minimally displaced fractures of the proximal part of the humerus. J Bone Joint Surg Am 1997;79:203–207
5. Goldman RT, Koval KJ, Cuomo F, Gallagher MA, Zuckerman JD. Functional outcome after humeral head replacement for acute three- and four-part proximal humerus fractures. J Shoulder Elbow Surg 1995;4:81–86
6. Ilchmann T, Ochsner PE, Wingstrand H, Jonsson K. Non-operative treatment versus tension-band osteosynthesis in three and four part proximal humerus fractures. Int Orthop 1998;22:316–320
7. Zyto K. Non-operative treatment of comminuted fractures of the proximal humerus in elderly patients. Injury 1998;29:349–352
8. Zyto K, Wallace WA, Frostick SP, Preston BJ. Outcome after hemiarthroplasty for three- and four-part fractures of the proximal humerus. J Shoulder Elbow Surg 1998;7:85–89
9. Rowles DJ, McGrory JE. Percutaneous pinning of the proximal part of the humerus. An anatomic study. J Bone Joint Surg Am 2001;83-A:1695–1699
10. Resch H, Povacz P, Frohlich R, Wambacher M. Percutaneous fixation of three- and four-part fractures of the proximal humerus. J Bone Joint Surg Br 1997;79:295–300
11. Chen CY, Chao EK, Tu YK, Ueng SW, Shih CH. Closed management and percutaneous fixation of unstable proximal humerus fractures. J Trauma 1998;45:1039–1045
12. Lyons FA, Rockwood CA Jr. Migration of pins in operations on the shoulder. J Bone Joint Surg Am 1990;72:1262–1267
13. Jaberg H, Warner JJ, Jakob RP. Percutaneous stabilization of unstable fractures of the humerus. J Bone Joint Surg Am 1992;74:508–515
14. Hawkins RJ, Bell RH, Gurr K. The three-part fracture of the proximal part of the humerus. Operative treatment. J Bone Joint Surg Am 1986;68:1410–1414
15. Cornell CN, Levine D, Pagnani MJ. Internal fixation of proximal humerus fractures using the screw-tension band technique. J Orthop Trauma 1994;8:23–27
16. Cornell CN. Tension-band wiring supplemented by lag-screw fixation of proximal humerus fractures: a modified technique. Orthop Rev 1994;suppl:19–23
17. Cuomo F, Flatow EL, Maday MG, Miller SR, Mclveen SJ, Bigliani LU. Open reduction and internal fixation of two- and three-part displaced surgical neck fractures of the proximal humerus. J Shoulder Elbow Surg 1992;1:287–295
18. Kristiansen B, Christensen SW. Plate fixation of proximal humeral fractures. Acta Orthop Scand 1986;57:320–323
19. Esser RD. Open reduction and internal fixation of three- and four-part fractures of the proximal humerus. Clin Orthop 1994; 299:244–251
20. Moda SK, Chadha NS, Sangwan SS. Open reduction and fixation of proximal humeral fractures and fracture-dislocations. J Bone Joint Surg Br 1990;72:1050–1052
21. Hessman MBF, Gehling H, Klingelhoeffer I, Gotzen L. Plate fixation of proximal humeral fractures with indirect reduction: surgical technique and results utilizing three shoulder scores. Injury 1999;30:453–462
22. Wijgman AJ, Roolker W, Patt TW, Raaymakers EL, Marti RK. Open reduction and internal fixation of three and four-part fractures of the proximal part of the humerus. J Bone Joint Surg Am 2002;84-A:1919–1925
22a. Ruch DS, Glisson RR, Marr AW, et al. fixation of three-part proximal humeral fractures: a biomechanical evaluation. J Orthop Trauma 2000;14:36–40
23. Skutek M, Fremerey RW, Bosch U. Level of physical activity in elderly patients after hemiarthroplasty for three- and four-part fractures of the proximal humerus. Arch Orthop Trauma Surg 1998;117:252–255
24. Egol KA, Zuckerman JD, Koval KJ. Proximal humerus fractures: pitfalls in diagnosis and management. J Musculoskel Med 1999; April:247–251
25. Wretenberg P, Ekelund A. Acute hemiarthroplasty after proximal humerus fracture in old patients. A retrospective evaluation of 18 patients followed for 2–7 years. Acta Orthop Scand 1997;68:121–123

7

Four-Part Fractures and Fracture-Dislocations

DOUGLAS MURRAY AND JOSEPH D. ZUCKERMAN

Four-part fractures represent 2 to 10% of all proximal humerus fractures and are associated with a higher energy mechanism of injury.[1-5] The displacement pattern of four-part fractures is secondary to the muscular attachments of the different segments. The humeral shaft is displaced medially and anteriorly by the pectoralis major. Retraction of both the greater and lesser tuberosities occurs due to the pull of the rotator cuff tendons, and the separation of these fragments results in a longitudinal tear in the rotator cuff usually along the rotator interval. Classically, the articular segment is displaced and rotated laterally (Fig. 7–1), although its position in a four-part fracture can be variable. Of significance is the loss of soft tissue attachments to the articular segment that compromises the blood supply to the humeral head, resulting in a significant risk of osteonecrosis. A fracture-dislocation is characterized by a dislocation of this articular segment either anteriorly or posteriorly along with this fracture pattern.[4]

The valgus-impacted four-part fracture has been described as a distinct type of four-part fracture pattern (Fig. 7–2).[6-9] Not specifically described in Neer's original classification, this pattern meets the criterion for displacement of all four segments, but the articular segment is impacted into valgus rather than completely separated from the shaft. This pattern is reported to account for 14 to 35% of all four-part fractures.[5,8,10,11]

The important distinction between the classical displaced four-part fracture and the valgus-impacted pattern is based on the impact on the blood supply to the articular surface (Fig. 7–3). In the classic displaced pattern, the articular surface is devascularized because it is detached from all soft tissue attachments. Neer reported that six of eight patients treated by open reduction for this type of four-part fracture developed osteonecrosis. This resulted in his recommendation that humeral head replacement should be performed for four-part fractures.[4] Subsequent studies have documented osteonecrosis in 20 to 75% of these fractures[12-16]; however, only 8 to 26% of the valgus-impacted four-part fractures develop osteonecrosis.[9,15,16] Jakob et al[17] theorized that without lateral displacement of the humeral head, an intact medial periosteum may preserve the blood supply to this fragment. This vascular preservation has been confirmed by radiographic analysis, direct specimen analysis, and perfusion studies.[9,18]

■ Clinical Evaluation

Information obtained from the patient's history will direct the treatment of proximal humerus fractures. Patients who sustain four-part fractures and fracture-dislocations are more often elderly with compromised bone quality, making stable internal fixation more difficult to obtain.[19] Other factors to consider in deciding treatment include the patient's activity level, medical status, and the ability to follow a structured postoperative rehabilitation program.[5,20-23]

The evaluation of the patient with four-part fracture or fracture-dislocation must include a complete evaluation of the patient, with a focused exam of the involved extremity and chest wall. Neurovascular injuries are reported to occur most commonly with anterior four-part fracture-dislocations.[4] Stableforth[5] reported vascular injuries in four of 81 (5%) four-part fractures.[5] Nerve injuries have been reported in 6 to 27% of four-part fractures and can involve the axillary, median, or ulnar

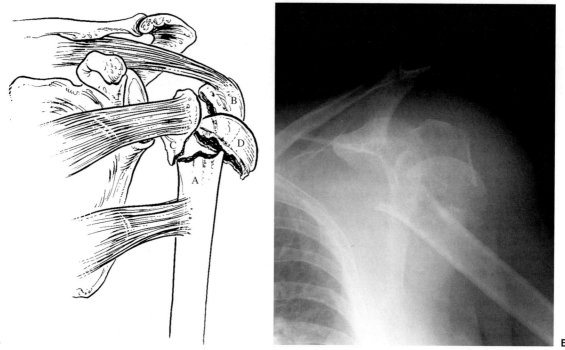

A

B

FIGURE 7–1 The "classic" four-part fracture is characterized by lateral displacement of the articular segment, medial displacement of the lesser tuberosity, and posterior/superior displacement of the greater tuberosity shown graphically **(A)** and radiographically **(B)**. The four identified fragments are as follows: A, shaft; B, greater tuberosity; C, lesser tuberosity; D, articular segment.

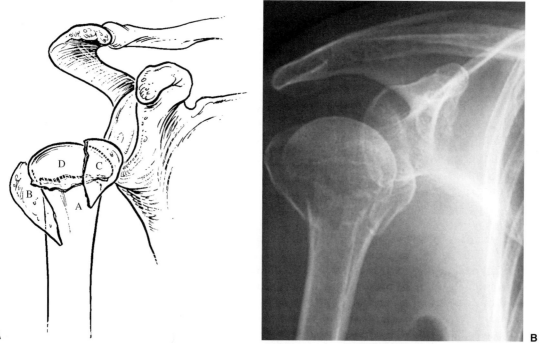

A

B

FIGURE 7–2 The "valgus-impacted" four-part fracture is characterized by a valgus and impacted position of the articular segment resulting in outward displacement of the tuberosities shown graphically **(A)** and radiographically **(B)**. The four identified fragments are as follows: A, shaft; B, greater tuberosity; C, lesser tuberosity; D, articular segment.

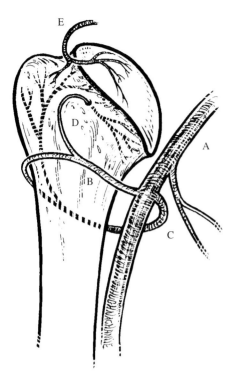

FIGURE 7–3 The blood supply to the humeral head originates form the axillary artery **(A)** and is derived from the anterior **(B)** and posterior **(C)** humeral circumflex arteries through the arcuate artery **(D)** and from the rotator cuff insertion **(E)**. It may be compromised with four-part fractures, resulting in risk for the development of osteonecrosis.

nerves or a combination of these nerves.[4,5,24] Neer documented 12 nerve injuries in his series of 44 four-part fractures. Five of the nerve deficits occurred after attempted closed reduction of a fracture-dislocation. Ten of the 12 resolved spontaneously.[24] Chest wall injuries including rib fracture, pneumothorax, and intrathoracic humeral head dislocation have been documented in association with four-part fractures that occur as a result of high-energy injuries.[5] Although four-part fractures and fracture dislocations are most commonly encountered in the elderly, these injuries do occur in young patients and are frequently secondary to high-energy injuries.

Radiographic/Imaging Studies

The standard trauma series is usually sufficient to evaluate four-part fracture patterns in the acute setting. Assistance is usually needed to position the patient for the axillary view. Computed tomography (CT) scans can be helpful to further delineate the fracture pattern and displacements, but are not routinely obtained. In our experience, two- and three-dimensional reconstructions have been of limited value.

■ Treatment

Nonoperative

Four-part fractures by definition represent significant displacement of all four segments of the proximal humerus. The deforming muscular forces causing displacement of each fragment makes an adequate closed reduction essentially impossible to maintain.[4,19] Closed reduction of four-part fracture-dislocations may also be of limited usefulness due to the limited chance of success and the increased risk of neurovascular injury associated with traction on the injured extremity. Neer reported 11 acceptable closed reductions out of 38 attempts of four-part fractures or fracture-dislocations, with unsatisfactory results in all 11 due to nonunion, malunion, or osteonecrosis.[4] A review of five series with a total of 97 four-part fractures treated nonoperatively documented only 5% satisfactory results.[4,5,12,14,20,25] Stableforth[5] reported greater functional disability and loss of sleep (due to pain) in patients treated nonoperatively compared with those who underwent hemiarthroplasty. Although valgus-impacted fractures have a lower risk of osteonecrosis, closed reduction will also be unsuccessful resulting in malunion.[5,9,17] In our experience, nonoperative treatment is reserved for selected patients who are poor operative risks or have very limited functional demands. For these patients, we do not attempt a closed reduction; rather, the degree of deformity is accepted (Fig. **7–4**). With a period of 4 to 6 weeks of immobilization, the goal in these patients is limited, painless below-shoulder motion, which may be indeed possible in spite of the residual deformity.

Operative

Operative management is the recommended treatment for four-part fractures including the classic pattern and the valgus-impacted pattern. Options include open reduction and internal fixation (ORIF) with or without bone grafting, closed reduction with percutaneous fixation, or humeral head replacement with tuberosity reconstruction.

Open reduction and internal fixation of four-part proximal humerus fractures is typically reserved for younger patients with good quality bone or for the valgus-impacted fracture pattern. Techniques utilized for fixation of four-part fractures and fracture-dislocations include AO/Association for the Study of Internal Fixation (ASIF) plates and screws,[3,26,27] cerclage wires or sutures,[16,27] lag screws,[16] intramedullary nails,[28] or a fixed-angle device.[29] Plates can be bent to create improved fixed-angled stability[29,30] or modified to minimize the prominence in the subacromial space.[26]

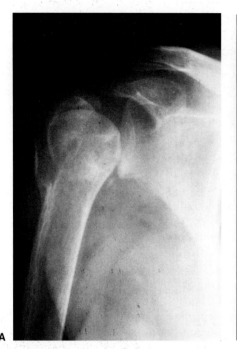
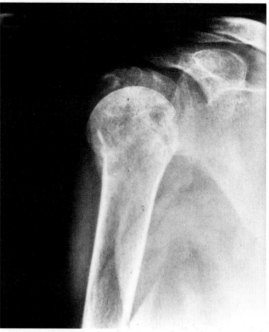

A   B

FIGURE 7–4 (A,B) Nonoperative treatment of this four-part fracture in this 72-year-old patient with significant medical comorbidities resulted in malunion but reasonable function for activities of daily living.

Evaluating the results of internal fixation of complex, comminuted proximal humerus fractures requires a careful analysis to confirm the distinction between three- versus four-part fractures, classic displaced versus valgus-impacted fractures, and young patients with better bone quality versus elderly patients with poor bone quality.[31] In addition, differentiating the outcomes of four-part fractures versus fracture-dislocations is also important because of the higher energy associated with fracture-dislocations and the greater potential for additional soft tissue injuries.

Neer[4] reported that open reduction with preservation of the humeral head failed in all eight four-part fractures or fracture-dislocations secondary to osteonecrosis in six and nonunion or infection in the other two. Other investigators have reported that malunion or other soft tissue injuries rather than osteonecrosis is the primary cause for failure of ORIF of these injuries. Lee and Hansen[13] did not identify osteonecrosis in their series of 19 four-part fractures and fracture-dislocations treated nonoperatively or by ORIF at an average follow-up of 23.6 months. Four of their patients did demonstrate evidence of revascularization of the humeral head following the transient appearance of osteonecrosis. Gerber et al[32] recommend attempting ORIF of four-part fractures in young patients as long as anatomic reduction can be obtained. Their results in patients who developed osteonecrosis in the absence of malunion were similar to the results of primary hemiarthroplasty. Wijgman et al[33] demonstrated satisfactory results in

17 of 20 four-part fractures treated with ORIF with cerclage wiring or a T-plate. All three poor results developed symptomatic osteonecrosis, but 10 of the 17 good or excellent results also developed osteonecrosis that had minimal impact on the outcome. Sturzenegger et al[16] demonstrated that limited internal fixation of three- and four-part fractures was associated with osteonecrosis in 10% of cases, compared with 30% of fractures treated with plate and screw fixation. They recommended minimal osteosynthesis as an alternative to primary prosthetic replacement.

Despite these findings, internal fixation for classic displaced four-part fractures is considered primarily in the younger patient if stable fixation and anatomic reduction can be obtained to allow early rehabilitation exercises.[31] A review of eight series reported in the literature identified 74 four-part fractures treated by ORIF and demonstrated a satisfactory result in only 36 patients (49%) (Table **7–1**). These reports did not necessarily differentiate between classic or valgus-impacted four-part fractures, which may certainly affect the outcome. Unsatisfactory results were associated with osteonecrosis, wound infection, stiffness, hardware impingement or loosening, malalignment, and axillary nerve palsy.[4,5,12,16,26,27,29]

Valgus-impacted four-part proximal humerus fractures may be more amenable to closed or open reduction and fixation. Jakob et al[17] reported satisfactory results in 14 of 19 patients with this type of fracture. Five patients were treated by closed reduction and Kirschner

TABLE 7–1 Results of Open Reduction and Internal Fixation (ORIF) in Eight Series

Series	Total Number of Patients in Series	Number of Four-Part Fractures Treated with ORIF	Operative Technique	Grading Scale for Satisfactory Result	Number of Satisfactory or Better Results for Four-Part ORIF	% Satisfactory or Better
Neer 1970	117	13	Various	Neer	0	0
Sturzenegger 1982	27	5	Buttress plate or minimal internal fixation	Saillant	4	80%
Paavolainen 1983	41	13	Screws with or without a plate	Neer	0	0
Stableforth 1984	81	3	Open reduction	"Based on restoration of function"	0	0
Yamano 1986	18	5	Hook plate	Flexion/ abduction >80	4	80%
Kristiansen 1987	188	5	Plate osteosynthesis	Neer	3	60%
Esser 1994	26	10	Modified cloverleaf plate	Bigliani	8	80%
Wijgman 2002	60	20	Cerclage wires or T-plate	Constant	17	85%
Totals	558	74			36	49%

wire (K-wire) fixation, and 14 were treated by open reduction and fixation by screws, K-wires, or cerclage wires. Osteonecrosis developed in all of the unsatisfactory results and in none of the satisfactory results. Resch et al[9] reported 20 good results in 22 valgus impacted fractures. The authors indicated that lateral displacement of the articular surface and severe osteopenia were contraindications to this procedure. In these patients, hemiarthroplasty was recommended. Careful surgical technique with minimal internal fixation resulted in only two cases of osteonecrosis in this series. Functional results correlated with anatomic reduction of the fragments. This technique utilized limited dissection through a deltopectoral approach. The articular fragment was elevated and the tuberosities reduced. Fixation consisted of a combination of percutaneous K-wires and suture repair of the tuberosities. Bone graft was used to fill any void that remained as a result of the initial impaction.

Percutaneous fixation for classic displaced four-part fractures has also been attempted but with less favorable results. Resch et al[15] reported good results for three-part or valgus-impacted four-part fractures treated with percutaneous reduction and fixation, but two of the five displaced four-part fractures required conversion to prosthetic replacement secondary to loss of reduction or osteonecrosis. Soete et al[34] reported similar results with three of their four four-part fractures developing osteonecrosis and unsatisfactory results.

Neer[4,35] originally recommended humeral head replacement for four-part fractures due to the high complication rate associated with nonoperative management

or ORIF; 31 of 32 four-part fractures and fracture-dislocations treated with humeral head replacement and reconstruction of the tuberosities and rotator cuff achieved excellent, good, or satisfactory results, with only one failure due to wound infection. With prosthetic replacement, pain relief is predictable, but functional outcome is unpredictable.[4,21,36–38] Isolating the results of four-part fractures and fracture dislocations in 10 studies treated by hemiarthroplasty (totaling 207 fractures), 79% achieved satisfactory or better results in fracture-dislocations treated with prosthetic replacement (Table 7–2).[4,5,22,37–43]

Many reports combine the results of hemiarthroplasty for all comminuted proximal humerus fractures together, but stratification of the results into fracture types demonstrates the inherent difficulties in reconstructing the more severely comminuted fractures. Goldman et al[21] reported better results with hemiarthroplasty for three-part fractures than for four-part fractures. Many authors have demonstrated the correlation of proper reconstruction of the rotator cuff and tuberosities with improved functional outcome.[20–22,40,44] Other factors associated with improved results are younger age,[21,22,41] male sex,[21] and compliance with the postoperative rehabilitation program.[20,23,40] Prosthetic reconstruction after failed ORIF or malunion following four-part humerus fractures is more technically challenging and is more commonly associated with complications and worse functional results than hemiarthroplasty for acute fracture.[38,45–47] This emphasizes the importance of acute fracture management to optimize outcomes.

TABLE 7–2 Results of Humeral Head Replacement (HHR) in 10 Series

Series	Total Number of Fractures	Number of Four-Part Fractures Treated with HHR	Grading Scale for Satisfactory Result	Number of Satisfactory or Better Results for Four-Part HHR	% Satisfactory or Better
Neer 1970	117	32	Neer	31	97%
Kraulis 1977	11	11	Neer	2	18%
Tanner 1983	49	14	Subjective patient satisfaction	14	100%
Stableforth 1984	81	14	"Based on restoration of function"	11	79%
Willems 1985	10	10	Neer	4	40%
Moeckel 1992	22	13	Hospital for Special Surgery (HSS) score	12	92%
Hawkins 1993	20	18	UCLA score	8	44%
Green 1993	28	28	Patient satisfaction from ASES evaluation	25	89%
Dimakopoulos 1997	38	38	Neer	32	84%
Prakash 2002	22	15	Subjective patient satisfaction	14	93%
Totals	398	193		153	79%

Preferred Operative Techniques

We prefer to perform humeral head replacement with tuberosity reconstruction for the vast majority of four-part fractures and fracture-dislocations. The exceptions are the treatment of valgus-impacted four-part fractures and fractures that occur in younger patients with good bone stock in whom an acceptable reduction and secure fixation can be achieved. We will describe techniques for hemiarthroplasty followed by our preferred approaches for ORIF.

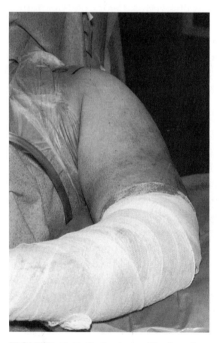

FIGURE 7–5 Patient positioning for proximal humeral replacement.

Humeral Head Replacement

The basic principles of prosthetic replacement for proximal humerus fractures include (1) utilization of a deltopectoral approach that preserves the origin and insertion of the deltoid muscle; (2) insertion of the proximal humeral prosthesis to restore humeral length and proper retroversion; and (3) secure fixation of the tuberosities to the prosthesis, to the humeral shaft, and to each other to allow early postoperative rehabilitation.

The success of humeral head replacement depends, in large part, on close attention to the technical details of the procedure and the utilization of meticulous surgical technique. The patient should be placed on the operating table in a supine position. The head of the operating table should be elevated ~30° in a modified beach chair position. A small bolster should be placed behind the involved shoulder. The patient should be moved to the side of the table so that the upper extremity can be placed into maximum extension without obstruction by the operating table (Fig. **7–5**). The patient should be secured to the operating table to minimize any changes in position intraoperatively. The entire upper extremity should be prepped and draped to allow full mobility during the procedure.

Surgical Approach   A straight deltopectoral incision is used that begins just lateral to the tip of the coracoid process and extends distally and laterally to the insertion of the deltoid (Fig. **7–6**). The subcutaneous tissues are divided, and medial and lateral flaps are elevated to expose the deeper muscular layers. The deltopectoral interval is identified by localization of the cephalic vein. The cephalic vein is usually retracted laterally

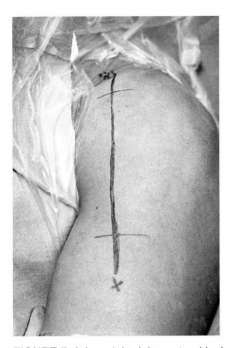

FIGURE 7–6 A straight deltopectoral incision is used.

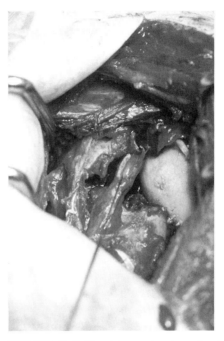

FIGURE 7–7 The biceps tendon should be identified, exposed, and tagged with a suture. Note the articular segment lateral to the biceps tendon.

with the deltoid muscle. In some instances, the cephalic vein is more easily retracted medially with the pectoralis major. In either case, care should be taken to preserve the cephalic vein throughout the procedure. The subdeltoid space is mobilized, as is the pectoralis major. The conjoined tendon muscles are identified, and the clavipectoral fascia is divided at the medial edge of the conjoined tendon muscles. The fracture hematoma is usually evident after dividing the clavipectoral fascia. The conjoined tendon muscles and the pectoralis major are retracted medially and the deltoid is retracted laterally. This can be most easily accomplished with the use of a self-retaining type of retractor. After the fracture hematoma has been evacuated, the deeper structures can be visualized. The biceps tendon should be identified and tagged with a suture (Fig. **7–7**). The biceps tendon provides an orientation to the greater and lesser tuberosities. The lesser tuberosity is located medial to the biceps tendon and the greater tuberosity is located superiorly and laterally. Each tuberosity should be tagged with a No. 2 suture for easier mobilization (Fig. **7–8**). These sutures should be placed at the tendon insertion site because this is generally the most secure area; placement of the sutures through the tuberosity itself can result in fragmentation. The lesser tuberosity is mobilized and retracted medially, while the greater tuberosity is retracted laterally and superiorly. This allows visualization of the articular segment. In four-part fractures this segment is generally devoid of soft tissue attachments and is easily removed. The

coracoacromial ligament should be identified at its coracoid attachment and followed to its acromial attachment. We feel it is important to preserve the coracoacromial ligament because of its contribution to anterosuperior stability.

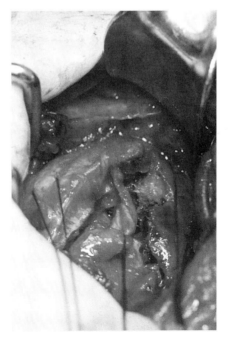

FIGURE 7–8 The lesser and greater tuberosities should be identified and sutures passed through the rotation cuff tendon adjacent to their attachment.

With the articular segment removed and the tuberosities retracted, the glenoid articular surface should be inspected. In the vast majority of situations, the articular surface of the glenoid is intact. It should be visualized to confirm the absence of preexisting degenerative changes or acute injury. The axillary nerve can usually be easily palpated at the anteroinferior aspect of the glenoid. Continuity of the axillary nerve can be confirmed by the "tug test," which consists of palpation of the nerve as it comes around the humeral neck on the underside of the deltoid and as it passes inferior to the glenoid. A gentle back and forth "tugging" motion confirms its continuity. At this point the humerus should be placed in extension to expose the proximal portion of the humeral shaft.

Humeral Shaft Preparation   After the humerus has been placed in extension, the proximal humeral shaft can be accessed easily (Fig. 7–9). A series of intramedullary broaches should be used to prepare the canal. Broaching should be continued until there is good cortical contact. At this point a trial component of appropriate size can be inserted. Because of the degree of proximal bone loss, it is necessary to place the prosthesis in a "proud" position; however, it is usually difficult to maintain the prosthesis in this position and to control rotation during trial reductions. To overcome this problem we have found it helpful to use a surgical sponge wrapped around the prosthesis (Fig. 7–10). This fills the canal and maintains the prosthesis in proper position. The

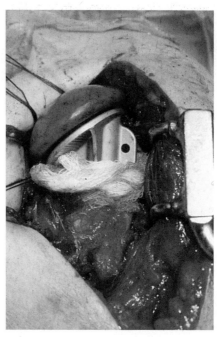

FIGURE 7–10 A sponge placed around the trial implant provides sufficient stability to maintain position during trial reductions.

desired position of retroversion is 20° to 35°. This can be modified if there is a preexisting chronic dislocation or fracture-dislocation.

The position of retroversion should be confirmed by comparing the position of the prosthesis with the transepicondylar axis. In addition, the position of the lateral or anterior flange of the prosthesis in relation to the adjacent humeral cortex should be marked and used to confirm proper position during cementing. The choice of head size should be guided by the size of the removed humeral head. With the humeral trial implant in place, the trial reduction can be performed.

The trial reduction is a critical part of the procedure because it defines the parameters needed to obtain a stable construct (Fig. 7–11). After the humeral head is reduced onto the glenoid, the greater and lesser tuberosities are pulled into position. The biceps tendon is allowed to fall between the tuberosities. Traction on the tuberosity sutures not only maintains the tuberosities in position but also provides a more realistic assessment of stability. The self-retaining retractor should be relaxed for an accurate assessment of soft tissue tension. Assessment of posterior, inferior, and anterior stability should be assessed by translating the humeral head in these directions. Up to 50% of posterior translation of the humeral head on the glenoid is acceptable; up to 50% of inferior translation is also acceptable; however, anterior translation should not

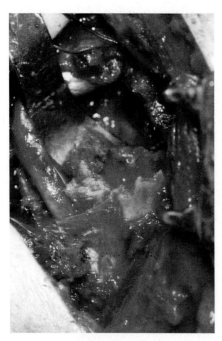

FIGURE 7–9 Extension of the humerus provides exposure and access to the upper portion of the shaft.

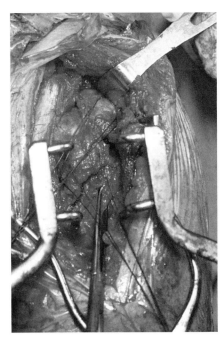

FIGURE 7–11 During the trial reduction the tuberosities are pulled back into position to provide soft tissue tension to assess stability.

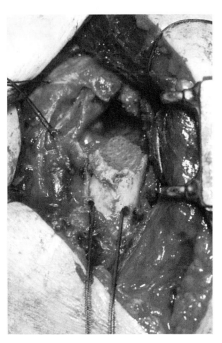

FIGURE 7–12 The drill holes in the humeral shaft should be placed adjacent to the bicipital groove and sufficiently distal to prevent extension into the fracture site.

exceed 25%. If these parameters are exceeded, the position of the component should be reevaluated to confirm that it has not subsided or rotated in the canal. If soft tissue laxity is excessive, a larger humeral head should be used. On the other hand, if soft tissue tension is excessive, a smaller humeral head may be necessary. In either situation, repeat assessment of stability is required to confirm that the proper components and position have been chosen. When the proper position and component sizes are confirmed, the trial prosthesis should be removed.

At this point two drill holes should be placed through the humeral cortex into the medullary canal. These holes should be placed about 1.5 to 2 cm distal to the level of the surgical neck component in proximity to the bicipital groove. Three No. 5 nonabsorbable sutures are passed through one drill hole into the medullary canal and then out through the second drill hole (Fig. **7–12**). These sutures will be used for tuberosity fixation. The medullary canal should be irrigated copiously, and any loose cancellous bone removed. The use of the cement restrictor is preferred to enhance cement distribution; however, we avoid any formal pressurization of the cement to decrease the possibility of humeral shaft fracture. The canal should be packed with a sponge to obtain adequate drying before cementing.

The cement is mixed and poured into a vented 60-cc Toomey-type syringe approximately 1 minute after mixing (Fig. **7–13**). This syringe should be vented by preparing a hole at the 30-cc mark. This hole allows air

to escape during insertion of the plunger so that a continuous column of cement is formed. Use of a shortened chest tube attached to the sponge enhances insertion of the cement more distally in the canal. The size of the chest tube should be based on the canal diameter; however, if this technique is utilized, the cement should be injected when it is relatively "wet" because of the resistance provided by the chest tube. The cement is then injected into the canal. During insertion of the prosthesis it is essential to maintain the prosthesis in the proper "proud" position as well as in the desired position of retroversion. The prosthesis should be held in position until the cement is completely set to avoid inadvertent subsidence or rotation into an unacceptable position. When the cementing is complete, the position should be confirmed. The modular head is then impacted into place, making certain that the taper is dry and free of any debris.

Tuberosity Fixation   Fixation of the tuberosities to the prosthesis and the shaft is a critical component of this procedure. Proper reattachment and secure fixation will enhance the probability of a successful outcome in terms of range of motion and overall function; however, careful attention must be given to the technical aspects of this portion of the procedure. Heavy (No. 5) nonabsorbable sutures should be used. These sutures are generally passed through the rotator cuff tendons just at their insertion into the tuberosities. The biceps tendon is allowed to fall between the tuberosities and is incorporated into the

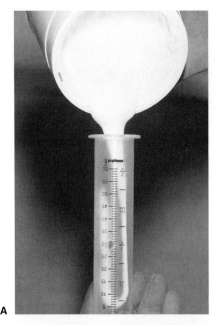

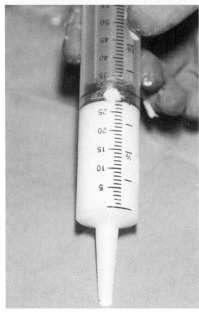

FIGURE 7–13 A vented 60-cc syringe **(A)** provides a continuous column of cement **(B)** for injection into the canal.

fixation. This results in a "functional tenodesis," but probably preserves at least a portion of its humeral head depressor function.

The principles of tuberosity fixation include (1) cerclage suture fixation, which brings the tuberosities into contact with each other; and (2) placement of longitudinal sutures to bring the tuberosities into a position below the prosthetic articular surface and into contact with the humeral shaft. This is analogous to the principles of fixation of the greater trochanter in hip surgery, in which longitudinal wires are used to advance the trochanter distally into the proper position, and transverse/

cerclage wires are used to secure the trochanter in this position.

At this point, the two cerclage sutures are passed using No. 5 nonabsorbable sutures (Fig. **7–14A**). The first is passed through the upper portion of the subscapularis tendon as it inserts into the lesser tuberosity, around the medial portion of the prosthesis, and through the supraspinatus tendon as it inserts into the greater tuberosity. The second cerclage suture is passed through the lower portion of the subscapularis tendon as it inserts into the lesser tuberosity, around the medial portion of the prosthesis, and through the infraspinatus tendon as it inserts into the greater tuberosity.

At this point the two longitudinal sutures, which have already been passed through the humeral cortex, are used. The first longitudinal suture should be placed in a figure-of-eight fashion through the supraspinatus tendon as it inserts into the greater tuberosity and then through the upper portion of the subscapularis tendon as it inserts into the lesser tuberosity (Fig. **7–14B**). The second longitudinal suture should be passed in similar fashion through the infraspinatus tendon as it inserts into the greater tuberosity and through the lower portion of the subscapularis tendon as it inserts into the lesser tuberosity. The suture tying sequence is important (Fig. **7–14C**). The first longitudinal suture should be tied first. This advances the tuberosities distally below the articular surface of the prosthesis and into contact with the humeral cortex, which is essential to obtain bone to bone healing. If necessary the second longitudinal suture can also be tied. Care should be taken to avoid excessive distal displacement of the greater tuberosity. When the tuberosities are confirmed to be in proper position, the superior cerclage suture is tied followed by the inferior cerclage suture. Cerclage fixation brings the tuberosities into contact with each other and maintains the position, obtained by the longitudinal sutures. The second longitudinal suture can then be tied if it was not tied previously (Fig. **7–14D**). If a third longitudinal suture was passed through the shaft, it should be tied at this time to augment the fixation. Tuberosity reattachment should be performed with the arm in approximately 20° of abduction, neutral flexion, and 10° to 20° of external rotation. When the tuberosity fixation is completed, the stability of the fixation should be carefully assessed. Range of motion in forward elevation, external rotation, internal rotation, and abduction should be performed to determine the specific limits of motion that will be allowed in the postoperative rehabilitation program. If there are concerns about the security of the fixation, the remaining suture passed through the shaft should be used to enhance the construct. In addition, we have found that bone grafting the tuberosities can enhance the healing potential. Cancellous bone from the humeral head should be placed in the area of

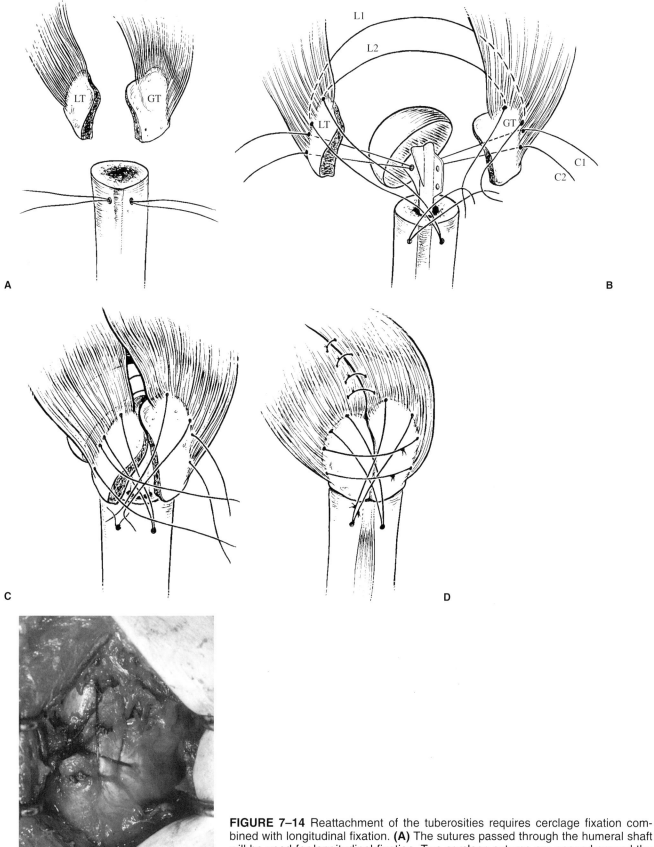

FIGURE 7–14 Reattachment of the tuberosities requires cerclage fixation combined with longitudinal fixation. **(A)** The sutures passed through the humeral shaft will be used for longitudinal fixation. Two cerclage sutures are passed around the medial aspect of the prosthesis. **(B)** The two longitudinal sutures are then passed in a figure-of-eight technique. **(C)** The longitudinal sutures are tied first, followed by the two cerclage sutures. **(D)** When tuberosity fixation is completed, the tuberosities should be in contact with each other, with the shaft and below the articular surface. **(E)** Rotator interval closure should also be performed.

contact between the shaft and the tuberosities as well as between the tuberosities.

Closure includes repair of the rotator interval with No. 1 or No. 2 nonabsorbable sutures (Fig. **7–14E**). This repair should be performed with the humerus in external rotation to decrease the possibility that rotator interval closure will restrict rotation. A closed suction drain is usually placed deep to the deltopectoral interval and brought out through the skin distally and laterally. The deltopectoral interval is repaired with absorbable suture, as is the subcutaneous tissue. This skin closure is performed with either sutures or staples. A sterile dressing is applied and the upper extremity is placed in a sling.

We feel it is very important to obtain a complete set of radiographs in the operating room (Fig. **7–15**). These should include an anteroposterior (AP) view of the shoulder with the humerus in internal rotation (on the chest) and maximum external rotation as defined by the intraoperative assessment. An axillary view should also be obtained. These radiographs provide excellent visualization of the position of the prosthesis as well as the position of the tuberosities.

Postoperative Rehabilitation   On the first postoperative day, the patient is started on a rehabilitation program that consists of active range of motion of the elbow,

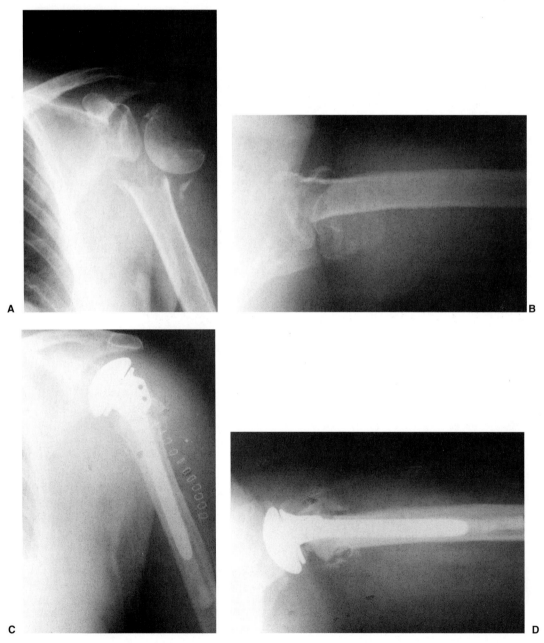

FIGURE 7–15 Preoperative **(A,B)** and postoperative radiographs **(C,D)** of a four-part fracture treated by humeral head replacement.

wrist, and hand, and passive range of motion of the shoulder. External rotation should be limited based on the intraoperative evaluation. This is important in avoiding any excess stress on the tuberosity repair that could compromise healing. Internal rotation is allowed to the chest. These exercises are continued for the first 8 weeks. Radiographs are obtained approximately 2 weeks following surgery to confirm the position of the tuberosities. Additional radiographs are obtained at 8 weeks following surgery to assess the degree of tuberosity healing. If tuberosity healing is sufficient, the sling is discontinued and an active range-of-motion program is begun. The patient is encouraged to use the involved upper extremity for activities of daily living. Passive range of motion is continued with gentle stretching to increase the overall range. At 8 weeks following surgery, isometric deltoid and internal and external rotator strengthening exercises are begun. Vigorous strengthening exercises are not begun until active forward elevation of at least 90° is obtained. Our experience has shown that patients can expect continued recovery during the first year following surgery, although most recovery will occur during the first 6 months.

ORIF: Displaced Four-Part

Treatment of a displaced four-part fracture with ORIF requires a thorough understanding of the anatomy of the injury and meticulous attention to surgical technique. Although many different internal fixation techniques have been described, our preferred approaches include the use of multiple tension band suture fixation (Fig. 7–16) or, more recently, the use of a Synthes (Pauli, Pennsylvania) proximal humeral locking plate (Fig. 7–17). We have used multiple tension band sutures in younger patients when significant comminution is not present. The Synthes proximal humeral locking plate can also be used, particularly when more comminution is present. In each situation we have found it necessary to add cancellous allograft (freeze-dried) to the construct to fill the metaphyseal defect that results from the impaction component of the injury. Regardless of the fixation method utilized, the goal of the procedure is to achieve an acceptable reduction and adequate fixation for healing and to initiate an early range of motion program. Achieving these goals is more difficult than in most proximal humeral fractures because of the complexity of the injury.

A deltopectoral approach is used beginning just lateral to the coracoid process and extending in a straight line toward the insertion of the deltoid. Skin subcutaneous tissues are divided and the subcutaneous flaps are developed to identify the deltopectoral interval. The interval is developed proximally and distally and the cephalic vein is usually retracted laterally. The subdeltoid space is mobilized. At this point, the fracture hematoma is evident below the clavipectoral fascia. In some cases, the clavipectoral fascia may be disrupted. The conjoined tendon muscles are mobilized and retracted medially. A self-retaining retractor can be used at this point to improve exposure. The biceps tendon is identified and tagged with a No. 1 Mersilene suture. By following the biceps tendon proximally, the lesser tuberosity and greater tuberosity fragments can usually be identified. The lesser tuberosity fragment is expected to be medial and inferior to the biceps tendon. The greater tuberosity fragment/fragments will be located posterior and superior to the biceps tendon. Number 2 Mersilene sutures are passed through the subscapularis tendon as it inserts into the lesser tuberosity.

In a similar fashion, sutures are passed through the supraspinatus and infraspinatus insertions into the greater tuberosity. The greater tuberosity may be fractured into two or more parts. It is important to place a suture into the rotator cuff tendon for each fragment. The rotator interval is usually separated because of displacement of the fragments. If it remains partially intact, it should be divided to the anterosuperior glenoid to enhance exposure. Traction on the sutures will displace the tuberosities and enhance visualization of the articular segment and the joint. The joint should be inspected to remove any bony fragments. In a classic displaced pattern, the articular segment is usually displaced laterally and is often perched on the lateral cortex of the proximal humerus. The fragment should be mobilized and reduced into position on the humeral shaft. The few remaining soft tissue attachments will permit proper orientation of the articular segment. The tuberosities should be reduced into position using the previously placed sutures. Intraoperative fluoroscopy is used to assess the reduction and alignment in the AP and axillary projections. The fluoroscopy will be used repeatedly during the procedure to assess the reduction as fixation is performed. When the articular segment is reduced on the shaft segment, there will usually be excessive shortening of the proximal humerus; therefore, it is important to determine the appropriate height of the articular segment by reducing the tuberosities into position and determining the "gap" that exists. This gap should be filled with cancellous allograft that will support the articular segment. It is important to emphasize that this assessment does not represent an exact science. The tuberosities cannot be reduced anatomically, but by reducing them into better position a reasonable assessment of the appropriate height of the articular segment can be obtained.

At this point a final decision is made concerning the type of internal fixation to be utilized. If multiple tension band sutures are to be utilized, attention is turned to the shaft component. Two drill holes are placed through the lateral humeral cortex. Five No. 5 Ethibond sutures are passed through the drill holes in an "in-and-out"

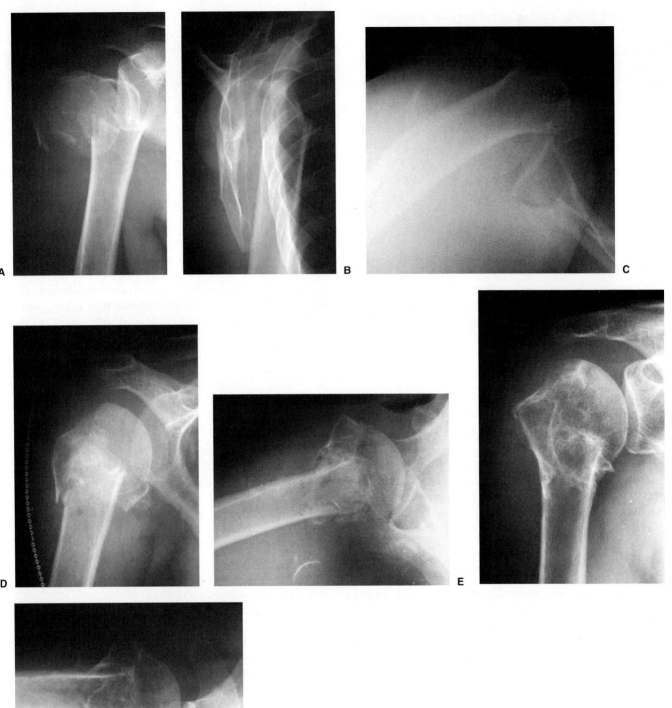

FIGURE 7–16 A 48-year-old man with a four-part fracture **(A–C)** underwent open reduction and internal fixation with No. 5 nonabsorbable tension band sutures combined with corticocancellous allograft **(D,E)**. At 2-year follow-up the fracture has healed, and he has regained excellent function with an American Shoulder and Elbow Surgeons (ASES) score of 92 **(F,G)**.

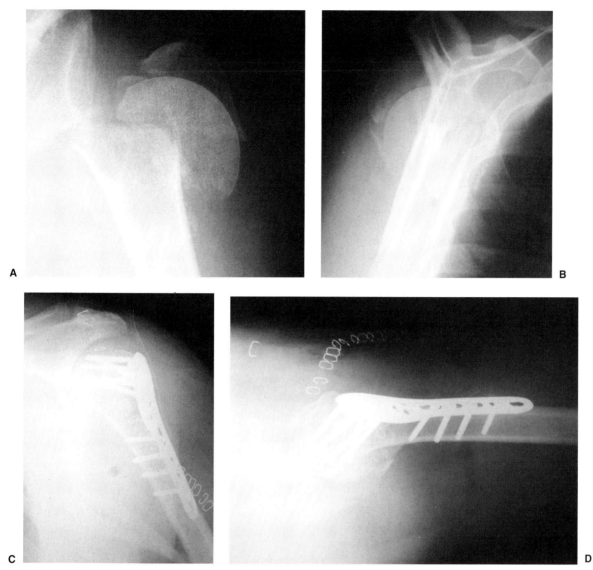

FIGURE 7–17 A 46-year-old man sustained a four-part fracture **(A,B)** as a result of a fall from a ladder. Open reduction and internal fixation with a locking plate **(C,D)** and tension band-suture fixation of the tuberosities to the plate.

fashion. These sutures will be used to reattach the tuberosities. Cancellous allograft is then used to fill the defect in the proximal humerus. It is packed onto the upper portion of the shaft segment to provide a "platform" for the articular segment. The articular segment is then reduced onto the shaft and oriented to the glenoid articular surface. At this point, the tuberosities are brought back into position by placing traction on the previously placed sutures. It is important to maintain the humerus in a secure position and avoid excessive movement as the tuberosities are reattached. This will prevent the articular segment from displacing. The No. 5 Ethibond sutures that were passed through the humeral shaft are then used to reattach the tuberosities. Two sutures are passed individually in a figure-of-eight fashion through the subscapularis insertion into the

lesser tuberosity across the rotator interval and through the supraspinatus insertion into the greater tuberosity. The third suture is passed in a horizontal fashion through the infraspinatus insertion into the greater tuberosity, and the fourth suture is passed in a horizontal fashion through the subscapularis insertion into the lesser tuberosity. These sutures are then tied in the same sequence. It is important to make certain that the greater tuberosity is reduced below the level of the articular surface to prevent encroachment on the subacromial space. After these sutures are tied, the fifth suture can be used to augment the fixation based on the intraoperative assessment. The tension-based sutures provide fixation of the tuberosities to each other and to the shaft. The humerus is then placed through a range of motion, assessing the security of the fixation, particularly at the extremes of rotation and abduction. It is also important to repair the rotator interval to enhance the security of the fixation. This is done with a No. 1 or No. 2 Mersilene suture. The mini–C-arm should be used to confirm the reduction, and final radiographs should be obtained consisting of AP view in internal and external rotation and an axillary view.

When a proximal humeral locking plate is to be used, the proper length plate is chosen (three or five holes) and the alignment guide is attached. It is applied to the humeral cortex lateral to the bicipital groove and positioned by placing the guidewire through the superior hole. This guidewire should be placed just above the articular surface to prevent plate impingement on the subacromial space. Additional K-wires are then placed for provisional fixation of the articular segment. It is important to consider the position and size of the tuberosities when reducing the articular segment to the shaft because they will be reduced and fixed later in the procedure and will have to "fit." The mini–C-arm should be used at this time and during subsequent steps to confirm the reduction, the position of the plate, and the location and length of the screws. If the reduction is acceptable and the plate is in good position, a distal screw can be placed for fixation to the humeral shaft. Proximal locking screws can then be placed and the K-wires exchanged for screws. The guide allows the screws to be placed in either a more anterior or posterior orientation depending on the position of the articular segment in relation to the plate. At this point cancellous allograft is packed into the defect between the humeral head and the shaft. The tuberosities are then brought back into position and fixed to the plate using multiple No. 5 nonabsorbable sutures passed through the peripheral holes in the plate. The rotator interval should be closed with a No. 2 nonabsorbable suture. The humerus is placed through a range of motion to confirm the security of the repair. The mini–C-arm should be used to confirm the reduction and the placement of the plate and screws. Final radiographs should also be obtained as described previously.

This approach changes somewhat based on whether a fracture-dislocation is present. Although a vast majority of four-part fracture-dislocations are treated by hemiarthroplasty (Fig. 7–18), when open reduction is preferred it is important to identify and reduce the articular segment. For anterior fracture-dislocations, mobilization of the lesser tuberosity usually allows visualization of the dislocated articular segment, which is usually in a subcoracoid position. In these injuries, the articular segment is usually free of any soft tissue attachments; therefore, it is important to handle the fragment carefully and maintain it within the operative site. In posterior fracture-dislocations, identification of the articular segment requires displacement of the lesser tuberosity

medially and the shaft laterally. The articular segment is usually located in a subacromial position posterior to the glenoid. Once again, careful handling of this fragment is essential. For fracture-dislocations, the articular segment is reduced onto the proximal portion of the shaft with bone grafting and fixation options as described.

ORIF: Valgus-Impacted Four-Part

The approach to the valgus-impacted four-part fracture is somewhat different (Fig. 7–19). Location of the biceps tendon allows identification of the lesser and greater tuberosity. In this fracture pattern, the articular surface has been impacted and, as a result, the tuberosities are displaced outwardly. The split between the greater and lesser tuberosity can be identified. This interval is then treated in an "open book" fashion to allow visualization of the impacted articular segment. Opening of the rotator interval will enhance visualization of the articular segment. An elevator is then used to restore the articular segment to proper position. In doing so, a bony void will be evident between the articular segment and the shaft. This represents the area of metaphyseal cancellous bone impaction from the injury. This defect is filled with corticocancellous allograft. Sufficient bone is placed to maintain the articular segment at the appropriate height. A few millimeters of overreduction is reasonable to compensate for the settling that inevitably occurs postoperatively. Drill holes are then placed through the lateral humeral cortex in a similar fashion as described previously. These sutures are then passed in horizontal mattress fashion through the subscapularis tendon insertion and through the supraspinatus and infraspinatus tendon insertions. Additional sutures are placed in a figure-of-eight fashion across the rotator interval to further enhance the fixation. By bringing the tuberosities into reduced position, the tension effect maintains the articular segment in reduced position.

Closure is performed in a standard fashion. A Hemovac drain may be appropriate and, if so, this is placed deep to the deltopectoral interval. The deltopectoral interval is closed with 0 Vicryl in simple interrupted sutures. The subcutaneous tissue is closed with 2-0 Vicryl in simple interrupted sutures, and the skin is closed with a subcuticular closure with 3-0 Prolene. Steri-Strips are applied. After application of sterile dressing, a full set of radiographs is obtained, including AP views in internal and external rotation and an axillary view. This provides a more detailed evaluation of the reduction and fixation.

The postoperative rehabilitation program is begun on postoperative day 1 and consists of active range of motion of the elbow, wrist, and hand, and passive-assisted range of motion of the shoulder including forward

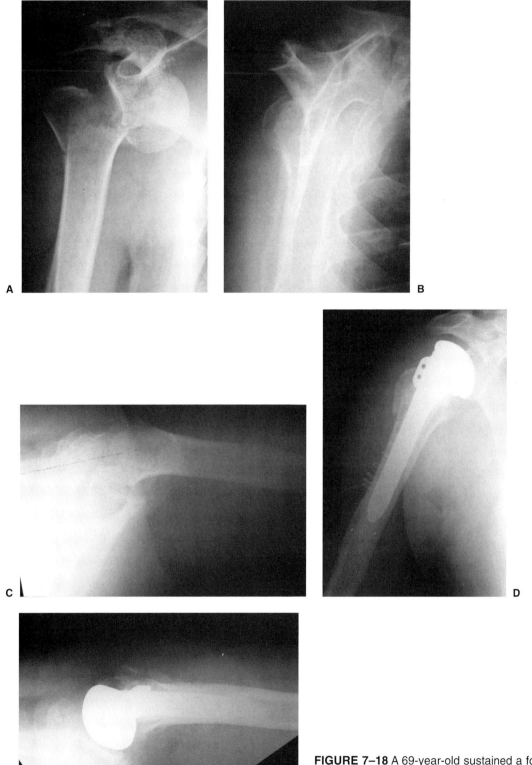

FIGURE 7–18 A 69-year-old sustained a four-part anterior fracture dislocation **(A–C)**. Operative management was delayed because the patient required stabilization of medical problems. Patient underwent proximal humeral replacement 5 days after injury **(D,E)**.

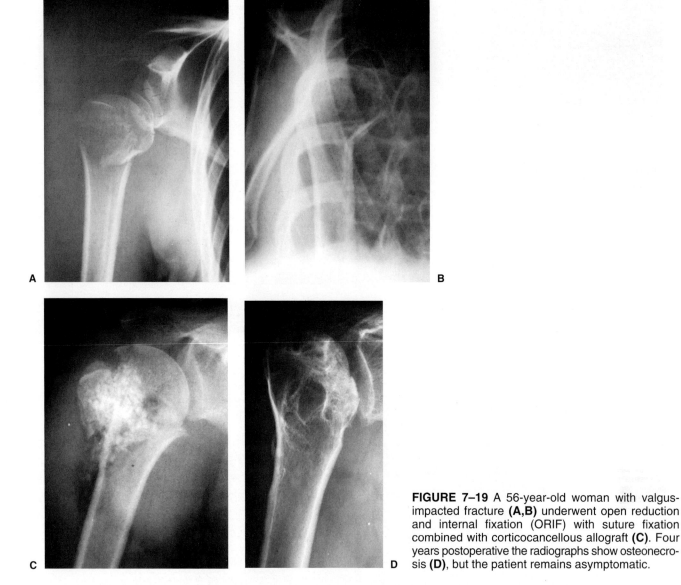

FIGURE 7–19 A 56-year-old woman with valgus-impacted fracture **(A,B)** underwent open reduction and internal fixation (ORIF) with suture fixation combined with corticocancellous allograft **(C)**. Four years postoperative the radiographs show osteonecrosis **(D)**, but the patient remains asymptomatic.

elevation without limitation, external rotation to a limit determined by the intraoperative assessment of fracture fixation, and internal rotation to the chest. These exercises are maintained for 6 or 7 weeks following surgery. The patient is reevaluated 2 weeks following the surgery with additional x-rays to confirm that the reduction has been maintained. At 6 weeks following the surgery, additional x-rays are obtained to assess the degree of healing. At this point, active range of motion is usually initiated focusing on forward elevation, external rotation, and internal rotation behind the back. Isometric deltoid and rotator cuff strengthening is begun approximately 2 weeks later. Stretching and resistive strengthening are initiated 12 weeks postoperatively.

Percutaneous Fixation

As discussed previously, closed reduction and percutaneous fixation technique have been used to treat four-part fractures and, specifically, valgus impacted types, with varying results. Surgeons with extensive experience with this technique for two- and three-part fractures have extended its use to these fractures with some success. Use of this approach requires an exacting technique both for closed reduction and internal fixation. Intraoperative C-arm visualization is essential throughout the procedure. Closed reduction can be obtained by a combination of closed and percutaneous manipulation. Percutaneous pins can often be used as a "joystick" to manipulate fragments into position. Fixation

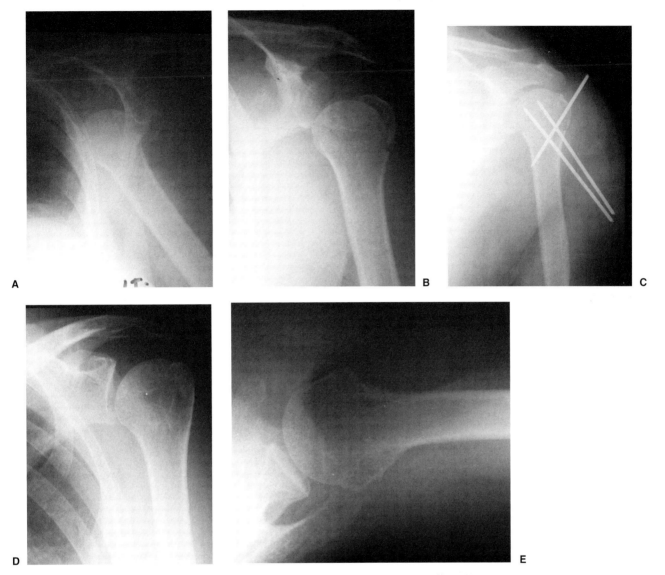

FIGURE 7–20 (A) A 60-year-old man sustained a proximal humeral fracture-dislocation. **(B)** Following closed reduction the valgus-impacted fracture pattern is evident. **(C)** Percutaneous reduction with elevation of the articular segment was performed followed by percutaneous pin fixation. **(D)** The pins were removed 6 weeks later. **(E)** One year postoperative, the fracture is well-healed with excellent alignment.

is achieved by use of percutaneous terminally threaded 3.5-mm Schantz pins (Fig. **7–20**) or a combination of percutaneous pins and screw fixation (Fig. **7–21**). When percutaneous pins are used, they should be cut off just below the skin surface. Postoperative mobilization should be performed carefully through a limited range to prevent skin irritation and the potential for migration. Postoperative radiographs should be obtained 7 to 10 days after surgery to evaluate the possibility of pin migration. Pins are generally removed 8 to 10 weeks after surgery when fracture healing has occurred and mobilization can be progressed.

The evaluation and treatment of four-part fractures and fracture-dislocations require a careful assessment of both the patient and the fracture. In some clinical situations, nonoperative management may be preferred when a limited-goals outcome is desired. The majority of "classic" four-part fractures will be treated by humeral head replacement with tuberosity reattachment. ORIF is preferred for valgus-impacted patterns and in young patients with "classic" fracture patterns. Closed reduction and percutaneous fixation techniques can be considered when the fracture pattern and the surgeon's experience are compatible.

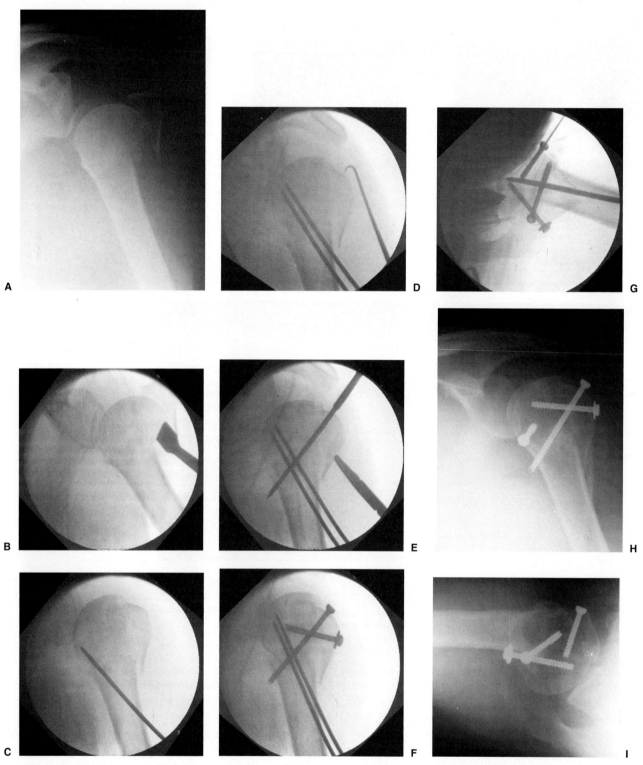

FIGURE 7–21 Percutaneous reduction of a valgus-impacted four-part fracture **(A)** in this 56-year-old man begins with percutaneous elevation of the articular segment with an elevator **(B)**, followed by fixation with the first of two pins **(C)**. The greater tuberosity is then reduced **(D)** and fixed in this case provisionally with a pin **(E)** and then with two screws **(F)**. The lesser tuberosity is then reduced and fixed in a similar manner **(G)**. At 1-year follow-up, the fracture is healed with good alignment **(H,I)**.

REFERENCES

1. Clifford PC. Fractures of the neck of the humerus: a review of the late results. Injury 1980;12:91–95
2. Knight RA, Mayne JA. Comminuted fractures and fracture-dislocations involving the articular surface of the humeral head. J Bone Joint Surg Am 1957;39-A:1343–1355
3. Kristiansen BK, Christensen SW. Plate fixation of proximal humeral fractures. Acta Orthop Scand 1986;57:320–323
4. Neer CS II. Displaced proximal humerus fractures. J Bone Joint Surg Am 1970;52:1077–1103
5. Stableforth PG. Four-part fractures of the neck of the humerus. J Bone Joint Surg Br 1984;66:104–108
6. de Anquin CE, de Anquin CA. Prosthetic replacement in the treatment of serious fractures of the proximal humerus. In: Bayley I, Kessel L, eds. Shoulder Surgery. Berlin: Springer-Verlag, 1982:207–217
7. Duparc J, Largier A. [Fracture-dislocations of the upper end of the humerus.] Rev Chir Orthop Reparatrice Appar Mot 1976;62:91–110 (French)
8. Jakob RP, Kristiansen T, Mayo K, Ganz R, Muller ME. Classification and aspects of treatment of fractures of the proximal humerus. In: Bateman JE, Welsh RP, eds. Surgery of the Shoulder. Philadelphia: BC Decker, 1984:330–343
9. Resch H, Beck E, Bayley I. Reconstruction of the valgus-impacted humeral head fracture. J Shoulder Elbow Surg 1995;4:73–80
10. Mills HJ, Horne G. Fractures of the proximal humerus in adults. J Trauma 1985;25:801–805
11. Mueller ME, Nazarian S, Koch P, Schatzker J. The Comprehensive Classification of Fractures in Long Bones. Berlin: Springer-Verlag, 1990
12. Kristiansen BK, Christiansen SW. Proximal humerus fractures. Acta Orthop Scand 1987;58:124–127
13. Lee CK, Hansen HR. Posttraumatic avascular necrosis of the humeral head in displaced proximal humerus fractures. J Trauma 1981;21:788–791
14. Leyshon RL. Closed treatment of fractures of the proximal humerus. Acta Orthop Scand 1984;55:48–51
15. Resch H, Povacz P, Frohlich R, Wambacher M. Percutaneous fixation of three- and four-part fractures of the proximal humerus. J Bone Joint Surg Br 1997;79:295–300
16. Sturzenegger M, Fornaro E, Jakob RP. Results of surgical treatment of multifragmented fractures of the humeral head. Arch Orthop Trauma Surg 1982;100:249–259
17. Jakob RP, Miniaci A, Anson PS, Jaberg H, Osterwalder A, Ganz R. Four-part valgus impacted fractures of the proximal humerus. J Bone Joint Surg Br 1991;73:295–298
18. Brooks CH, Revell WJ, Heatley FW. Vascularity of the humeral head after proximal humeral fractures. An anatomical cadaver study. J Bone Joint Surg Br 1993;75:132–136
19. Horak J, Nilsson BE. Epidemiology of fracture of the upper end of the humerus. Clin Orthop 1975;112:250–253
20. Compito CA, Self EB, Bigliani LU. Arthroplasty and acute shoulder trauma. Clin Orthop 1994;307:27–36
21. Goldman RT, Koval KJ, Cuomo F, Gallagher MA, Zuckerman JD. Functional outcome after humeral head replacement for acute three-and four-part humeral fractures. J Shoulder Elbow Surg 1995;4:81–86
22. Green A, Barnard WL, Limbird RS. Humeral head replacement for acute, four-part proximal humerus fractures. J Shoulder Elbow Surg 1993;2:249–254
23. Neer CS II. Recent results and techniques of prosthetic replacement for four part proximal humerus fractures. Orth Trans. 1986;10:475
24. Neer CS II, McIlveen SJ. [Humeral head replacement with reconstruction of the tuberosities and the cuff in 4-fragment displaced fractures. Current results and techniques] Rev Chir Orthop Reparatrice Appar Mot 1988;74(suppl 2):31–40 (French)
25. Svend-Hansen H. Displaced proximal humerus fractures. Acta Orthop Scand 1974;45:359–364
26. Esser RD. Treatment of three- and four-part fractures of the proximal humerus with a modified cloverleaf plate. J Orthop Trauma 1994;8:15–22
27. Paavolainen P, Bjorkenheim JM, Slatis P, Paukku P. Operative treatment of severe proximal humeral fractures. Acta Orthop Scand 1983;54:374–379
28. Adedapo AO, Ikpeme JO. The results of internal fixation of three- and four-part proximal humerus fractures with the Polarus nail. Injury 2001;32:115–121
29. Yamano Y. Comminuted fracture of the proximal humerus treated with a hook plate. Arch Orthop Trauma Surg 1986;105:359–363
30. Sehr JR, Szabo RM. Semitubular blade plate for fixation in the proximal humerus. J Orthop Trauma 1988;2:327–332
31. Cofield RH. Comminuted fractures of the proximal humerus. Clin Orthop 1988;230:49–57
32. Gerber C, Hersche O, Berberat C. The clinical relevance of post-traumatic avascular necrosis of the humeral head. J Shoulder Elbow Surg 1998;7:586–590
33. Wijgman AJ, Roolker W, Patt TW, Raaymakers EL, Marti RK. Open reduction and internal fixation of three and four-part fractures of the proximal part of the humerus. J Bone Joint Surg Am 2002;84-A:1919–1925
34. Soete PJ, Clayson PE, Costenoble VH. Transitory percutaneous pinning in fractures of the proximal humerus. J Shoulder Elbow Surg 1999;8:569–573
35. Neer CS II. Articular replacement for the humeral head. J Bone Joint Surg Am 1955;37-A:215–228
36. Kay SP, Amstutz HC. Shoulder hemiarthroplasty at UCLA. Clin Orthop 1988;228:42–48
37. Kraulis J, Hunter G. The results of prosthetic replacement in fracture dislocations of the upper end of the humerus. Injury 1976;8:129–131
38. Tanner MW, Cofield RH. Prosthetic arthroplasty for fractures and fracture-dislocations of the proximal humerus. Clin Orthop 1983;179:116–128
39. Dimakopoulos P, Potamitis N, Lambiris E. Hemiarthroplasty in the treatment of comminuted intraarticular fractures of the proximal humerus. Clin Orthop 1997;341:7–11
40. Hawkins RJ, Switlyk P. Acute prosthetic replacement for severe fractures of the proximal humerus. Clin Orthop 1993;289:156–160
41. Moeckel BH, Dines DM, Warren RF, Altchek DW. Modular hemiarthroplasty for fractures of the proximal part of the humerus. J Bone Joint Surg Am 1992;74:884–889
42. Prakash U, McGurty DW, Dent JA. Hemiarthroplasty for severe fractures of the proximal humerus. J Shoulder Elbow Surg 2002;11:428–430
43. Willems WJ, Lim TEA. Neer arthroplasty for humerus fractures. Acta Orthop Scand 1985;56:394–395
44. Torino AJ, van de Werf GJIM. Hemiarthroplasty of the shoulder. Acta Orthop Belg 1985;51:625–631
45. Dines DM, Warren RF, Altchek DW, Moeckel B. Posttraumatic changes of the proximal humerus: malunion, nonunion, and osteonecrosis. Treatment with modular hemiarthroplasty or total shoulder arthroplasty. J Shoulder Elbow Surg 1993;2:11–21
46. Frich LH, Sojbjerg JO, Sneppen O. Shoulder arthroplasty in complex acute and chronic proximal humeral fractures. Orthopedics 1991;14:949–954
47. Norris TR, Green A, McGuigan FX. Late Prosthetic shoulder arthroplasty for displaced proximal humerus fractures. J Shoulder Elbow Surg 1995;4:271–280

8

Humeral Head Impression Fractures and Head-Splitting Fractures

ANDREW L. CHEN, STEPHEN A. HUNT, AND JOSEPH D. ZUCKERMAN

■ Humeral Head Impression Fractures

The diagnosis and treatment of impression fractures of the proximal humerus remain a challenge for the treating physician. The treatment of such lesions has been the subject of investigation for centuries, with reports of treatment of head impression fractures dating as early as 1741.[1] The armamentarium of treatment options has since expanded, with successful management predicated on the recognition of these often challenging injuries, as well as a full understanding of the indications for specific approaches to treatment.

Impression fractures of the proximal humerus occur with impaction of the humeral head against the glenoid rim at the time of shoulder dislocation. This can occur with an acute, first-time dislocation, but is more common with recurrent dislocations. The location of the humeral head impression fracture is dependent on the direction of glenohumeral dislocation. Anterior dislocations, which occur much more frequently than posterior dislocations,[2,3] result in the classic Hill-Sachs impression fracture on the posterolateral aspect of the anteriorly dislocated humeral head as it impacts the anterior glenoid rim (Fig. 8-1).[3,4] This defect has been observed in up to 100% of patients with recurrent anterior instability,[5] 80% with primary anterior dislocation,[4,6] and 25% of patients with anterior shoulder subluxation.[7] Although posterior dislocations account for only 1.5% of dislocations of the glenohumeral joint,[2] they account for most chronic shoulder dislocations because of the significant number that are missed at the time of initial evaluation.[3,8] Impaction of the anteromedial aspect of the posteriorly dislocated humeral head on the posterior glenoid rim results in the so-called reverse Hill-Sachs

lesion (Fig. 8-2).[9] This chapter addresses humeral head impression fractures that occur in association with chronic (dislocated for more than 3 weeks' duration) shoulder dislocations.

Clinical Evaluation

History
Patients presenting with impression fractures of the humeral head typically have sustained a chronic glenohumeral dislocation. These patients usually report a traumatic episode, such as a motor vehicle accident or fall from a height, a history of a seizure episode, or much less commonly an electrical shock. Because the internal rotators of the shoulder are inherently more powerful than the external rotators, seizures have classically been associated with posterior glenohumeral dislocations, although anterior dislocations have been reported to account for up to one half of all seizure-related shoulder dislocations.[10,11] Multiply injured patients may sustain glenohumeral dislocations that are unrecognized due to other, more obvious or life-threatening injuries, or an inability to communicate their symptoms.

Unrecognized glenohumeral dislocations are generally associated with substantial pain following the acute episode and limitation of shoulder motion that is typically attributed to pain inhibition. Patients with anteromedial humeral head defects associated with posterior glenohumeral dislocation typically complain of an inability to raise or externally rotate the arm. Patients with posterolateral impression fractures associated with chronic anterior dislocations may complain of a limitation of internal rotation; however, this is generally not as dramatic or consistent as the findings associated with

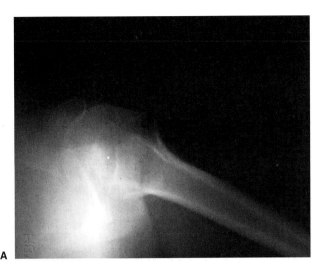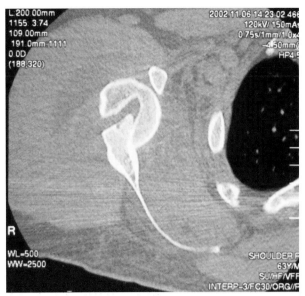

FIGURE 8–1 Hill-Sachs impression fractures are located on the posterolateral aspect of the humeral head and can be visualized with different imaging techniques including an axillary radiograph **(A)** and a computed tomography (CT) scan **(B)**.

posterior dislocation. With resolution of the shoulder discomfort—generally by 2 to 3 weeks after injury—the patient may initiate shoulder motion for activities of daily living (ADLs) at waist level; this resolution of pain and gradual functional return is often mistakenly attributed to recovery by the patient and treating physician, thus perpetuating the misconception that full functional recovery will occur. In reality, pain relief is due to resolution of inflammation from the initial injury as well as soft tissue healing, whereas the limited return of motion is secondary to the enlarging humeral head defect from the "windshield-wiper" effect of the glenoid rim within the impression fracture.

Alternatively, the patient with a chronic shoulder dislocation may report relief of pain following the traumatic episode, but with persistent limitation of motion. Such patients may be mistaken for having a posttraumatic frozen shoulder that fails to improve with efforts at rehabilitation.[3,8,11]

Physical Examination

A thorough neurovascular evaluation should be performed in patients with suspected impression fractures. Because many of the patients with impression fractures due to chronic glenohumeral dislocations are elderly, the relative incidence of neurovascular injury is higher than in younger patients who sustain acute dislocations. This may be due in part to the loss of elasticity and calcification of soft tissue structures that occurs with age.

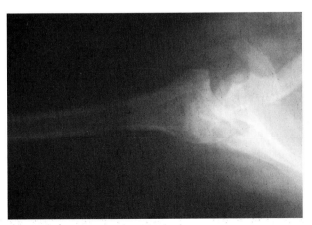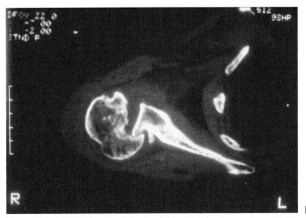

FIGURE 8–2 Reverse Hill-Sachs impression fractures are located on the anteromedial aspect of the humeral head as visualized on an axillary radiograph **(A)** and CT scan **(B)**.

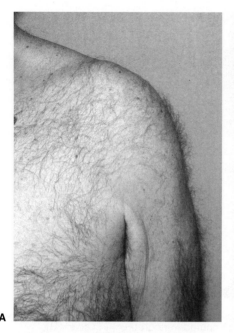

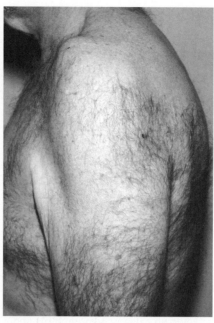

FIGURE 8–3 A 64-year-old man 1 month after posterior glenohumeral dislocation. Frontal view **(A)** shows loss of lateral contour of the shoulder, and side view **(B)** shows flattening anteriorly and fullness posteriorly.

An association between nerve injury—in particular axillary nerve—and shoulder dislocation has previously been established, with up to 45% of patients with anterior shoulder dislocation and 29% of patients with posterior shoulder dislocation sustaining electromyographically demonstrable nerve injury.[1,11,12] Similarly, injuries to the axillary artery in association with shoulder dislocations have been well documented.[13–15]

The patient with a posterolateral impression fracture due to chronic anterior glenohumeral dislocation may be surprisingly functional, with excellent functional capacity at waist level, minimal pain, and limited but functional range of shoulder motion. The shoulder is usually held in mild abduction and external rotation. Physical examination reveals squaring of the posterior acromion, loss of the lateral deltoid prominence, and anterior shoulder fullness, which are best observed with the patient seated and observed from behind or from the side. In thin patients, the humeral head may be palpable as a firm mass in the deltopectoral region. In heavier patients, these changes may be much less evident. Range of motion typically reveals limited adduction and internal rotation. Alternatively, the patient may present with severe functional limitations and restricted motion in all planes, similar in presentation to frozen shoulder. These patients are usually evaluated earlier in the course of chronic dislocation, potentially before significant enlargement of the humeral head defect has occurred from continued motion against the anterior glenoid rim.

The patient with an anteromedial impression fracture due to chronic posterior glenohumeral dislocation tends to have a more characteristic presentation.[16] By observing the seated patient from the front and side, the physician may appreciate subtle but consistent findings, including a loss of the anterior contour of the shoulder, prominence of the coracoid process due to posterior displacement of the humeral head, and a posterior fullness of the shoulder (Fig. 8–3). The arm is typically held in an internally rotated and adducted position, with loss of passive and active external rotation, and significant limitation of glenohumeral abduction. Long-standing chronic dislocation may also be associated with a surprisingly functional range of motion for activities at waist level. This is secondary to enlargement of the anteromedial humeral head defect by the "windshield-wiper" effect that occurs with shoulder motion.

Radiographic Evaluation
Standard Radiographs
The shoulder trauma series consists of anteroposterior (AP), scapular lateral ("Y view"), and axillary projections. These three orthogonal views allow for the identification of surface defects or fractures of the humeral head, as well as the presence of glenohumeral dislocation. Chronic dislocations are frequently unrecognized either because of a failure to seek medical attention or a failure to obtain proper radiographs.

The scapular AP is useful to evaluate the position of the humeral head in relation to the glenoid, particularly when anterior dislocation is present (Fig. 8–4). The radiographs should be scrutinized for evidence of associated fractures of the proximal humerus or glenoid, as multiple authors have documented the presence of associated fractures of the shoulder in up to 50% of patients with glenohumeral dislocations.[8,11,17]

The scapular lateral (Fig. 8–5) may be useful for the identification of posterolateral impression defects, and

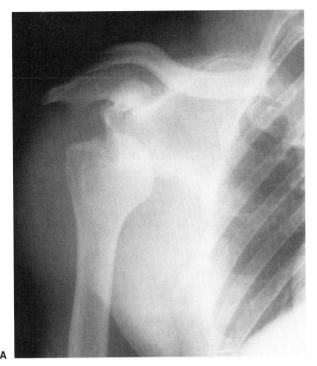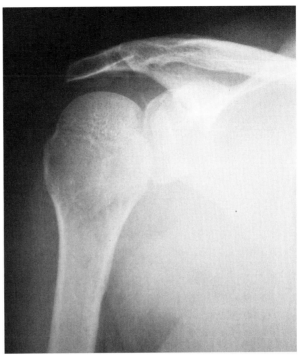

A   B

FIGURE 8–4 Scapular anteroposterior (AP) radiographs of a chronic anterior dislocation **(A)** and posterior dislocation **(B)**. Note the anteriorly dislocated humerus is externally rotated and the posteriorly dislocated humerus is internally rotated.

the direction of glenohumeral dislocation; however, the presence of multiple overlapping structures, such as the posterior thorax and scapular body, frequently obscures osseous details and thus limits its clinical utility.

The axillary projection is invaluable in determining the direction of glenohumeral dislocation, size, and location of impression fractures of the humeral head, degree of glenoid bone loss, and identification of associated fractures of the glenoid, coracoid, or acromion (Fig. **8–6**). A standard axillary radiograph is obtained with the patient supine and the shoulder abducted at least 40° with the beam centered in the axilla. A Velpeau axillary view may be obtained in patients who are unable to position the

shoulder for a standard axillary view due to pain or limitation of motion. It is obtained by having the patient lean backward 30° over the x-ray table with the shoulder in adduction and internal rotation (sling position). The beam is then centered on the glenohumeral joint from a cephalad to caudad direction, with the film cassette placed on the x-ray table behind the patient. Although helpful, the Velpeau axillary does not provide as much information as the standard axillary projection.

Of the three orthogonal projections of the shoulder trauma series, the axillary radiograph is most valuable for guiding treatment that is based on the percentage of articular involvement of the humeral head defect.

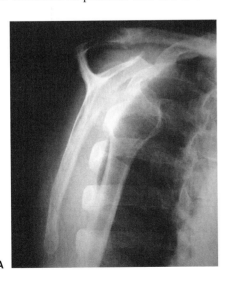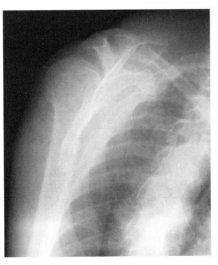

A   B

FIGURE 8–5 Scapular lateral radiograph of a chronic anterior dislocation **(A)** and posterior dislocation **(B)**. In both views the glenoid is clearly visualized because of the displacement of the humeral head.

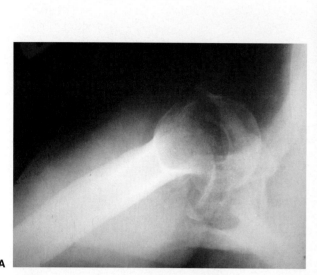
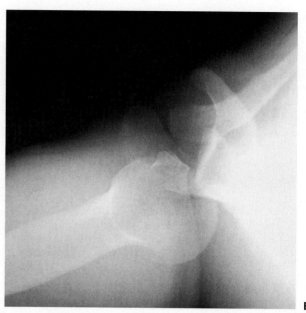

A   **B**

FIGURE 8–6 (A) Axillary radiograph of a chronic anterior dislocation showing the humeral head locked on the anterior glenoid rim. **(B)** The posterior dislocation shows the humeral head locked on the posterior glenoid rim.

Special Imaging Studies

Computed axial tomography (CT) images are useful in treatment planning to further characterize humeral head impression fractures and to evaluate glenoid bone loss. As the treatment of humeral head impression fractures is based largely on defect size (and chronicity of the injury), it is often helpful to obtain CT images to quantify the degree of head involvement. Some authors recommend performing a CT scan only if the humeral defect is greater than 20% of the articular surface to more precisely define and characterize the defect, and to determine if associated glenoid injury is present.[18,19] We prefer to obtain a CT scan for all patients with chronic glenohumeral dislocations because of the additional information it provides. Two-dimensional sagittal and coronal oblique reconstructions may aid in fracture characterization but are not essential.

Although magnetic resonance imaging (MRI) can be useful for evaluation of concomitant injuries to the rotator cuff, this is not a common finding in patients with chronic dislocation. As such, MRI is not generally obtained; however, if a patient presents with a constellation of symptoms and signs not completely explained by the osseous injury, MRI may be helpful.[3,20] In such cases, estimation of the humeral head defects may be performed on the axial MRI, thus obviating the need for an additional CT scan.

Ancillary Studies

Electromyography and nerve conduction studies should be obtained in cases of suspected nerve injury. An association between traumatic shoulder injuries and nerve injuries has previously been established, with up to 45%

of patients with anterior shoulder dislocation sustaining nerve injuries, most commonly to the axillary nerve.[1,11,12] These studies should be performed preoperatively to document that the deficit is injury related. Arteriography should be performed in cases of suspected vascular compromise, as axillary artery injuries in association with shoulder dislocations and proximal humerus fractures have been well documented.[13–15]

Treatment

As the management of humeral impression fractures remains a challenge to the treating surgeon, it is essential that the physician maintain a thorough understanding of the available treatment options in the context of an organized, disciplined treatment algorithm. Satisfactory pain relief and optimization of functional recovery are the main goals of treatment; it is therefore incumbent upon the treating physician to establish with the patient and family reasonable expectations for each treatment approach. The desire to perform aggressive, often technically demanding interventions should be tempered by the patient's general health and functional requirements, as well as the anticipated degree of recovery and the patient's ability to participate in a postoperative rehabilitation program.

The management of impression fractures of the proximal humerus necessitates consideration of many factors. Patient factors, such as age and medical comorbidities, affect whether the patient should be considered a surgical candidate. Injury-related factors, such as defect size, displacement, and chronicity, influence the selection of operative procedure. The availability of specialized equipment and implants, and the expertise of the surgeon may determine whether appropriate referral should be made to centers familiar with treating these often complex and challenging fractures.

Nonoperative

Nonoperative treatment of humeral head impression fractures in association with chronic dislocation may be undertaken in patients with minimal pain and functional disability (Fig. 8–7). Elderly patients with low functional demands may demonstrate excellent adaptation following resolution of the acute shoulder injury. These patients may have small or large anteromedial or posterolateral surface defects and may have adapted sufficiently to perform basic ADL, usually in conjunction with a functional contralateral upper extremity.[21,22] Nonoperative treatment of impression fractures may also be

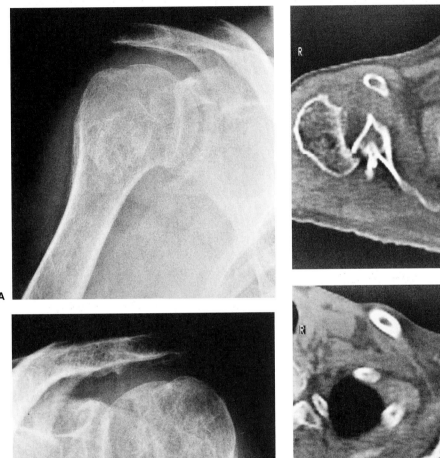
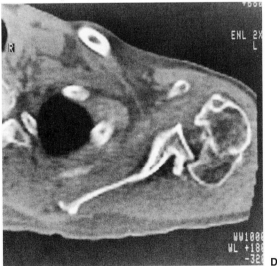

FIGURE 8–7 (A,B) A 69-year-old man with bilateral chronic posterior glenohumeral dislocations. **(C,D)** CT scans show reactive bone formation about the posterior glenoid consistent with chronic dislocations.

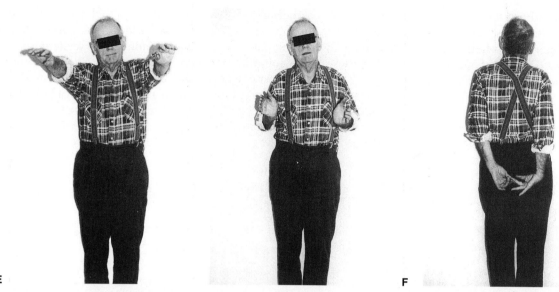

E   F   G

FIGURE 8–7 *(Continued)* **(E–G)** The patient had limitation of range of motion, but he was reasonably comfortable and functional for activities of daily living; therefore, nonoperative management was the preferred treatment. (Adapted from Zuckerman JD. *Comprehensive Care of Orthopaedic Injuries in the Elderly*. Baltimore: Urban & Schwarzenberg, 1990:287–288, with permission.)

desirable in patients with an unacceptably high medical risk, patients with uncontrollable seizures, or patients physically or mentally unable to comply with postoperative instructions or rehabilitation. In these cases, supportive measures should be instituted, including a brief period of sling immobilization, nonnarcotic analgesia, and gradual mobilization of the shoulder with physical therapy based on the degree of deficit present.

Patients with chronic dislocations in whom nonoperative management is preferred should be started on pendulum exercises as well as a progression of active-assisted and active range-of-motion exercises. Exercises should be performed gently with the goal of regaining functional range of motion for ADLs at waist level. Forceful stretching should be avoided to minimize the risk of additional injury. Strengthening exercises are generally limited to isometrics and gentle resistive strengthening. In these patients, we are trying to achieve a "limited goals" outcome.

Several authors have reported their results of nonoperative treatment of humeral impression fractures associated with chronic dislocations. In 1952 McLaughlin[16] reported a series of 16 patients with chronic posterior dislocations of the shoulder associated with anteromedial impression fractures. Three were managed nonoperatively and all experienced unfavorable outcomes, with severe restriction of shoulder motion, an inability to raise the arm above the horizontal, disabling pain, and muscular atrophy.[16] Hawkins and coworkers[8] reported on seven patients with an average follow-up of 5.5 years who were treated nonoperatively for anteromedial humeral defects in association with chronic posterior shoulder dislocations. Only two were able to raise their hands above

head level, although pain ratings and functional losses did not progress beyond immediate postinjury levels. Rowe and Zarins[3] noted that of patients with humeral head defects associated with chronic shoulder dislocations, patients with anteromedial defects (posterior dislocations) had higher functional scores and functional range of motion than their counterparts with posterolateral defects (anterior dislocations). They attributed this difference to the position of the humeral head defect on the glenoid rim. They felt that the adducted and internally rotated position of the posteriorly dislocated shoulder was more functional than the abducted and externally rotated position of the anteriorly dislocated shoulder.[3]

Operative

The surgical management of humeral head impression fractures in association with chronic dislocations requires consideration of many factors that will determine the procedure to be performed (Table 8–1). Advanced patient age may steer the surgeon toward prosthetic replacement in the presence of a large defect, particularly if underlying degenerative changes are evident. Other patient factors that should be considered include hand dominance, functional capacity, vocational and avocational requirements, medical comorbidities, and ability to comply with postoperative instructions and rehabilitation.

Injury-related factors that influence the surgical decision-making process include the size and location of the humeral impression defect; the bone quality and quantity of the humeral head; the presence of underlying degenerative changes of the glenohumeral articulation;

TABLE 8–1 Factors Affecting the Surgical Management of Impression Fractures of the Proximal Humerus

Patient factors
    Age
    Hand dominance
    Vocational and avocational activities
    Medical comorbidities
    Functional requirements
    Functional adaptation
    Ability to comply with postoperative regimen or rehabilitation

Injury-related factors
    Location of defect
    Size of impression fracture or degree of head involvement
    Displacement
    Chronicity
    Bone quality/quantity

Other factors
    Expertise of surgeon
    Availability of specialized equipment/instruments
    Availability of implants

and the chronicity of the injury, that is, the length of time since dislocation.

Of particular importance is the ability of the surgeon to treat humeral head impression fractures. The surgeon should be familiar and comfortable with the management of such injuries. Specialized equipment, such as special shoulder retractors and table positioners, may facilitate the procedure. Implants, such as proximal humeral prostheses in a variety of head and stem sizes, should be available. Finally, physical or occupational therapy should be available to facilitate postoperative recovery and maximize functional outcomes.

Anteromedial Impression Fractures

Most authors addressing the treatment of anteromedial impression fractures associated with chronic posterior shoulder dislocation have based their treatment approach on the size of the humeral impression defect.[3,8,11,16,21–24] Calculation of the degree of articular involvement is based on the axillary radiograph or CT images. The percentage of articular involvement is determined by measuring the arc of the area of impaction divided by the total arc of the intact articular surface, multiplied by 100 (Fig. 8–8). Treatment recommendations based on this calculation reflect the propensity of the anterior glenoid rim to "fall into" the humeral head defect with the shoulder in adduction and internal rotation. In addition, the chronicity of the injury must be considered, as associated articular cartilage degeneration and osseous compromise are directly related to the duration of dislocation.

With anteromedial impression fractures involving up to 40% of the humeral articular surface, there are many options available to the treating surgeon. These include disimpaction and bone grafting, subscapularis tendon transfer, lesser tuberosity transfer, and allograft reconstruction. When the defect is greater than 40% of the articular surface, prosthetic replacement is indicated. Articular defects associated with a dislocation of less

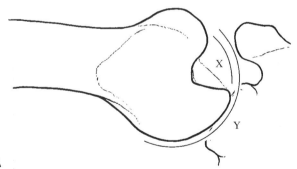

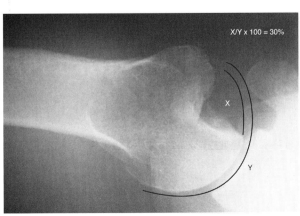

X/Y x 100 = 30%

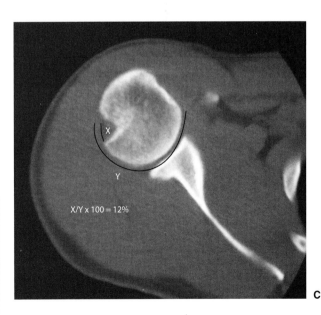

X/Y x 100 = 12%

FIGURE 8–8 (A) The size of the impression fracture is an important factor to determine treatment. It should be described as the percent of articular involvement-based measurements of the arc of the area of impaction (X) divided by the total arc of the articular surface (Y). **(B,C)** Impression fractures can vary greatly in size.

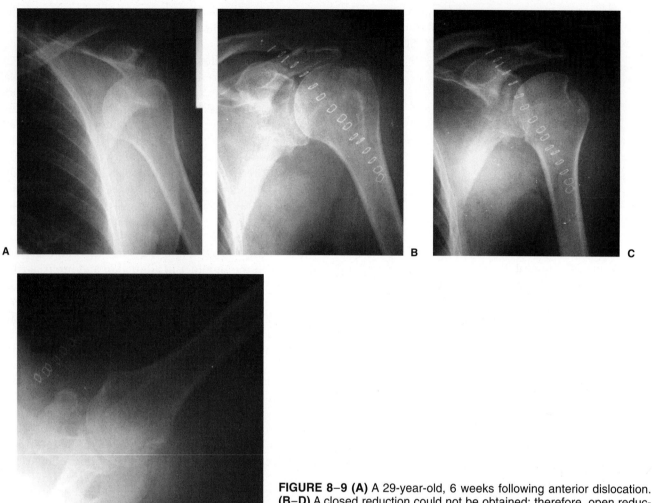

FIGURE 8–9 (A) A 29-year-old, 6 weeks following anterior dislocation. **(B–D)** A closed reduction could not be obtained; therefore, open reduction was performed. The posterolateral impression fracture was small and the shoulder was stable after reduction and repair of the anterior soft tissues.

than 3 weeks' duration may be amenable to disimpaction combined with bone grafting, as the impacted articular cartilage is usually viable. Defects associated with dislocations of between 3 weeks' and 6 months' duration can usually be treated by nonprosthetic reconstruction, because the remaining articular cartilage maintains viability. Dislocations present for more than 6 months are usually associated with articular cartilage degeneration and usually require prosthetic replacement; however, it is important to recognize that these are only guidelines, and each case has to be individualized. *In certain situations, closed or even open reduction may be attempted for a chronic dislocation. If the shoulder is stable through a functional range of motion and the cartilage appears viable, no further intervention may be needed* (Fig. **8–9**).

Disimpaction and Bone Grafting

The ideal candidate for this procedure has a defect less than 3 weeks old involving less than 40% of the articular

surface and has good bone quality and quantity to allow for secure fixation. The remaining articular cartilage should be intact. Because of these factors, this procedure is ideal for use in younger patients, but may also be used effectively in older patients who fulfill the above criteria.

A standard deltopectoral approach is used, with care taken to maintain the integrity of the coracoacromial arch. The proximal humerus is exposed to the level of the lesser tuberosity and bicipital groove. We prefer to open the rotator interval from its lateral extent to the anterosuperior glenoid. By retracting the subscapularis and supraspinatus, the defect can be palpated and the preoperative findings confirmed. Any change in operative plan can be determined at this time. When disimpaction and bone grafting is chosen, the subscapularis and capsule are divided 1 cm medial to its insertion with additional release of the anteroinferior capsule from the humeral neck. This allows visualization of the glenoid after removal of the fibrous tissue that develops after the initial injury. The humeral head is dislocated posteriorly with the posterior glenoid rim filling the impression fracture. Gentle rotation of the humerus is preferred to disengage the humeral head. A flat Darrach elevator is inserted between the humeral head and the glenoid and is used to "shoehorn" the humeral head into the reduced position. When this is accomplished the defect can be fully appreciated. A humeral head retractor can be inserted to allow for inspection of the posterior labrum and capsule. Although disruption of the posterior capsulolabral complex is often present, repair of these structures is not usually necessary to prevent recurrent instability.[8,21]

Once inspection of the humeral defect has determined that the impacted articular cartilage is salvageable, the humerus is internally rotated to locate a position on the lateral humeral cortex opposite the defect. A 1-cm cortical window is created using an osteotome, and the articular surface is disimpacted indirectly using a bone tamp. With external rotation visualization of the disimpacted articular surface will be possible. The humerus should be externally rotated at this time to provide visualization of the disimpaction. A small curved osteotome or elevator may be used to facilitate the disimpaction process by directly elevating the articular surface fragments.

Once disimpaction is complete, the subchondral void created by the disimpaction process is grafted. We prefer allograft cancellous bone, although autogenous cancellous bone obtained from the iliac crest has been described.[21] Two cancellous screws are then placed through the lesser tuberosity, directed posteriorly and deep to the defect to buttress the disimpacted defect.

The shoulder is then placed through a range of motion and the grafted area is monitored closely as it encounters the glenoid. Specific positions to be avoided postoperatively for the first 6 weeks until bony consolidation occurs are noted. Following wound closure, the patient is placed into a prefabricated shoulder orthosis that maintains the upper extremity in 15° abduction, 10° extension, and 10° of external rotation. Rehabilitation is begun on postoperative day 1 and consists of gentle passive external rotation, abduction, and forward elevation. After 4 to 6 weeks, the brace is replaced by a sling, and the patient begins a program of active shoulder motion. The sling is worn for 1 or 2 weeks, at which time rehabilitation program is progressed.

Although no large clinical series using this technique has been reported, Gerber[21] has reported success achieving excellent bony consolidation and articular restoration in a small group of patients.

Subscapularis Tendon or Lesser Tuberosity Transfer

Prerequisites for theses techniques include defects of less than 40% of the articular surface, adequate bone quality and quantity to allow for secure fixation, and intact articular cartilage of the remainder of the humeral head.

Subscapularis tendon transfers are ideally suited for patients with small anteromedial defects (less than 20%) (Fig. 8–10). A standard deltopectoral approach is utilized, with inspection of the defect by opening the rotator interval as described previously. If a subscapularis transfer is to be performed, the subscapularis tendon is elevated directly from its insertion on the lesser tuberosity. The humeral head is reduced as previously described. The anteromedial defect is debrided to provide a clean, cancellous bed of bleeding bone. Transosseous drill holes are then made at the base of the defect, and the subscapularis tendon is secured using multiple nonabsorbable sutures passed in horizontal mattress fashion. In addition, sutures are passed through the articular cartilage and into the tendon to protect the glenoid margin from falling into the medial edge of the defect with internal rotation.

Larger defects (20 to 40%) are better addressed with transfer of the lesser tuberosity (Fig. 8–11). This technique utilizes the approach described above. The lesser tuberosity is then osteotomized, with care taken to preserve the medial wall of the bicipital groove to prevent destabilization of the tendon. The subscapularis and underlying capsule are mobilized to the glenoid neck, with release of adhesions and scar. The humeral head is reduced as previously described. The anteromedial defect is debrided to provide a clean bed of cancellous bleeding bone. The lesser tuberosity is fashioned to match the humeral impression defect and secured using two cancellous lag screws directed into the humeral head. Sutures are passed through the edge of the articular surface to secure the tendon as described previously.

Following either procedure, the patient is placed in a shoulder orthosis with the arm in 15° of abduction, 10° of extension, and 10 to 20° of external rotation. Rehabilitation is begun on postoperative day 1 and consists of gentle passive external rotation, abduction, and forward elevation. At 4 to 6 weeks, the brace is replaced by a sling for 2 weeks and a program of full active-assisted and active shoulder motion is begun. By the 12th week, resistive strengthening exercises are initiated.

McLaughlin[16] first reported his results with subscapularis tendon transfer for the treatment of anteromedial impression defects in association with posterior shoulder dislocations. Since then, successful treatment of such defects using the same technique has been reported by Hawkins et al[8] and Rowe and Zarins.[3] Successful results have also been reported with lesser tuberosity transfer for the treatment of larger anteromedial defects, with restoration of excellent shoulder motion.[8,24]

Allograft Reconstruction

Allograft reconstruction of anteromedial impression defects can be considered for patients with excellent

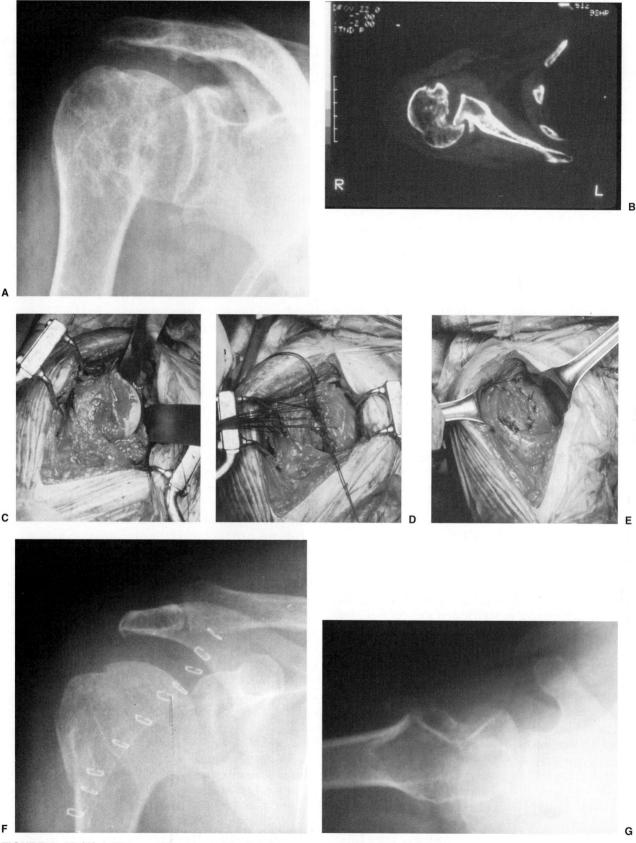

FIGURE 8–10 (A) A 63-year-old woman with chronic posterior dislocation. **(B)** CT scan indicates ~30% humeral head defect. **(C–E)** Intraoperative photographs show the humeral head defect **(C)** after elevation of the subscapulous insertion, which was then transferred into the defect **(D,E)** and secured with sutures to bone. **(F,G)** Postoperative radiographs confirm a concentric reduction.

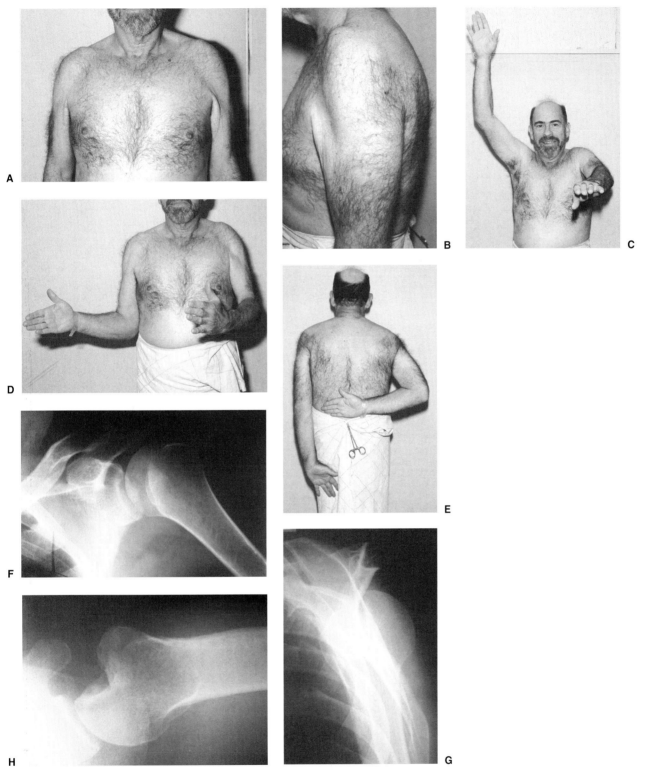

FIGURE 8-11 (A,B) A 64-year-old man with chronic posterior dislocation of left shoulder. **(C–E)** There is significant limitation of range of motion. **(F–H)** A closed reduction was performed under general anesthesia in the operating room; however, the shoulder was very unstable.

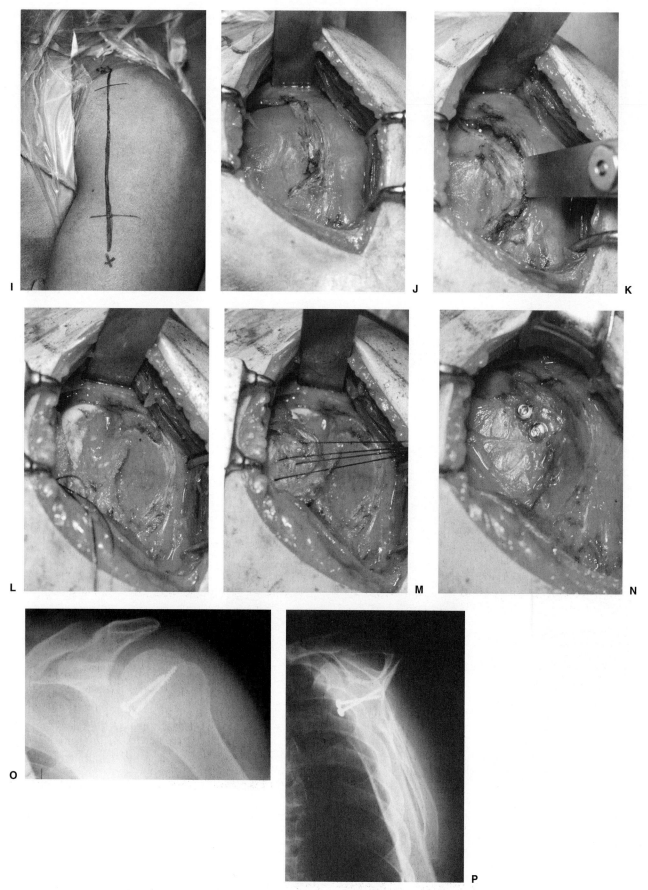

FIGURE 8–11 *(Continued)* **(I)** A lesser tuberosity transfer was performed through a deltopectoral approach. The tuberosity was outlined **(J)** and osteotomized with a saw **(K)** and mobilized **(L)**. It was transferred into the defect **(M)** and secured with two cancellous screws **(N)**. Postoperative radiographs **(O–Q)** and CT scan

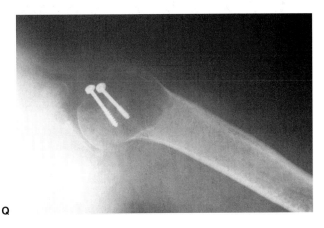

Q

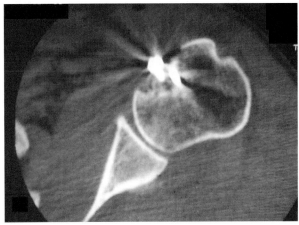

R

FIGURE 8–11 *(Continued)* **(R)** show the reduced humeral head and the lesser tuberosity filling the defect.

bone stock and less than 50% humeral head involvement (Fig. **8–12**).[21,23] It is therefore best suited for the younger patient with a large humeral head defect in whom prosthetic replacement would be less than ideal. A preoperative CT scan is essential to delineate the size of the defect, estimate the humeral head size, and evaluate the humeral bone stock. A size-matched, fresh-frozen humeral head or femoral head allograft is generally utilized. Prosthetic replacement should also be considered a possibility if intraoperative findings indicate significant degenerative changes to the humeral head.

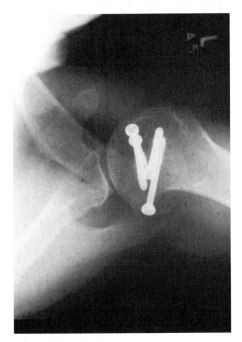

FIGURE 8–12 A Patient with both anterior and posterior humeral head defects secondary to instability underwent anterior and posterior humeral head allografts utilizing screw fixation.

A standard deltopectoral approach is used as described previously and the subscapularis tendon is divided 1 cm medial to its insertion. Fibrous tissue within the joint is removed and the humeral head is carefully reduced. The anteromedial defect is then evaluated. An oscillating saw is used to convert the impacted defect into a wedge-shaped defect, with walls of bleeding cancellous bone. The dimensions of the wedge are then measured, and a matched allograft wedge about 2 mm wider than the true defect is fashioned. The allograft wedge is then impacted within the defect and secured using one or two retrograde or antegrade countersunk cancellous screws. A standard closure is performed.

The patient is placed in a prefabricated shoulder orthosis as described in neutral rotation for 6 weeks. Rehabilitation is begun on postoperative day 1 and consists of gentle passive external rotation, abduction, and forward elevation. When the brace is discontinued, active-assisted and active range-of-motion exercises are performed with gentle stretching to regain motion. Strengthening begins 10 to 12 weeks postoperatively with isometric deltoid and rotator cuff exercises followed by resistive internal rotation exercises.

The use of allograft reconstruction for anteromedial defects of the humeral head was described by Gerber and Lambert[23] in 1996. In this series, three of the four patients with locked posterior dislocation had satisfactory results. The poor outcome was secondary to humeral head osteonecrosis that developed 6 years postoperatively, which the authors attributed to the patient's alcohol abuse rather than the surgery itself.[23] In his second report, Gerber[21] documented similar results, although warned against the use of allograft reconstruction in patients with osteopenia. Although these series were based on limited numbers of patients, the results of allograft reconstruction compare favorably with the previously described humeral-head preserving techniques.

Prosthetic Replacement: Hemiarthroplasty and Total Shoulder Arthroplasty

The primary indications for humeral hemiarthroplasty include defects greater than 40 to 50% of the articular surface and the presence of significant articular cartilage damage (Fig. 8–13). If glenoid damage is present due to preexisting degenerative changes, chronic dislocation for more than 6 months, or associated glenoid rim erosion contributing to the instability, resurfacing of the glenoid (i.e., total shoulder arthroplasty) should be considered. Significant glenoid bone loss may necessitate bone grafting.

Prosthetic replacement of the shoulder is performed through a standard deltopectoral approach with a subscapularis tenotomy. The joint is debrided of fibrous tissue, and the glenoid is inspected. The humeral head is reduced and brought through a range of motion. The degrees of internal rotation necessary for the posterior glenoid rim to engage the anteromedial defect is measured. Hawkins and co-workers[8] maintain that this approach assists in determining the precise degree of component version necessary to provide immediate postoperative joint stability. In our experience, appropriate component version is usually near neutral. After resection of the humeral head to create the desired amount of version, the glenoid is carefully inspected to evaluate the integrity of the articular cartilage and the presence and degree of bone loss. If a glenoid component is to be inserted, the glenoid should be prepared and an all-polyethylene component cemented in place. The humeral shaft is then sequentially reamed to accommodate an appropriately sized humeral component. A modular component should be utilized to adjust the soft tissue tension. Eccentricity of the head may also assist in achieving a stable construct. If necessary, component version may also have to be changed to enhance stability. In cases of long-standing posterior dislocations, the posterior soft tissues may be so stretched that a stable construct is difficult to achieve. In this setting, we prefer an "internal" posterior capsular plication using a purse-string suture technique. If this is needed, postoperative immobilization in an orthosis is utilized. After closure of the subscapularis tendon, the amount of external rotation is documented because this determines the parameters of the early postoperative rehabilitation program.

A sling is used for postoperative immobilization as long as the construct is stable. If there are concerns about the stability, a shoulder orthosis should be used postoperatively maintaining the arm in 15° abduction, and 10° extension at 0 to 10° of external rotation. Rehabilitation is begun on the first postoperative day and varies based on the postoperative immobilization utilized. When a sling is used, passive and assisted forward elevation, external rotation, and internal rotation to the chest wall are begun. At 4 weeks following surgery, a program of active shoulder motion is initiated, including internal rotation behind the back. Isometric strengthening exercises are started at the same time; resistive strengthening exercises are usually initiated 10 to 12 weeks postoperatively after active range of motion has progressed. When a shoulder orthosis is utilized, the previously described protocol is followed.

Hawkins et al[8] reported their results of prosthetic replacement (humeral hemiarthroplasty and total shoulder replacement) in patients with large anteromedial impression fractures. Satisfactory results were obtained in 11 of 16 patients, with the best results in patients who underwent total shoulder arthroplasty. Five of six of these patients achieved excellent results, with an average active forward elevation of 152°, external rotation to 40°, and internal rotation to T12. The authors therefore recommend total shoulder arthroplasty for the treatment of large, chronic anteromedial surface defects not amenable to humeral head–sparing procedures. They used case-specific "dialing-in" of the degree of retroversion to achieve joint stability.[8] Although Gerber[21] agrees with the use of total shoulder replacement to address large, chronic anteromedial humeral defects, he maintains that the normal axis of rotation should be restored at the time of prosthetic replacement, as this would more closely approximate normal joint kinematics.

Posterolateral Impression Fractures

As with the treatment of anteromedial humeral impression fractures, the surgical treatment of posterolateral surface defects is based on the size of the humeral impression defect, the chronicity of the injury, the integrity of the articular cartilage of the humeral head and glenoid, and the quantity and quality of the remaining bone.[3,11,21,24] The calculation of the degree of articular involvement is based on the axillary radiographic projection and axial CT images, in which the percentage of articular involvement is determined as described previously. Treatment recommendations based on this calculation are based on the propensity of the anterior glenoid rim to engage the humeral head defect with the shoulder in abduction and external rotation.

For posterolateral impression fractures involving less than 20% of the articular surface, surgery to address the humeral defect is usually not necessary, and operative treatment is directed toward open reduction of the dislocation and stabilization of the anterior capsulolabral complex. For posterolateral impression fractures involving 20 to 40% of the humeral articular surface, surgical options include infraspinatus tendon transfer, disimpaction and bone grafting, and allograft reconstruction. If the defect is greater than 40 to 50% of the articular surface, prosthetic replacement (hemiarthroplasty or total shoulder replacement) is indicated because the previously mentioned surgical options are insufficient to

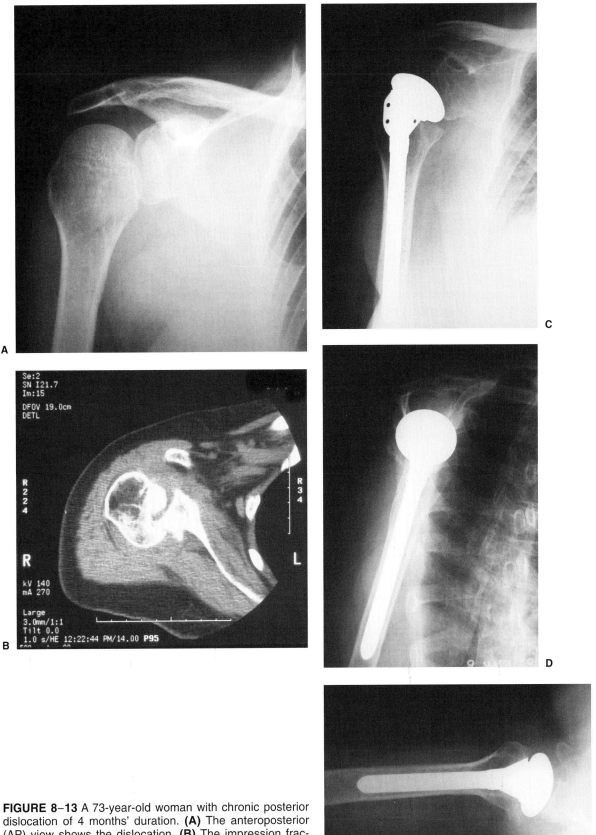

FIGURE 8–13 A 73-year-old woman with chronic posterior dislocation of 4 months' duration. **(A)** The anteroposterior (AP) view shows the dislocation. **(B)** The impression fracture and articular injury is evident on the CT scan. Proximal humeral head replacement was performed **(C,D)** with excellent position on the axillary view **(E)**.

restore stability. In addition, when dislocation is present for more than 6 months, there is usually significant articular cartilage degeneration of the humeral head and glenoid; in this situation a total shoulder arthroplasty may be required even when humeral head defects of less than 40 to 50% are present.

The treatment of posterolateral impression fractures associated with chronic anterior dislocations begins with an open reduction of the dislocation. Prior to the procedure, assessment of the size of the defect and chronicity of the dislocation determines the anticipated procedure that. Although some intraoperative decisions may be required (i.e., hemiarthroplasty vs. total shoulder replacement), for the most part, the preoperative assessment should determine the operative plan.

A deltopectoral approach is used. After development of the interval and mobilization of the deltoid and pectoralis major, the coracoid process and conjoined tendon muscles are identified. The humeral head is displaced anteriorly and inferiorly. The conjoined tendon muscles should be mobilized and retracted medially to expose the proximal humerus. The lesser tuberosity and bicipital groove should be identified. The subscapularis tendon is divided 1 cm medial to its insertion into the lesser tuberosity. The rotator interval is divided toward the anterior glenoid with care taken to make certain that all overlying tissues are elevated from the subscapularis. The anteroinferior capsule is released from the humeral neck. These steps allow exposure of the humeral head and palpation of the glenoid. Prior to reduction, any fibrous tissue within the joint should be removed. Gentle manipulation of the humerus starting with internal rotation combined with lateral displacement will allow the humeral head to be disengaged from the anterior glenoid. When the humeral head is reduced, a Fukuda retractor should be inserted to expose the glenoid for inspection of the articular cartilage. This retraction maneuver also places tension on the posterior capsule and rotator cuff and can relieve some of the contracture that has developed. At this point the specific procedure indicated can be performed. For long-standing dislocations with large humeral head defects in which prosthetic replacement is planned, the humeral head osteotomy is frequently performed during the exposure. This facilitates mobilization of the proximal humerus and the necessary soft tissue releases for a stable reduction after the prosthesis is inserted.

Infraspinatus Tendon/Greater Tuberosity Transfer
Infraspinatus tendon transfer is performed to prevent the anterior glenoid rim from "falling into" the posterolateral impression defect with abduction and external rotation of the shoulder.[25,26] It is best suited for smaller defects (less than 25%) that are felt to be at

risk for recurrent anterior instability. This procedure requires a separate posterior approach in conjunction with a deltopectoral approach. Therefore, planning of patient positioning is essential. We prefer the sitting position with exposure of the anterior and posterior aspects of the shoulder rather than the lateral position. Using a posterior axillary incision the deltoid fibers are split to expose the underlying infraspinatus and teres minor. The infraspinatus is dissected directly from its insertion into the greater tuberosity along with the underlying capsule. This exposes the humeral head defect. The edge of the tendon is then placed into the defect and secured in position with No. 2 nonabsorbable transosseous sutures passed through the greater tuberosity. For somewhat larger defects, the infraspinatus and a portion of the greater tuberosity can be osteotomized and transferred into the defect as described for the lesser tuberosity transfer. Fixation is then achieved with two cancellous screws. The posterior and anterior exposures are closed in standard fashion and a sling is used for postoperative immobilization. Rehabilitation is started on the first postoperative day, consisting of active range of motion of the elbow, wrist, and hand. Assisted shoulder motion is permitted, including forward elevation and abduction. External rotation is usually limited to neutral, and combinations of abduction and external rotation are avoided. The sling is discontinued 6 weeks postoperatively and a full active range-of-motion program is begun along with isometric strengthening. Resistive strengthening exercises and stretching are gradually incorporated into the rehabilitation regimen 10 to 12 weeks postoperatively.

Disimpaction and Bone Grafting
This procedure is best suited for defects less than 3 weeks old involving less than 45% of the articular surface in which good bone quality and quantity will allow secure fixation and with intact articular cartilage. It is preferred for younger patients, but may also be used effectively in older patients who meet these criteria.

The previously described approach is utilized. After the humeral head is reduced the defect is inspected to confirm that the impacted articular cartilage is salvageable. The humerus is then internally rotated and adducted to locate a position lateral to the lesser tuberosity directly opposite the defect. A 1-cm cortical window is created using an osteotome, and the articular surface is disimpacted indirectly using a bone tamp. The humerus should be externally rotated at this time to provide visualization during the disimpaction process. A small curved osteotome or elevator may be used to facilitate the disimpaction process by directly elevating articular surface fragments. Once disimpaction is complete, the subchondral void created by the disimpaction process is grafted using cancellous allograft. Two cancellous screws are then placed perpendicular to the grafted area to provide support for the construct.

The shoulder is placed through a range of motion and the disimpacted area is visualized as it comes into contact with the anterior glenoid. These positions are specifically avoided postoperatively until bony consolidation occurs at about 6 weeks. The patient is maintained in a sling for 6 weeks, with rehabilitation started on the first postoperative day consisting of passive range-of-motion exercises, including forward elevation, external rotation as determined by the intraoperative findings, and internal rotation to the chest wall. At 6 weeks, the patient is allowed active range of motion of the shoulder, although abduction and external rotation are limited for 8 weeks postoperatively when osseous consolidation is expected.

Gerber[21] has reported success with this technique in selected patients, achieving excellent bony consolidation and articular restoration. Thus far there has not been an outcome study reported using this technique.

Allograft Reconstruction

Allograft reconstruction of posterolateral impression defects is considered for large defects in a younger patient in whom prosthetic replacement would be less than ideal (Fig. **8–12**).[21,27] A preoperative CT scan is essential to delineate the osseous architecture, estimate the humeral head size, and evaluate the humeral bone stock. A size-matched, fresh-frozen humeral head or femoral head allograft is used to fill the defect. Of course if significant articular cartilage damage is evident at the time of surgery, prosthetic replacement may be preferred.

The previously described deltopectoral approach is used. In some cases it may be possible to perform this procedure through a single anterior approach, although a combined anterior and posterior approach may be necessary. An oscillating saw is used to convert the impacted defect to a true wedge, with exposed cancellous bone. The dimensions of the wedge are measured, and a matched allograft wedge, 2 mm wider than the true defect, is fashioned. The allograft wedge is then impacted within the defect and secured using two cancellous screws. Alternatively, screws can be placed from anteriorly and into the graft if it is large enough to obtain secure fixation.

Postoperatively, the patient is placed in a sling for 6 weeks. Rehabilitation is begun on the first postoperative day and consists of passive forward elevation, external rotation to neutral, and internal rotation to the chest. External rotation beyond 0° is avoided for 6 weeks until osseous consolidation has occurred. Active range of motion is initiated at 6 weeks followed by stretching at 10 to 12 weeks.

Gerber[21] documented successful results with the use of allograft reconstruction to address posterolateral humeral defects, with an average postoperative elevation of 145° and Constant score of 70%. Although this series was based on a small number of patients, the results of allograft reconstruction compare favorably with the previously described humeral head–preserving techniques.

Prosthetic Replacement: Hemiarthroplasty and Total Shoulder Arthroplasty

Humeral hemiarthroplasty should be performed in older patients with posterolateral defects that involve more than 40 to 50% of the articular surface and in patients with significant articular cartilage degeneration. If glenoid degenerative changes are present or if associated glenoid erosion contributes to the instability, resurfacing of the glenoid in addition to proximal humeral replacement (i.e., total shoulder arthroplasty) is indicated. Chronic anterior dislocation of more than 6 months' duration usually results in significant osteopenia. In this situation manipulation of the humeral head during open reduction can result in pressure collapse of the humeral head necessitating prosthetic replacement.[28] Dislocations of more than 6 months' duration are also usually associated with significant articular cartilage compromise that will necessitate prosthetic replacement as the preferred treatment (Fig. **8–14**).

Prosthetic replacement of the proximal humerus with or without glenoid resurfacing is performed through the deltopectoral approach described. To maximize anterior stability after prosthetic replacement, the humeral component should be placed in 10 to 15° more retroversion (i.e., 35 to 50°). When glenoid replacement is necessary, it is important to be certain that the component is well supported by bone and secure fixation is obtained. The version of the glenoid component cannot and should not be altered significantly. Secure fixation with good bony support is very important.

Rehabilitation is begun on postoperative day 1, including assisted forward elevation, external rotation based on the intraoperative assessment following repair of the subscapularis tendon, and internal rotation to the chest wall. Isometric deltoid and external rotation can be started within a few days after surgery. A sling is worn for 4 weeks postoperatively, after which active shoulder motion is begun. Stretching and resistive strengthening are begun at 10 to 12 weeks postoperatively.

Flatow et al[28] reported their results with total shoulder arthroplasty for the treatment of large posterolateral defects associated with chronic anterior dislocation. Of nine patients, eight had satisfactory results with an average forward elevation to 147° and active external rotation to 70°, and all were able to perform ADLs. Pritchett and Clarke[29] reported their results of total shoulder arthroplasty to address chronic anterior shoulder dislocations, observing that increasing the amount of retroversion up to 50° could compensate for the chronic dislocation and prevent recurrent instability after prosthetic replacement.

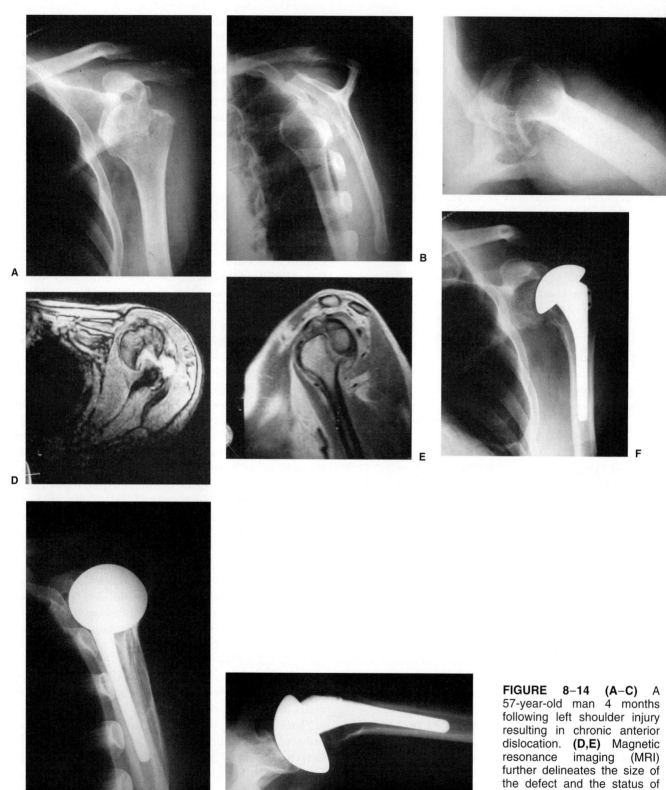

FIGURE 8–14 (A–C) A 57-year-old man 4 months following left shoulder injury resulting in chronic anterior dislocation. **(D,E)** Magnetic resonance imaging (MRI) further delineates the size of the defect and the status of the soft tissues. **(F–H)** Following proximal humeral replacement, a stable articulation was obtained.

Preferred Approach

For patients with chronic glenohumeral dislocations in association with anteromedial or posterolateral humeral head impression fractures, we reserve nonoperative treatment for elderly patients with low functional demands who may demonstrate reasonable adaptation following resolution of the acute shoulder injury, patients with unacceptably high medical risks, patients with uncontrollable seizures, and patients physically or mentally unable to comply with postoperative instructions or rehabilitation. In these cases, as discomfort subsides, rehabilitative exercises are initiated with gradual mobilization of the shoulder, resulting in a reasonable functional outcome in a "limited goals" context.

For patients with chronic posterior dislocation and anteromedial impression fractures up to 40%, we perform an open reduction in conjunction with a lesser tuberosity transfer. In our experience, transfer of the lesser tuberosity and its attached subscapularis tendon provides excellent stability. Although osteoarticular allograft reconstruction has been described with encouraging results, we have no experience with it and existing series are small.[21] For anteromedial impression fractures greater than 40%, or in cases with significant articular cartilage degeneration, we perform prosthetic replacement. Glenoid resurfacing is also performed if significant glenoid articular cartilage degeneration is present.

For patients with chronic anterior dislocation and posterolateral impression fractures up to 20%, we perform an open reduction. For somewhat larger defects, we transfer a portion of the greater tuberosity and attached infraspinatus tendon. In younger patients with posterolateral impression fractures up to 40 to 50%, we consider the use of osteoarticular allograft reconstruction. Although the experience with this technique is limited,[21] in our experience osteoarticular allograft reconstruction is a good alternative for a large posterolateral impression fracture in a younger patient in whom prosthetic replacement is less desirable. For posterolateral impression fractures greater than 40%, or in cases with significant articular cartilage degeneration, we perform prosthetic replacement. Glenoid resurfacing is also performed if significant glenoid articular cartilage degeneration is present.

Summary

The diagnosis and treatment of impression fractures of the proximal humerus remain a challenge for the treating physician. Successful management is predicated on the recognition of these injuries, as well as a thorough understanding of the available treatment options in the context of an organized, disciplined treatment algorithm. Satisfactory pain relief and optimization of functional recovery are the main goals of treatment; it

is therefore incumbent upon the treating physician to establish with the patient and family reasonable expectations for each treatment discussed. The enthusiasm to perform aggressive, often technically challenging procedures should be tempered by assessment of the patient's functional requirements, and realistic expectations of functional recovery.

■ Head-Splitting Fractures

The true head-splitting fracture of the proximal humerus is an uncommon injury. More commonly it occurs as a component of other fractures of the proximal humerus including those involving the anatomic or surgical neck, the tuberosities, or a combination of these. Unless significant displacement is present, the head-splitting component of these fractures may be diagnostically challenging, particularly if the fracture plane is oblique to standard radiographic projections of the shoulder. In this context, special imaging studies are necessary to understand the characteristics of the fracture. Treatment goals are stable fixation of the proximal humerus and restoration of articular congruity; if this cannot be established, prosthetic replacement should be considered. In the younger patient (less than 40 years of age), every effort should be made to restore the articular surface and to preserve proximal humeral bone stock for possible future reconstruction.

Clinical Evaluation

History
Patients with head-splitting fractures of the proximal humerus often report a history of significant trauma, such as an industrial or motor vehicle accident, although older patients with osteopenic bone may sustain such injuries by lower energy mechanisms, such as a fall from a standing position. As head-splitting fractures occur with direct impact of the humeral head upon the glenoid, patients usually report falling directly onto the injured shoulder, rather than onto an outstretched upper extremity.[30] The patient usually complains of severe pain at rest associated with a loss of function of the involved extremity. Attempted motion of the injured shoulder by the patient typically accentuates the pain and may elicit a sensation of crepitation.

Physical Examination
The patient with an acute head-splitting fracture usually presents with the involved extremity held tightly adducted and internally rotated across the chest, often supported by the contralateral hand. Patients who sustain high-energy trauma should undergo a complete trauma evaluation and assessment of hemodynamic

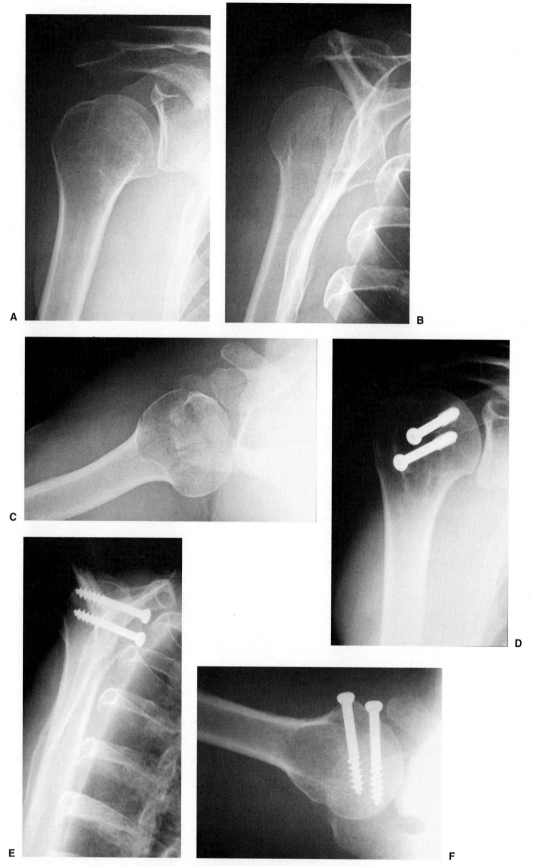

FIGURE 8–15 A 58-year-old with head-splitting fracture as a result of a fall directly on the shoulder. **(A)** Note the double subchondral density on the AP view. **(B,C)** The humeral head is perched on the posterior glenoid at the site of the head-splitting component. **(D–F)** Open reduction and internal fixation (ORIF) with two cancellous screws was performed to obtain an anatomic reduction.

stability. A thorough neurovascular evaluation should be performed in all patients. As many of the patients are elderly, the relative incidence of neurovascular injury is higher than in younger patients, and may be due in part to age-related loss of elasticity and calcification of soft tissue structures.[15,31-34]

Attempts at passive or active range of motion are typically limited in all planes of motion by pain. Crepitation may be appreciated with minimal shoulder motion (i.e., during removal of a sling or clothing) or position changes of the body. Because of the discomfort experienced by the patient, further evaluation of strength or associated injury, such as to the rotator cuff, is often impossible.

Radiographic Evaluation
Standard Radiographs
The shoulder trauma series consists of anteroposterior, scapular lateral ("Y view"), and axillary projections. The anteroposterior radiograph should be scrutinized for evidence of associated fractures of the proximal humerus involving the tuberosities or surgical neck. Head-splitting fractures may be identified depending on the degree of displacement and the portion of the head that is involved. The "double-density" sign indicates a head-splitting component and represents the overlapping densities of subchondral bone of two separate fragments (Fig. 8–15).

The scapular lateral view may be useful for the identification or further delineation of head-splitting fractures in the coronal plane. The axillary projection is particularly useful, as it provides further characterization of these fractures. It may be necessary to position the patient for this radiograph because of the associated pain. The standard axillary view provides much more information about the fracture than the Velpeau axillary. Of the three radiographs of the trauma series, the anteroposterior view and the axillary are most helpful in understanding the fracture anatomy.

Other Imaging Studies
Computed tomography is useful for further evaluation of head-splitting fractures, particularly when the head-splitting component is not well visualized on the three standard radiographic projections of the shoulder (i.e., the fracture plane is oblique in all three views) (Fig. 8–16). Axial CT images may confirm the diagnosis, allow for assessment of comminution, and aid in preoperative planning. CT is also useful in evaluating bone quality and quantity, both of which may affect operative considerations. Two-dimensional sagittal and coronal oblique reconstructions may aid in fracture characterization, but we have not found them to be essential. Magnetic resonance imaging can be useful for evaluation of concomitant injuries to the rotator cuff, but in general it is not utilized.

Treatment
The management of head-splitting fractures of the proximal humerus is dependent on many factors, including age, medical comorbidities, chronicity, and the functional requirements of the patient. In addition, the availability of implants and expertise of the surgeon are also important factors that determine treatment options.

Nonoperative
Nonoperative treatment of true head-splitting fractures may be undertaken in patients with minimal displacement and low functional demands. The majority of patients that fall into this category are elderly, often with medical comorbidities that may render the risk of operation greater than the possible benefit. In these cases, supportive measures should be instituted, including non-narcotic oral analgesics and gradual mobilization of the shoulder with physical therapy as dictated by the stability and healing of the fracture. When head-splitting fractures occur in combination with other fractures of the proximal humerus, the decision of operative versus nonoperative management is often determined by the overall fracture pattern and the patient factors identified.

Operative
The operative treatment of head-splitting fractures is based on the age of the patient, degree of displacement, the presence of other fractures of the proximal humerus, and the bone quantity and quality. Preoperative CT scans can be invaluable in determining the plane(s) of injury and the fragments involved. In general, the primary goal is to restore the integrity of the articular surface either by anatomic reduction and fixation or by prosthetic replacement.

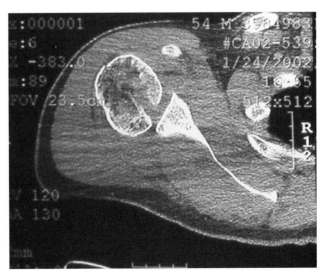

FIGURE 8–16 CT scan of a significant head-splitting fracture that was not well visualized on standard radiographs.

Operative reduction and fixation of head-splitting fractures is preferred in younger patients in whom prosthetic replacement is less desirable. With greater degrees of displacement, comminution, and the presence of associated proximal humeral fractures, the surgeon may be more inclined to perform prosthetic replacement. In the presence of significant osteopenia, in which secure fixation may not be possible, primary consideration should be given to prosthetic replacement.

Operative Reduction and Fixation

For the patient with adequate bone stock and a displaced, head-splitting fracture, either in isolation or in combination with a more complex proximal humerus fracture, operative reduction and fixation is indicated. It may be possible to accomplish this using percutaneous reduction and fixation techniques as determined by the skill and experience of the surgeon. These techniques are described in Chapters 6 and 7. Open reduction and internal fixation can be performed using a variety of techniques (Fig. 8–17).

A standard deltopectoral approach is utilized for exposure of the proximal humerus. For an isolated head-splitting fracture, the rotator interval is opened to assess the degree of articular incongruity. It is often difficult to reduce the fragments with this exposure. If

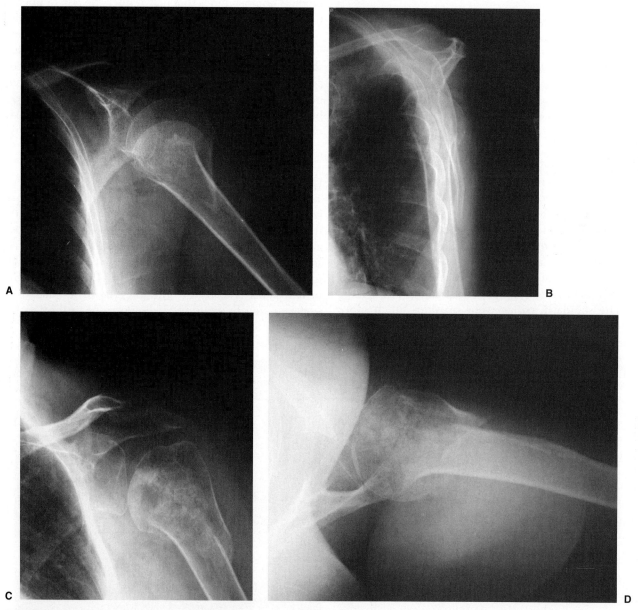

FIGURE 8–17 A 48-year-old man sustained a shoulder injury from a fall on the ice. Scapular AP **(A)** shows the typical "double density" of a head-splitting fracture, which is not evident on the scapular lateral **(B)**. **(C,D)** Six months following ORIF, with multiple tension band sutures combined with cancellous allograft, the patient had regained very good range of motion, with an American Shoulder and Elbow Surgeons (ASES) score of 89.

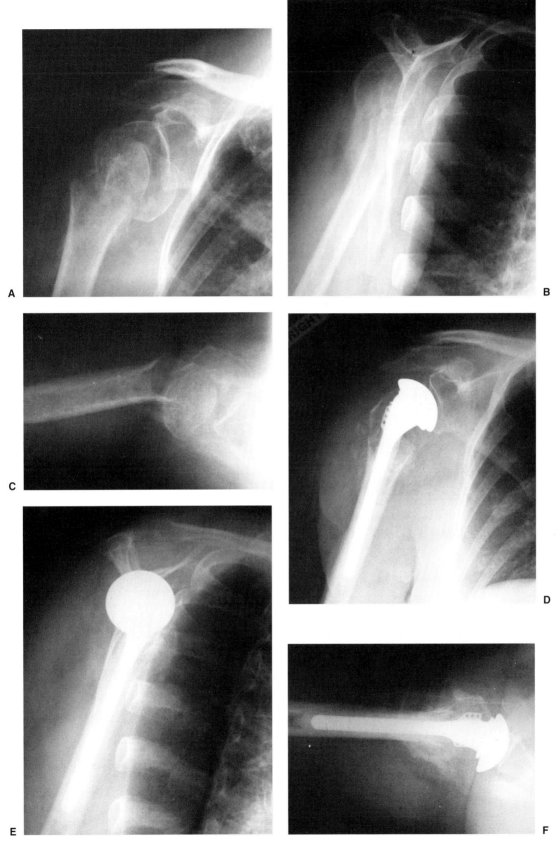

FIGURE 8–18 (A–C) This 71-year-old woman sustained a complex proximal humerus fracture with a significant head-splitting component 6 weeks earlier. **(D–F)** Proximal humeral replacement was performed because of the comminution, bone quality, age of the fracture, and patient age and activity level.

reduction can be accomplished, however, two cannulated cancellous screws should be placed for fixation, oriented as close to perpendicular to the fracture line as the articular surfaces will allow (Fig. **8–15**). If reduction cannot be accomplished through the rotator interval, the subscapularis tendon should be divided for wider exposure of the joint, thereby allowing reduction of the fragments and fixation.

When the head-splitting fracture is a component of a more complex proximal humerus fracture, the methods of reduction and fixation are determined by the overall fracture pattern with particular attention to restoration of the articular surface.

Sling immobilization is utilized and rehabilitation is begun on the first postoperative day consisting of assisted range of motion for forward elevation, external rotation, and internal rotation to the chest. Progression of rehabilitation is determined primarily by progression of healing on serial radiographs. Active range of motion is instituted at approximately 6 weeks when the sling is discontinued.

Hemiarthroplasty

Prosthetic replacement should be utilized in older patients in which the head-splitting fracture is a component of a more complex proximal humerus fracture, that is, a four-part fracture (Fig. **8–18**). In this context the procedure performed is as described in Chapter 7 for four-part fractures.

Outcome

Because true isolated head-splitting fractures are so uncommon, the literature is limited to case reports and only one clinical series that specifically evaluates the results of surgical treatment of these injuries.[30,35,36] Chesser et al[30] reported a series of eight cases of head-splitting fractures. Despite having a reasonable number of cases in this series, the variability of timing and type of treatment prevented useful conclusions about the treatment of these fractures. Others have included head-splitting fractures in their outcome data of proximal humerus fractures, often demonstrating poorer results[37]; however, it is difficult to draw strong conclusions about the short- and long-term outcomes of operative treatment of these fractures from the sparse reports in the literature.

REFERENCES

1. Blom S, Dahlback L. Nerve injuries in dislocations of the shoulder joint and fractures of the neck of the humerus: a clinical and electromyographic study. Acta Chir Scand 1970;136:461–466
2. Cave E, Burke JF, Boyd RJ. Trauma Management. Chicago: Year Book Medical Publishers, 1974
3. Rowe C, Zarins B. Chronic unreduced dislocations of the shoulder. J Bone Joint Surg Am 1982;64:494–505
4. Calandra J, Baker C, Uribe J. The incidence of Hill-Sachs lesions in initial anterior shoulder dislocations. Arthroscopy 1989;5:254–257
5. Taylor D, Arciero R. Pathologic changes associated with shoulder dislocations. Am J Sports Med 1997;25:306–311
6. Norlin R. Intraarticular pathology in acute, first-time anterior shoulder dislocation: an arthroscopic study. Arthroscopy 1993;9:546–549
7. Rowe C, Zarins B. Recurrent transient subluxation of the shoulder. J Bone Joint Surg Am 1981;63:159–168
8. Hawkins RJ, Neer CS II, Pianta RM, Mendoza FX. Locked posterior dislocation of the shoulder. J Bone Joint Surg Am 1987;69:9–18
9. Cole BJ, Warner JP. Anatomy, biomechanics, and pathophysiology of glenohumeral instability. In: Iannotti JP, Williams GR, eds. Disorders of the Shoulder: Diagnosis and Management. Philadelphia: Lippincott, 1999:207–232
10. Bennet G. Old dislocations of the shoulder. J Bone Joint Surg Am 1936;18:594–606
11. Schulz TJ, Jacobs B, Patterson RL Jr. Unrecognized dislocations of the shoulder. J Trauma 1969;9:1009–1023
12. de Laat EA, Visser CP, Coene LN, Pahlpatz PV, Tavy DL. Nerve lesions in primary shoulder dislocations and humeral neck fractures. A prospective clinical and EMG study. J Bone Joint Surg Br 1994;76:381–383
13. Antal C, Conforty B, Engelberg M. Injuries to the axillary artery due to anterior dislocation of the shoulder. J Trauma 1973;13:564–566
14. Kirker JR. Dislocation of the shoulder complicated by rupture of the axillary vessels. J Bone Joint Surg Br 1952;34:72–73
15. Zuckerman JD, Flugstad DL, Teitz CC, King HA. Axillary artery injury as a complication of proximal humeral fracture. Two case reports and a review of the literature. Clin Orthop 1984;189:234–237
16. McLaughlin HL. Posterior dislocation of the shoulder. J Bone Joint Surg Am 1952;24-A:584–590
17. Wilson J, McKeever FM. Traumatic posterior (retroglenoid) dislocation of the humerus. J Bone Joint Surg Am 1949;31:160–172
18. Kirtland S, Resnick D, Sartoris DJ, Pate D, Greenway G. Chronic unreduced dislocations of the glenohumeral joint: imaging strategy and pathologic correlation. J Trauma 1988;28:1622–1631
19. Mullaji A, Beddow FH, Lamb GHR. CT management of glenoid erosion in arthritis. J Bone Joint Surg Br 1994;76:384–388
20. Neviaser RJ, Neviaser TJ, Neviaser JS. Anterior dislocation of the shoulder and rotator cuff rupture. Clin Orthop 1993;291:103–106
21. Gerber C. Chronic locked anterior and posterior dislocations. In: Warner J, Iannotti JP, Gerber C, eds. Complex Revision Problems in Shoulder Surgery. Philadelphia: Lippincott, 1997
22. Griggs SM, Holloway B, Williams GR Jr, Iannotti JP. Treatment of locked anterior and posterior dislocations of the shoulder. In: Iannotti JP, Williams GR, eds. Disorders of the Shoulder: Diagnosis and Management. Philadelphia: Lippincott, 1999:335–359
23. Gerber C, Lambert SM. Allograft reconstruction of segmental defects of the humeral head for the treatment of chronic locked posterior dislocation of the shoulder. J Bone Joint Surg Am 1996;78:376–382
24. Neer CS II. Shoulder Reconstruction. Philadelphia: WB Saunders, 1990
25. Willis JB, Meyn MA, Miller EH. Infraspinatus transfer for recurrent anterior dislocation of the shoulder. Presented at the annual meeting of the American Academy of Orthopaedic Surgeons, Las Vegas, Nevada, February 27, 1981
26. Weber BG. Operative treatment for recurrent dislocation of the shoulder: preliminary report. Injury 1969;1:107–109
27. Miniaci A, Hand C, Berlet G. Segmental humeral head allografts for recurrent anterior instability of the shoulder with large Hill-Sachs defects: a 2 to 8 year follow up. Presented at the 20th

annual meeting of the American Shoulder and Elbow Surgeons, October 8–10, 2003

28. Flatow E, Miller SR, Neer CS II. Chronic anterior dislocation of the shoulder. J Shoulder Elbow Surg 1993;2:2–10

29. Pritchett JW, Clark JM. Prosthetic replacement for chronic unreduced dislocations of the shoulder. Clin Orthop 1987;216:89–93

30. Chesser TJ, Langdon IJ, Ogilvie C, Sarangi PP, Clarke AM. Fractures involving splitting of the humeral head. J Bone Joint Surg Br 2001;83:423–426

31. Hayes M, Van Winkle N. Axillary artery injury with minimally displaced fractures of the neck of the humerus. Clin Orthop 1983;289:156–160

32. de Laat EA, Visser CP, Coene LN, Pahlpatz PV, Tavy DL. Nerve lesions in primary shoulder dislocations and humeral neck fractures.

A prospective clinical and EMG study. J Bone Joint Surg Br 1994;76:381–383

33. Blom S, Dahlback L. Nerve injuries in dislocations of the shoulder joint and fractures of the neck of the humerus: a clinical and electromyographic study. Acta Chir Scand 1970;136:461–466

34. Kirker JR. Dislocation of the shoulder complicated by rupture of the axillary vessels. J Bone Joint Surg Br 1952;34:72–73

35. Richards RH, Clarke NMP. Locked posterior fracture-dislocation of the shoulder. Injury 1989;20:297–300

36. Rowe CR, Zarins B. Chronic unreduced dislocations of the shoulder. J Bone Joint Surg Am 1982;64:494–505

37. Moda SK, Chadha NS, Sangwan SS, Khurana DK, Dahiya AS, Siwach RC. Open reduction and fixation of proximal humeral fractures and fracture-dislocations. J Bone Joint Surg Br 1990;72:1050–1052

9

Complications of Proximal Humeral Fractures

JOSEPH D. ZUCKERMAN AND DOUGLAS MURRAY

Complications associated with proximal humerus fractures can occur at the time of injury or during treatment. The operative or nonoperative management of these complications is determined by the symptoms attributed to the complication itself. Thorough evaluation of the patient with a complication following a proximal humerus fracture must include an assessment of the patient's activity level, the degree of dysfunction associated with the complication and its effect on the patient, the patient's expectations of treatment, and the patient's ability to participate in the treatment plan. Early complications of operative management include loss of fixation and problems related to internal fixation devices. Bony and soft tissue abnormalities about the shoulder should be evaluated and their contribution to the symptoms and dysfunction assessed. Bony abnormalities include nonunion, malunion, incongruity of the articular surface, osteonecrosis, and heterotopic bone formation. Soft tissue abnormalities include contracture, infection, rotator cuff injury, and neurovascular compromise.

■ Early Failure of Fixation and Implant Complications

Fractures that undergo open or closed reduction and internal fixation can develop problems associated with the fixation devices utilized. The problems can vary from a change in position of an implant (i.e., backing out of a percutaneously placed pin or screw) to complete loss of fixation with redisplacement of the fracture to migration of an implant into the soft tissues adjacent or distant to the shoulder. When complications of this type arise, it is essential to carefully evaluate the significance

of the problem and the contributing factors to determine the appropriate treatment.

Failure of fixation can occur as a result of different factors including (1) improper insertion, (2) inability to obtain secure fixation, (3) too early or too aggressive postoperative mobilization program, and (4) patient noncompliance with postoperative instructions. Follow-up radiographs should be obtained early in the postoperative period, particularly after initiation of a mobilization program. The nature and degree of loss of fixation or loss of reduction usually determines the treatment required. Minor changes—backout of a pin or screw or a slight change of fracture alignment—may benefit from modification of the postoperative program. A period of immobilization may allow fracture healing to progress sufficiently to prevent further displacement. Although this may compromise recovery of range of motion, it is preferable to a more significant loss of fixation that may result in malunion or nonunion requiring revision surgery. Stiffness in the presence of a healed fracture with acceptable alignment is preferable to an early revision procedure.

When there is significant loss of fixation with displacement of the fracture, early revision is usually required (Fig. 9–1). Although each clinical situation should be evaluated individually, there are a few general principles to follow: first, the reason for the early loss of fixation should be evaluated carefully, so these factors can be controlled and prevented following the revision procedure; second, the procedure to be performed should have the best chance of a successful outcome and should minimize the need for another procedure; and third, for any procedure performed, patient compliance with the postoperative program is essential. If there is a question about whether the patient will be compliant, especially if

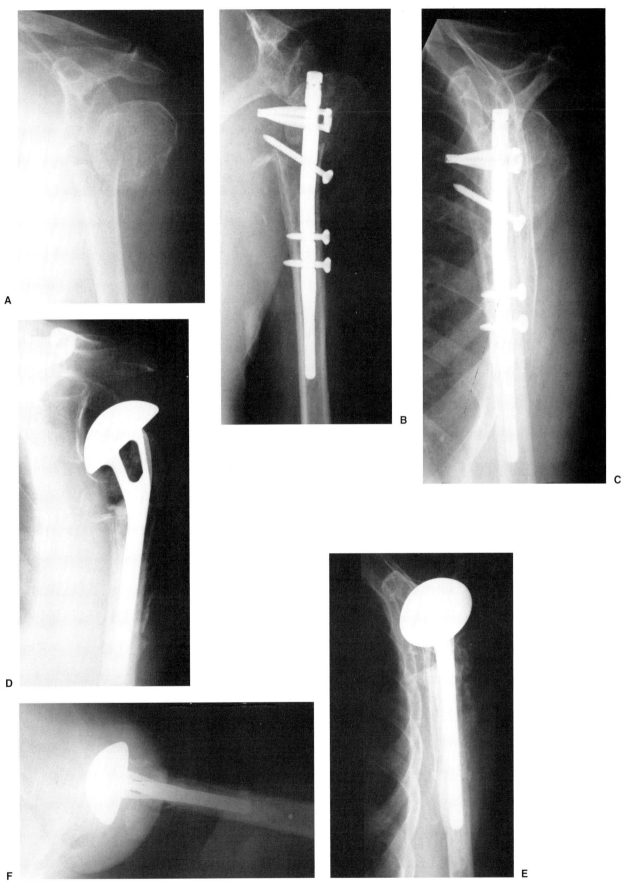

FIGURE 9–1 A 73-year-old with a displaced, comminuted surgical neck fracture **(A)** underwent intramedullary fixation **(B,C)**. Fracture reduction was not obtained and fixation was further compromised by the comminution. **(D–F)** Revision to proximal humeral replacement was performed 5 weeks after the initial surgery.

noncompliance contributed to the initial problem, addition procedures should probably be avoided.

There are a multitude of specific fixation problems that can develop depending on the type of fixation device utilized, which makes it impossible to address each potential clinical situation to be encountered. In general, however, revision open reduction and internal fixation (ORIF) should be considered in younger patients in whom there is a high likelihood of obtaining secure fixation with a revision procedure. The revision procedure should utilize a different type of fixation method than the original, unsuccessful method. If assessment of the failed fixation makes it unlikely that revision fixation can be obtained, proximal humeral replacement should be considered as the preferred approach (Fig. **9–1**). It is also important to note that early revision surgery requires meticulous handling of soft tissues to avoid additional problems, specifically the increased risk for heterotopic ossification, which is discussed later in this chapter.

Whenever internal fixation devices are utilized about the proximal humerus, there is the potential for hardware complications. Early implant loosening can occur, resulting in migration of an implant into the soft tissues (Fig. **9–2**). This usually occurs locally, but migration to

remote areas of the body has been reported. Improper placement of implants can cause problems particularly if there is violation of the articular surface (Fig. **9–3**). Settling of the fracture can also result in intraarticular migration of implants early, and in some cases, later in the healing process.[1]

Frequent postoperative radiographs should be obtained to monitor the position of the implants. Percutaneous pins should be removed when fracture healing has progressed sufficiently. Smooth pins should not be used, and care should be taken to avoid excessive advancement and backing out of the pins during insertion. When this occurs, a "track" remains, which facilitates migration. Unrecognized, intraarticular implants can result in rapid destruction of articular cartilage (Fig. **9–4**). It is essential to obtain a full set of radiographs to properly evaluate the location of the implants (Fig. **9–3**). These should be obtained in the operating room prior to completion of the procedure. At the time of follow-up evaluation, if there is any concern about intraarticular location of the implants, proper radiographic evaluation should be performed. In addition to appropriate orthogonal views, it may be necessary to obtain fluoroscopically positioned radiographs to confirm proper position of the implants.

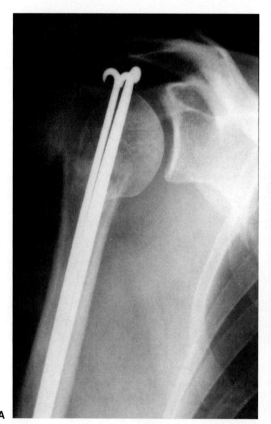

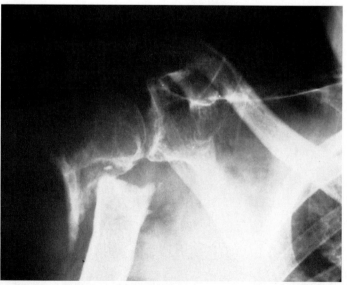

A   B

FIGURE 9–2 This 59-year-old man underwent Rush rod fixation of a surgical neck fracture. **(A)** The rods backed out, causing encroachment on the subacromial space and necessitating premature hardware removal 6 weeks postoperatively. **(B)** The fracture was not healed and a nonunion developed.

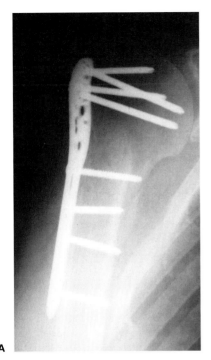
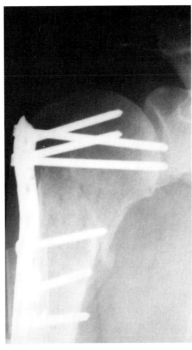

A

B

FIGURE 9–3 (A) A 57-year-old man underwent locking plate fixation of a surgical neck fracture. He was unable to regain active range of motion and had persistent pain. **(B)** Follow-up radiographs showed that two of the screws were intraarticular in location, a finding that was not evident on earlier radiographs.

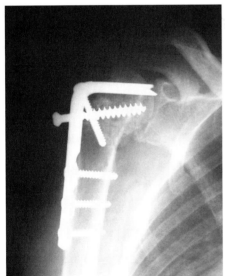
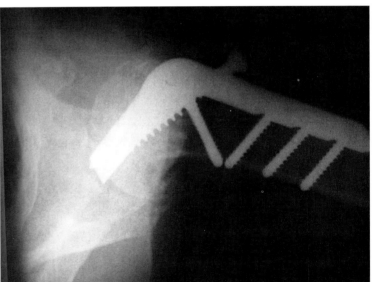

A

B

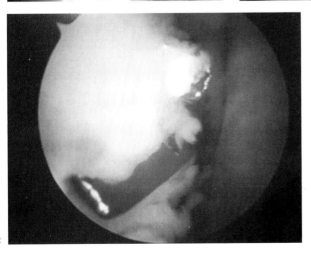

C

FIGURE 9–4 This 66-year-old woman underwent blade plate fixation of a surgical neck fracture. Initial x-rays confirmed proper position of the implant. The patient developed pain and crepitus 4 weeks following the surgery. **(A,B)** X-rays showed the tip of the blade plate was in an intraarticular location. **(C)** Arthroscopic images show the protruding portion of the plate. The patient improved following plate removal.

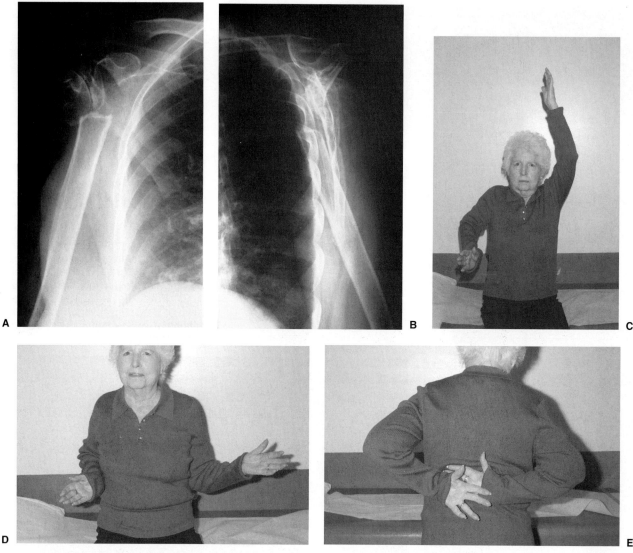

FIGURE 9–5 An 81-year-old woman 16 months following right surgical neck fracture that was treated nonoperatively. **(A,B)** Radiographs show an atrophic nonunion. The patient had minimal discomfort. **(C–E)** In spite of a significant loss of active motion, the patient did not feel that the symptoms and disability were sufficient to consider operative management.

Incomplete radiographs will fail to identify problematic hardware, leading to unnecessary problems.

Nonunion

Nonunion most commonly occurs following surgical neck fractures, less frequently with greater tuberosity fractures, and uncommonly following three- or four-part proximal humeral fractures. Surgical neck nonunion can occur as a result of different factors. One of the most common is distraction or motion at the fracture site. Distraction can occur due to soft tissue interposition or, much less commonly, with the use of a hanging arm cast.[2] Motion at the surgical neck fracture site is often due to (1) inadequate immobilization, (2) too early mobilization, and (3) inadequate fixation.[3,4]

Treatment of a surgical neck nonunion is determined by the symptoms associated with the nonunion. Nonoperative management may be most appropriate if the patient has minimal symptoms or disability (Fig. **9–5**). If the symptoms and disability are significant, operative management should be considered, and will typically consist of ORIF (using a variety of devices) or proximal humeral replacement.[5–8] Preoperative assessment must include the patient's age and activity level, the quality of the bone of the proximal humerus, and the size of the nonunited head fragment. Methods of operative management typically include tension band fixation with modified Enders rods, blade plate fixation, or other plate and screw devices (Fig. **9–6**).[5,6,8] Regardless of which method is utilized, bone grafting is a necessity.

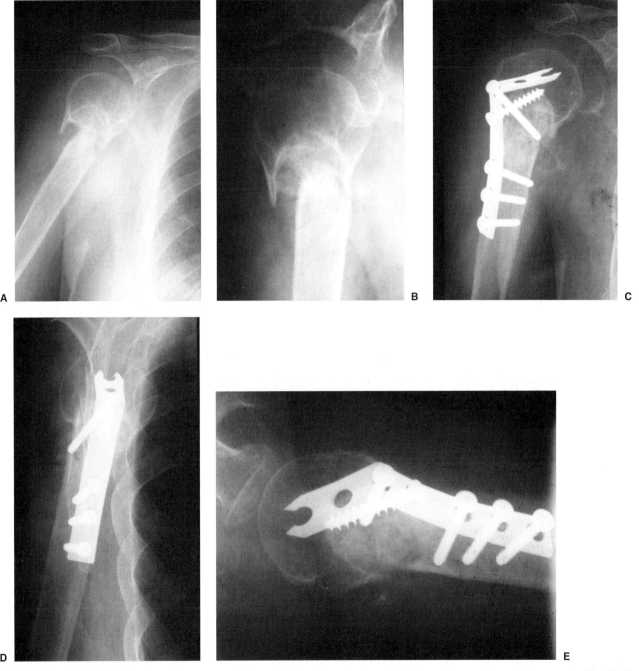

FIGURE 9–6 (A,B) A 58-year-old woman with surgical neck nonunion following nonoperative management. **(C–E)** Open reduction and internal fixation (ORIF) with a modified blade plate and bone grafting was performed.

The techniques of proximal humeral replacement varies based on the level of the nonunion and the size of the proximal fragment.[7] When the proximal fragment is small, the tuberosities should be osteotomized and reattached to the prosthesis (Fig. 9–7). Mobilization of the tuberosities is essential to obtain a tension-free reattachment. When the proximal fragment is larger, it may be possible to resect the articular surface and pass the prosthesis through the proximal segment ("skewering technique") and into the shaft. When this technique is used, it is essential to compress the fragments, avoid cement interposition at the nonunion site, and add bone graft to aid in achieving union (Fig. 9–8). If the "skewering" technique is utilized, mobilization of the proximal fragment is equally important to minimize the stresses on the nonunion site. Specific mobilization techniques should be performed in a step-by-step sequence. Both treatment approaches—ORIF and

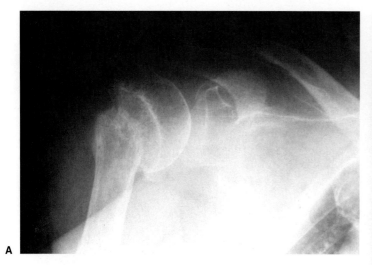

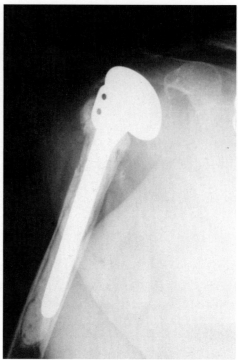

FIGURE 9–7 A 66-year-old with surgical neck nonunion. **(A)** The proximal fragment is small and osteopenic. **(B)** Proximal humerus replacement combined with tuberosity osteotomy and reconstruction was performed.

prosthetic replacement—can be technically demanding. Successful results have been achieved using both techniques.[5-8]

Greater tuberosity nonunions can occur due to medial displacement of the fragment onto the articular surface where it is bathed in synovial fluid (Fig. **9–9**). The synovial fluid lyses the fracture hematoma and interferes with the healing process. Inadequate initial radiographic evaluation can lead to a missed diagnosis, especially if the fragment is displaced posteriorly and not visualized on the anteroposterior (AP) radiographs. Patients with a greater tuberosity nonunion often present with pain and limitation of motion. Because the nonunited fragment results in a functional rotator cuff tear, weakness is also common.

Treatment of the nonunited displaced greater tuberosity is more difficult than an acute repair because of the contracted rotator cuff tissues, formation of adhesions in the subacromial space, and the quality of the bony fragment. Operative management utilizes a superior approach with development of the interval between the anterior and middle portions of the deltoid and elevation of the deltoid from the anterior acromion. A more limited deltoid splitting approach can be considered, but displacement of the fragment and the difficulties of mobilization generally require a more extensive exposure. In situations when a posterior portion of the greater tuberosity is displaced into a posterior and medial position, a posterior deltoid splitting approach may be necessary for adequate visualization and

mobilization. Regardless of the approach utilized, the ability to rotate the humerus significantly enhances the exposure even when relatively small incisions are utilized.

After exposure of the fragment, the first step is mobilization. This requires lysis of adhesions with subacromial space release of fibrous tissues that developed adjacent to the fragment. It is often necessary to release the coracohumeral ligament at the base of the coracoid for enhanced mobilization. The fibrous tissues that fill the gap between the fragment and the intact greater tuberosity should be resected. This allows visualization of the articular surface. Fibrous tissue should be removed from the area of the intact greater tuberosity to expose the area that corresponds to the site of the fracture. Cancellous bone should be exposed along with the portion of the greater tuberosity located anterior and posterior to the fracture site. It is often helpful to enlarge the bed slightly to allow overreduction of the fragment and minimize the possibility of any residual prominence.

Intraarticular mobilization is necessary, and usually consists of release of the capsule at the glenoid margin to enhance lateral advancement of the fragment. It is essential to achieve adequate mobilization of the fragment for an anatomic reduction with minimal tension. If the fragment originated from the anterior portion of the greater tuberosity, when it is reduced the arm should be able to be placed in a sling at the side without excessive tension on the repair. If a more posterior portion of the tuberosity was involved, ideally the arm should also be able to be placed in a sling without excessive tension

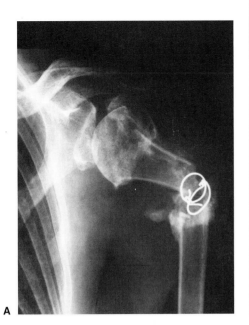

A

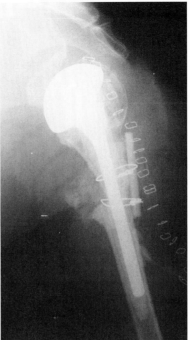

B

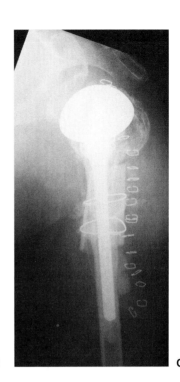

C

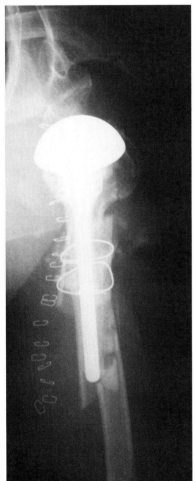

D

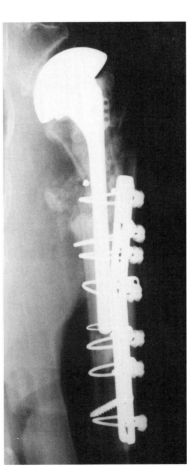

E

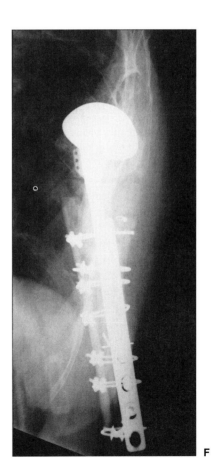

F

FIGURE 9–8 (A) An 81-year-old underwent ORIF of proximal humeral shaft fracture with inadequate cerclage fixation, resulting in nonunion. **(B,C)** Proximal humeral replacement was performed with the prosthesis used to "skewer" the proximal fragment to obtain "intramedullary" fixation combined with fibular strut grafting and cancellous autograft. **(D)** Two weeks following surgery the patient fell, sustaining a distal periprosthetic fracture requiring ORIF with a plate and fibular strut graft. **(E,F)** Three months later both the nonunion and the fracture have healed.

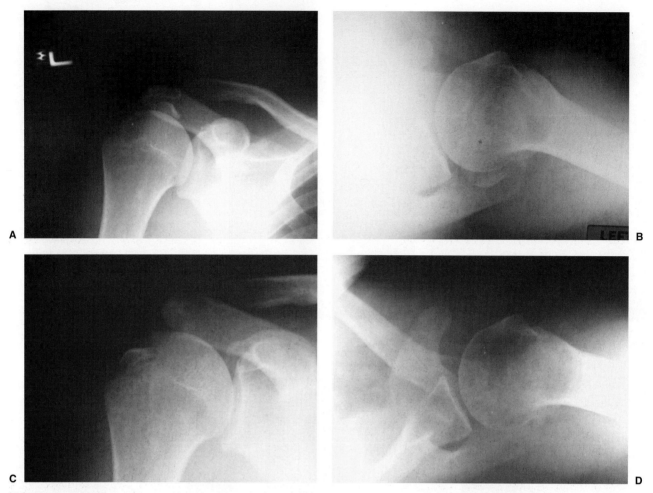

FIGURE 9–9 (A,B) A 43-year-old man with a greater tuberosity nonunion 6 months after an unrecognized injury. **(C,D)** Open reduction with soft tissue releases was performed, allowing the fragment to be reduced into its bed.

on the repair. If this is not possible, however, it is often beneficial to use a modified sling or an orthosis that maintains the humerus in varying degrees of external rotation. This reduces the tension on the repair. Fixation of the fragment is usually accomplished with figure-of-eight repair using No. 5 nonabsorbable suture passed through the rotator cuff insertion and through the humeral cortex distal to the bed. If the fragment is small and bone quality is poor, however, it can be excised and the tendon repaired directly to bone with nonabsorbable sutures passed through bone tunnels. This is the equivalent of a tendon to bone rotator cuff repair. When the repair is completed, range of motion should be assessed to determine the parameters of the postoperative therapy program. There should be minimal tension on the fragment with the arm at the side. If this cannot be achieved, it will be necessary to modify the position of immobilization.

Postoperatively, a passive range-of-motion program is initiated based on the parameters identified intraoperatively. Radiographs are obtained 1 week following the surgery to confirm that the fragment remains in position.

A passive range-of-motion program is utilized for 6 weeks, after which time radiographs are obtained. If there is any concern about healing, a longer period of immobilization is utilized; however, at 6 weeks an active range-of-motion program can usually be instituted. At 10 to 12 weeks, stretching and strengthening exercises can be added.

Malunion

Malunion following proximal humeral fractures can involve the articular surface, the tuberosities, the shaft, or a combination of these segments. This bony deformity is typically associated with soft tissue abnormalities, and both factors contribute to the loss of motion. Evaluation with a complete set of standard radiographs can be supplemented with a computed tomography (CT) scan to determine the relationship of the malunited fragments to the articular surface and the shaft.[9] The operative treatment of malunion is reserved for patients with persistent symptoms after nonoperative treatment fails to relieve pain or improve function and when there is

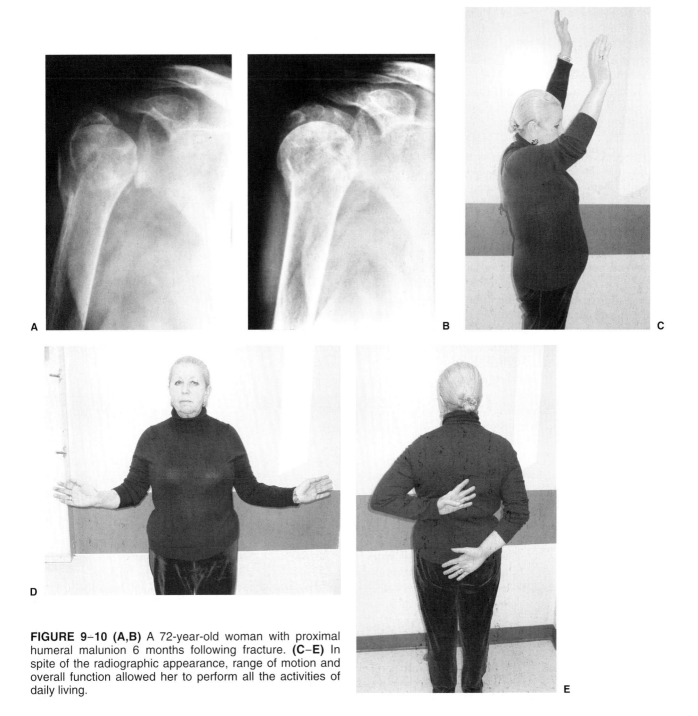

FIGURE 9–10 (A,B) A 72-year-old woman with proximal humeral malunion 6 months following fracture. **(C–E)** In spite of the radiographic appearance, range of motion and overall function allowed her to perform all the activities of daily living.

strong evidence that the malunion is the primary source of the symptoms. Some patients are able to regain very good range of motion and overall function in spite of radiographs that show significant malunion (Fig. **9–10**). For these patients, nonoperative management is the treatment of choice. The large spectrum of symptoms associated with proximal humeral malunions mandate that each case be considered individually.

Operative management for symptomatic malunion must address both osseous and soft tissue abnormalities.

These have been classified by Beredjiklian et al.[10] Type I osseous deformity is a greater tuberosity malunion of at least 1 cm; type II involves an intraarticular incongruity with a step-off greater than 5 mm; and type III is malalignment of the articular segment. Soft tissue abnormalities include type I, soft tissue contracture; type II, rotator cuff tear; and type III, subacromial impingement. The same authors document that operative management for malunion is challenging. In their series they reported 69% satisfactory results with a 28% complication rate.[10]

Tuberosity malunion usually involves the greater tuberosity because this fracture is much more common than lesser tuberosity fractures. The deforming forces of the rotator cuff on the greater or lesser tuberosity can cause additional displacement after initial radiographs may have shown acceptable position. Malunions also result from inadequate initial radiographic assessment of isolated greater tuberosity fractures or following closed reduction of two-part greater tuberosity anterior fracture-dislocations. A posteriorly displaced greater tuberosity fragment may not be visualized on AP radiographs. An axillary view is essential to evaluate this type of displacement. For those greater tuberosity fractures treated operatively, malunion can result from inadequate reduction or loss of reduction postoperatively.

The patient with a malunited greater tuberosity may complain of pain, loss of motion, and weakness. A displaced tuberosity can result in a mechanical block of motion. If the fragment is displaced superiorly and medially, subacromial impingement will result in pain and a loss of abduction and forward elevation (Fig. **9–11**). Displacement posteriorly will limit external rotation. A malunited tuberosity can also be the functional equivalent of a rotator cuff tear. Shortening of the rotator cuff interferes with the length tension relationship of the musculotendinous construct, thereby reducing function.

Treatment of a malunited greater tuberosity should be based on an assessment of the associated symptoms. If stiffness is the primary problem, it is important to confirm whether the patient was compliant with a structured, supervised rehabilitation program. Although it is somewhat unlikely that stiffness associated with significant deformity superiorly or posteriorly will respond to an exercise regimen, lesser degrees of malunion may respond very well to a therapy program. However, patients with an obvious mechanical block to motion experiencing pain and stiffness will not respond to nonoperative management. When the symptoms of pain and stiffness and the associated dysfunction are significant, operative management is indicated. Operative management primarily consists of osteotomy of the malunited fragment, mobilization, and reduction into an anatomic position to obtain bony union (Fig. **9–11**). In some instances, resection of the fragment and rotator cuff repair may be necessary if adequate mobilization cannot be obtained; however, this is a less attractive option than osteotomy, reduction, and fixation.

The approach to a greater tuberosity malunion is similar to that described for nonunion. After exposure of the subacromial space through a superior approach, we perform an acromioplasty to increase the space within the subacromial region both for exposure as well as to avoid any subacromial encroachment postoperatively. Identification of the malunited fragment may be difficult, and intraoperative radiographs can be beneficial.

The fragment can usually be identified by exposing the intact greater tuberosity anteriorly and posteriorly. The area corresponding to the origin of the fragment should be exposed. The bed is usually covered with fibrous tissue and/or bone depending on the amount of time since the injury, and it may not be easily identified. When the anterior and posterior margins of the fragment are identified, the rotator cuff can be incised longitudinally in these areas. This allows visualization of the articular surface. The junction between the fragment and the articular surface can either be visualized or at least palpated with a small elevator. Identification of this junction and the lateral extent of the fragment determine the direction and angle of the osteotomy to be performed. The osteotomy should be performed with a sharp osteotome. Care should be taken to avoid any compromise of the articular surface. In addition, it is essential that the osteotomy include an adequate fragment of bone, even if it has to be reduced in size at the time of reduction.

Once the fragment is osteotomized, the attached tendon should be tagged with sutures to begin the mobilization process. Extramuscular and intraarticular releases are performed to allow the fragment to be advanced laterally to a cancellous bed that should correspond to its origin. It may be necessary to reduce the size of the fragment so it can be reduced. Slight overreduction is preferred to prevent any residual prominence. We prefer fixation with figure-of-eight tension band suture using a No. 5 nonabsorbable suture. These sutures are passed through the lateral humeral cortex distal to the bed. The drill holes for these sutures should be placed distal enough to prevent the possibility of propagation of the drill hole into the cancellous bed. When the fixation of the fragment is completed, the anterior and posterior incisions in the rotator cuff should be repaired. The shoulder should be placed through a range of motion and the stability of the fixation assessed. This will determine the parameters for the postoperative rehabilitation program. The fragment ideally should be securely fixed in position so that the arm can be placed in a standard sling. For posterior fragments, however, it may be necessary to maintain some degree of external rotation to decrease tension on the repair. Modifications of the postoperative immobilization should be determined based on these intraoperative assessments.

Postoperatively, radiographs are obtained 1 to 2 weeks following the surgery to confirm that the fragment remains reduced. A passive range-of-motion program is utilized for the first 6 weeks. At that time, if radiographs confirm adequate healing, rehabilitation is progressed to an active range-of-motion program. If there is any question about healing, a longer period of immobilization should be utilized with continuation of passive range-of-motion exercises. A more vigorous stretching and

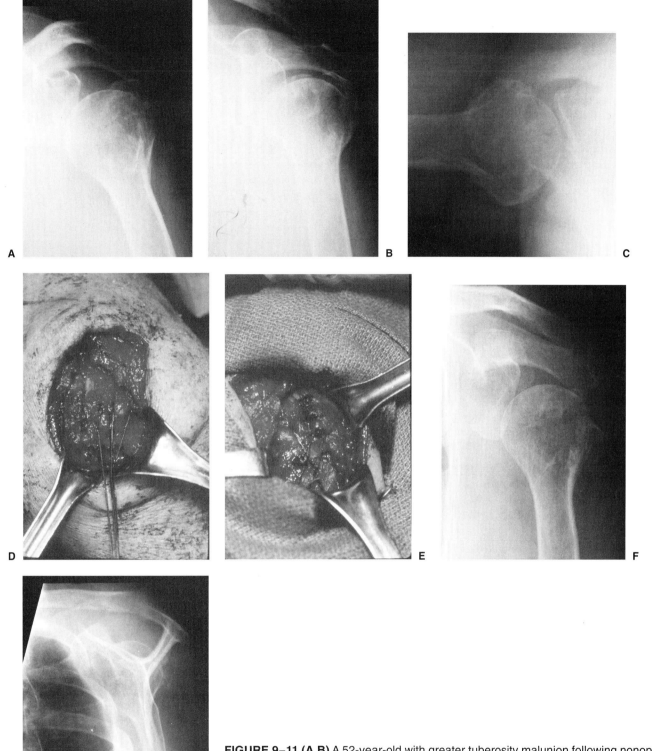

FIGURE 9–11 (A,B) A 52-year-old with greater tuberosity malunion following nonoperative management, resulting in painful, limited range of motion. The tuberosity is displaced superiorly into the subacromial space. **(C)** Axillary view does not show significant posterior displacement. **(D,E)** Treatment consisted of osteotomy, mobilization, and reattachment using tension band suture fixation. **(F,G)** Postoperative radiographs show the tuberosity in fixed position.

strengthening program is not initiated until at least 12 weeks following the surgery.

Surgical neck malunion most commonly occurs following two-part fractures. The deforming forces acting on this fracture are the pectoralis major displacing the humeral shaft anteriorly and medially and the rotator cuff abducting the humeral head. Nonoperative management of surgical neck fractures can result in significant malunion if the degree of initial displacement or angulation is not appreciated. Inadequate closed reduction or displacement of an initially acceptable closed reduction can also result in malunion. It is important to note that some degree of nonanatomic alignment is compatible with acceptable function. As apex anterior or posterior angulation approaches and exceeds 30°, however, motion becomes more limited and pain is frequently encountered. Operative management of two-part surgical neck fractures can also result in malunion if an adequate reduction is not obtained or, more commonly, reduction cannot be maintained with the fixation utilized. The poor bone quality frequently associated with these fractures is an important factor contributing to loss of reduction.

A complete radiographic evaluation is required to determine the multiplanar deformity of the surgical neck malunion. The deformity typically consists of varying degrees of apex anterior angulation, internal rotation, and varus. The varus deformity limits abduction and places the greater tuberosity into a prominent superior position. Forward elevation is limited by the amount of apex anterior angulation. A complete understanding of the nature of the malunion is essential to determine an appropriate treatment plan.

Operative management of surgical neck malunion should be considered in patients who have significant pain and functional limitations that interfere with their ability to perform daily activities. In surgical neck malunions, the articular surface is usually uninvolved. Therefore, corrective osteotomy, restoration of alignment, and internal fixation are preferred.[5,11] The type of fixation chosen should be based on the location of the osteotomy and the bone quality. In general, we prefer to use plate and screw fixation with either a blade plate or a locking plate (Fig. **9–12**). The procedure is performed using a deltopectoral approach. The soft tissue layers should be developed particularly at the deeper layers to enhance the "gliding" needed to regain range of motion. Adequate mobilization of the proximal fragment is very important. This is usually accomplished by mobilization of the subacromial space and the subdeltoid space. In some situations, however, release of the coracohumeral ligament area and excision of the coracoacromial ligament may be necessary. If there is concern about intraarticular adhesions, the rotator interval should be opened and intraarticular release is performed. It is important to mobilize the proximal fragment to avoid stresses at the osteotomy site, which could interfere with healing.

After mobilization of the proximal humerus, the area of malunion should be exposed. It is important to correlate the intraoperative findings with the preoperative radiographic evaluation. To accomplish this, it is often necessary to obtain intraoperative radiographs to confirm the location and direction of the osteotomy. A single-plane osteotomy may be sufficient but usually a wedge-shaped osteotomy is necessary to obtain the required correction. The rotational component of the malunion can be corrected by rotating the fragments after the osteotomy. Rotational alignment can be determined by evaluation of the biceps tendon as it passes through the bicipital groove into the distal fragment. For fixation of the osteotomy, we prefer a blade plate or a locking plate. A guidewire should be placed in the proximal fragment, and biplanar intraoperative imaging used to confirm proper location. Compression at the osteotomy site is essential. If a wedge osteotomy is performed, the bone removed should be utilized to bone graft the site. A complete set of radiographs should be obtained intraoperatively to confirm reduction of the malunion and proper placement of the fixation device. Intraoperative assessment of fixation stability should be used to determine the parameters for the postoperative rehabilitation program.

Postoperatively, the patient is maintained in a sling and started on an assisted range-of-motion program, including forward elevation and internal and external rotation. Active range of motion can be initiated approximately 6 to 8 weeks following the surgery when there is evidence of healing of the osteotomy. More vigorous stretching can be performed 10 to 12 weeks following the surgery when healing has progressed.

More complex malunions occur following three- and four-part fractures. In these situations, articular incongruity, degenerative changes, and osteonecrosis can be present, making proximal humeral replacement with osteotomy and reconstruction of the tuberosities the recommended management (Fig. **9–13**); however, outcomes following proximal humeral replacement in this context have been less satisfactory than when the procedure is performed for acute fractures.[12] This is particularly true if the patient has had previous ORIF and when tuberosity osteotomy is required.[13,14] Osteotomy and internal fixation of three- or four-part malunions has limited indications. It is generally considered in young patients with good bone quality in whom adequate fixation and healing can be obtained and in whom prosthetic replacement is less desirable.

Proximal humeral replacement for three- and four-part malunions utilizes the techniques described previously. An anterior deltopectoral approach is used with mobilization of the subacromial and subdeltoid spaces. The

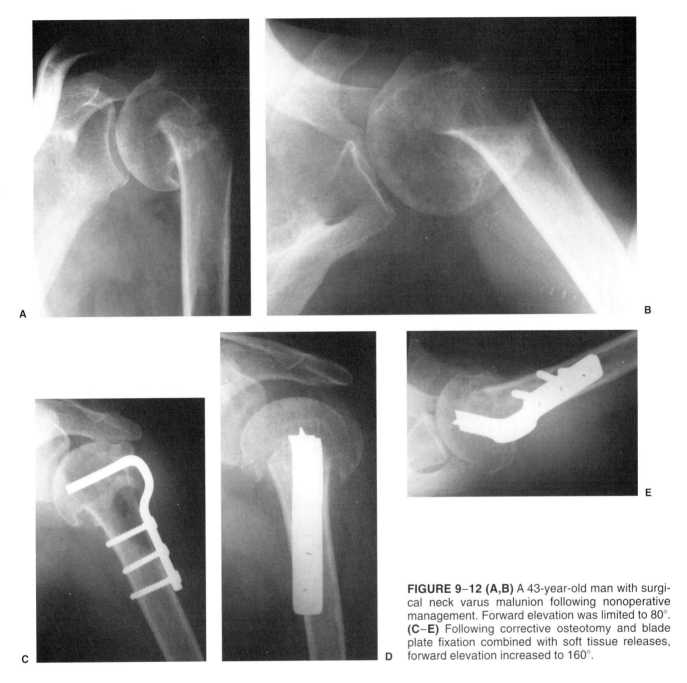

FIGURE 9–12 (A,B) A 43-year-old man with surgical neck varus malunion following nonoperative management. Forward elevation was limited to 80°. (C–E) Following corrective osteotomy and blade plate fixation combined with soft tissue releases, forward elevation increased to 160°.

proximal humeral anatomy must be carefully identified. The biceps tendon should be identified and tagged. This facilitates identification of the tuberosities. The lesser tuberosity with the subscapularis attached should be identified. It should be osteotomized with an adequate amount of bone to facilitate reattachment. This allows visualization of the articular surface and the greater tuberosity. Osteotomy of the greater tuberosity should include the entire tuberosity, which includes its superior and posterior portions. Based on the anatomy of the malunion, this may result in two fragments: a superior portion and a more posterior portion. Each one must be tagged at the rotator cuff tendon insertion.

The articular surface identified can then be visualized. It should be osteotomized at a level that preserves as much shaft as possible. Extramuscular and intraarticular mobilization of the tuberosities is performed to allow tension-free reattachment. At this point, the reconstruction consists of the technique described in Chapter 7 for a four-part fracture. It is important to emphasize the need for adequate mobilization of tuberosities with secure fixation to the prosthesis, the shaft, and to each other. The removed articular surface should be used to bone graft the tuberosity reattachment site to enhance healing. In some long-standing malunions, there may be significant degenerative changes of the glenoid, although in our

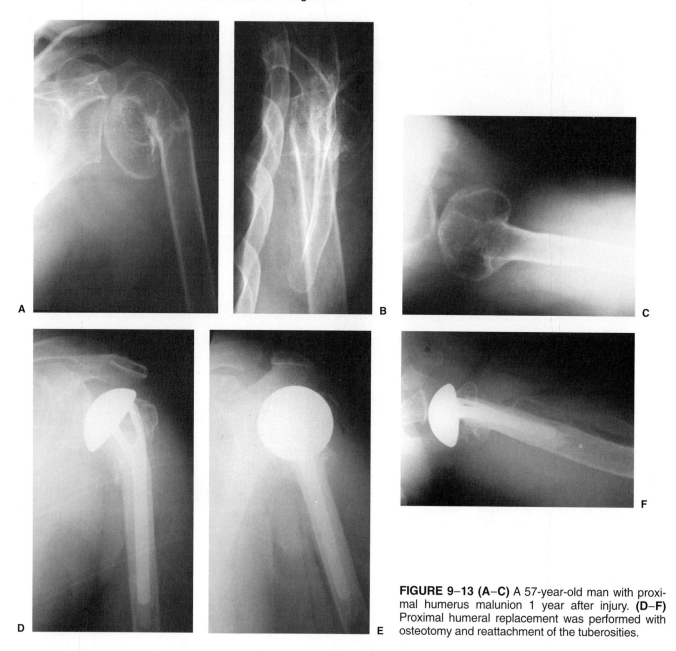

FIGURE 9–13 (A–C) A 57-year-old man with proximal humerus malunion 1 year after injury. **(D–F)** Proximal humeral replacement was performed with osteotomy and reattachment of the tuberosities.

experience this has been uncommon. When present, placement of a glenoid component is indicated.

Osteonecrosis

Osteonecrosis occurs more commonly after three- and four-part fractures and fracture-dislocations than less complex injuries. The arcuate artery, a terminal branch of the anterior circumflex humeral artery, provides the main blood supply to the humeral head. The rotator cuff insertions and the medial periosteal blood vessels provide secondary blood supply.[15,16] Osteonecrosis can develop from disrupting the blood supply at the time of fracture or as a result of additional devascularization secondary to operative management.

Four-part fractures that disrupt the soft tissue attachments to the articular surface have the greatest risk for osteonecrosis. Neer[3] reported osteonecrosis in six of eight four-part fractures, and therefore, advocated prosthetic replacement. Although this was a very small series, it resulted in significant treatment recommendations. Subsequent reports have documented a 20 to 75% incidence of osteonecrosis depending on the pattern of displacement and the fracture involved.[17–21] Valgus-impacted fractures without lateral displacement of the articular surface do not develop osteonecrosis as frequently because the intact medial periosteal hinge often maintains the blood supply to the articular surface.[22,23]

Less comminuted fractures of the proximal humerus have lower rates of osteonecrosis because the soft tissues with their associated vascular supply remain attached to the articular segment. The incidence in three-part fractures and fracture-dislocations has reported to vary from 3 to 25%.[3,24,25] Sturzenegger et al[21] found that ORIF of three-part fractures with plates and screws resulted in a higher incidence of osteonecrosis than those treated with limited internal fixation. Lee and Hansen[18] also reported that following ORIF, osteonecrosis may not be apparent for up to 2 years following surgery. When osteonecrosis develops following ORIF, collapse of the articular surface can result in prominence of the internal fixation device, which results in secondary damage to the glenoid articular surface.[1] Even though the incidence of osteonecrosis following three- and four-part fractures can be significant, it is important to understand that it is not always associated with significant symptoms. Gerber et al[26] reported that osteonecrosis of the articular surface with anatomically reduced tuberosities provided results equivalent to humeral head replacement performed for acute fractures. Wijgman et al[25] reported that 17 of 22 patients with osteonecrosis following ORIF of three- or four-part fractures maintained good or excellent Constant scores irrespective of the radiographic changes present.

Symptomatic osteonecrosis of the humeral head following proximal humeral fracture can be treated in different ways. The most important consideration is the degree of pain and disability. Mild symptoms can be treated nonoperatively with antiinflammatory medication, nonnarcotic analgesics, and a therapy program to maintain or improve range of motion. When the degree of pain and disability is significant, however, operative management is indicated and will usually consist of humeral head replacement or total shoulder replacement based on the degree of involvement of the glenoid. An important component of the preoperative assessment is an understanding of the degree of deformity of the proximal humerus that may be present. This is particularly important with respect to the position of the tuberosities and the surgical neck and shaft. If the tuberosities are in near-anatomic position and there is no significant shaft malalignment, prosthetic replacement can be performed without corrective osteotomies. If there is significant deformity of the proximal humerus, however, then corrective osteotomies will be necessary. This adds to the complexity of the procedure and increases the potential for complications. Significant residual displacement of the tuberosities requires osteotomies and mobilization to allow reattachment with minimal tension. This decreases the risk of fixation failure and redisplacement postoperatively. The decision to proceed with glenoid resurfacing is based on both the preoperative assessment of the symptoms and the intraoperative assessment of the glenoid articular surface (Fig. **9–14**). The results of prosthetic replacement for osteonecrosis following fracture depend primarily on the degree of proximal humeral deformity and the need for corrective osteotomies. Proximal humeral replacement for chronic fracture problems (osteonecrosis and other complications) has less satisfactory outcomes and a greater incidence of complications compared with prosthetic replacement for acute proximal humeral fractures.[12]

Nerve Injury

Neurologic injury associated with proximal humeral fractures can occur as a result of the injury, a closed reduction maneuver, or operative management. Assessment of nerve function at the time of the initial evaluation is essential, although it can be difficult due to the pain associated with the injury. Every effort must be made, however, to obtain a complete neurologic assessment at the time of injury that includes the axillary, suprascapular, and musculocutaneous nerves and terminal branches of the brachial plexus.[27,28]

Clinically significant nerve injuries have been reported in 9 to 50% of proximal humeral fractures[3,28–30]; however, Visser et al[31] performed a prospective electromyographic (EMG) study in patients following proximal humerus fractures and documented that 67% of patients had evidence of nerve injuries, with most patients having more than one nerve affected. Of these nerve injuries, 86% involved the axillary nerve and 72% involved the suprascapular nerve; 82% of displaced fractures had an associated nerve deficit; however, 59% of nondisplaced fractures also had EMG evidence of nerve compromise. In this study, all deficits resolved, but recovery of shoulder function was prolonged.[31] Fracture-dislocations are more commonly associated with nerve injury (77%) than simple glenohumeral dislocations (48%). Fracture-dislocations also have a greater incidence of multiple nerve involvement and the potential for more significant nerve injury.[32,33]

Several studies have documented an increased incidence of nerve palsy following proximal humeral fracture in elderly patients. Although permanent nerve palsies occur in up to only 8% of patients sustaining these fractures, they are reported in up to 50% of cases when the fracture and the nerve injury are secondary to blunt trauma to the lateral aspect of the shoulder.[27,31,34] This combination of factors results in direct injury to the nerve. Nerve injury can occur as a result of treatment by closed manipulation or operative management. The risk of nerve injury with closed reductions is relatively small. It generally occurs in association with repeated attempts at closed reduction.[3] Operative management carries an increased risk of nerve injury, although the incidence remains relatively small.[12] In each of these situations, it is essential to document neurologic function at the time of injury and prior to any closed manipulation or operative

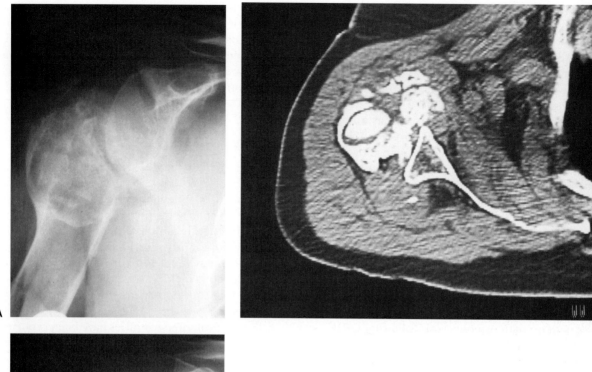

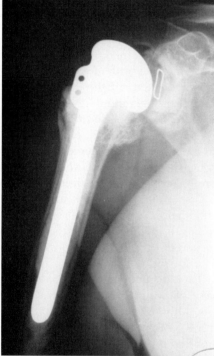

FIGURE 9–14 (A,B) This 69-year-old woman developed osteonecrosis 2 years following ORIF with tension band suture of a four-part proximal humerus fracture. There were significant glenoid degenerative changes. **(C)** Patient underwent total shoulder replacement with resolution of pain and excellent function.

management. With this approach, nerve compromise as a result of the injury can be clearly differentiated from nerve injury as a result of treatment.

Axillary nerve injury generally recovers completely within 4 to 6 months in the vast majority of cases. Other nerve injuries generally recover in a somewhat longer period of time.[35] With persistent deficits, initial baseline electrodiagnostic studies should be obtained 4 weeks following the injury. A follow-up study should be obtained 3 months following the injury if there is no clinical

evidence of improvement.[36] Complete recovery can take up to 12 months, but operative treatment should be considered if there is no clinical or electrodiagnostic evidence of recovery within 6 months after injury.[36,37]

A complete axillary nerve deficit with associated deltoid paralysis most commonly requires nerve grafting in the area of the quadrilateral space. This is the area where the nerve becomes tethered as a result of a traction injury. Direct nerve repair, decompression, and nerve transfer are less commonly used techniques. Grafting is typically recommended because the zone of injury usually involves several centimeters of the nerve. The anatomy of the axillary nerve makes it difficult to mobilize sufficiently to perform a direct repair.[36,38] The monofascicular pattern of the nerve and the relatively short length of the nerve are factors that have resulted in a satisfactory outcome in 66 to 93% of patients undergoing grafting procedures.[35–39] The best results of nerve grafting have resulted when the procedure is performed within 6 months of injury; however, functional improvement can be expected if the procedure is performed within 12 months of injury.[38–40] Several authors have documented that in the presence of combined axillary and suprascapular nerve injuries, a repair of both nerves is required to obtain a good functional result.[40,41]

Nerve grafting is not beneficial in the patient presenting more than 2 years after complete axillary nerve palsy due to muscle wasting. For these patients, muscle transfers should be considered primarily in those patients in whom significant shoulder disability affects all activities.[36] Young patients may fatigue easily but can demonstrate a functional range of motion despite the palsy (Fig. 9–15). For these patients, additional muscle transfer procedures would not be expected to result in significant improvement. The muscle transfers utilized for complete deltoid paralysis include transfer of the trapezius insertion from the acromion to the humerus or bipolar transposition of latissimus dorsi.[36]

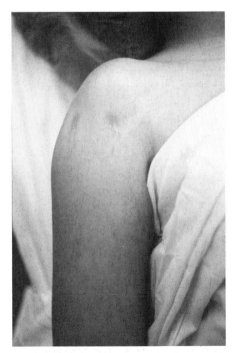

FIGURE 9–15 A 36-year-old woman with axillary nerve deficit following proximal humerus fracture treated by open reduction and pinning. Deltoid atrophy is noted. Three years following the surgery the nerve has not recovered, although the patient has regained a functional range of motion.

Vascular Injury

Vascular injuries associated with proximal humeral fractures occur much less commonly than nerve injuries. Careful examination at the time of injury with particular emphasis on the strength of the distal pulse in each upper extremity should be performed. Collateral vasculature about the shoulder makes it feasible to maintain a radial pulse in the presence of an axillary artery injury. If vascular compromise is suspected, Doppler examination can determine the magnitude and the quality of the distal arterial pulse. Vascular specialists should be promptly consulted to determine whether an arteriogram is indicated. Localization of the vascular injury determines the appropriate treatment.[1,42,43]

The axillary artery is susceptible to injury with surgical neck fractures (Fig. 9–16).[1,44] Fracture fragments can cause direct injury to the artery itself, or a branch of the axillary artery can be entrapped within the fracture, resulting in stretching or avulsion of the artery. The humeral circumflex and subscapular arteries originate on the axillary artery near the level of the surgical neck of the humerus, creating a tether on the artery at this level. Vascular injury can occur at the time of injury, even if the fracture appears nondisplaced at the time of evaluation.[45] Brachial plexus deficits are commonly encountered in association with vascular injuries due to the proximity of the cords to the branches of the axillary artery. The combination of a decreased distal pulse and a brachial plexus injury should increase the suspicion for arterial injury.

The treatment of arterial injury associated with proximal humeral fractures represents a combined effort of the vascular specialist and the orthopaedic surgeon. Stable internal fixation of the fracture should be obtained prior to vascular repair. This protects the repair from additional injury from fracture fragments or from displacement of the fragments. If the diagnosis of the vascular injury has been delayed and limb viability is at risk, it may be necessary for the vascular surgeon to achieve temporary flow first followed by stabilization of the fracture. The vascular specialist can then perform a definitive repair after limb viability has been addressed.

Joint Stiffness

Loss of motion is the most common "complication" following proximal humerus fractures. Some degree of loss of motion is associated with virtually all of these fractures, so it may be inappropriate to consider this a complication. As the degree of loss of motion increases and function becomes more compromised, however, stiffness becomes a more obvious complication. The etiology of postfracture stiffness is multifactorial. It is

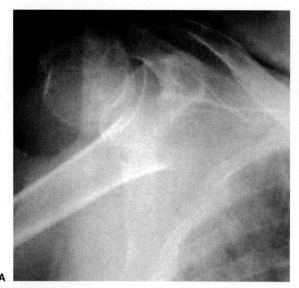

A

FIGURE 9–16 (A) This 68-year-old woman sustained a displaced surgical neck fracture while intoxicated. Following closed reduction, clinical findings included a reduced Doppler pressure of the radial artery of the affected extremity.

B

(B) Angiogram showed the axillary artery to be in the fracture site, necessitating vascular repair combined with open reduction and fracture fixation.

important to differentiate stiffness secondary to soft tissue contracture from loss of motion associated with malunion. Even in cases of malunion, secondary soft tissue contracture also contributes to stiffness and may be the primary etiology.

Treatment of postfracture stiffness should be directed at the underlying cause. In the absence of bony deformity a structured, supervised therapy program should be instituted. In many cases, this results in improved range of motion, particularly if the patient was not compliant during the early stages of therapy; however, in those patients who are compliant with therapy but do not improve, soft tissue releases should be considered. These can generally be performed arthroscopically with a combination of capsular release, as well as lysis of adhesions within the subacromial space. When significant stiffness is associated with malunion, it may be necessary to correct the malunion in combination with soft tissue releases to obtain improvement. It is also important to determine whether articular incongruity is contributing to the stiffness. In this context, when degenerative changes are present, prosthetic replacement in combination with soft tissue releases should be considered.

Heterotopic Ossification

Heterotopic ossification is an uncommon complication following proximal humeral fractures. It most commonly occurs following operative management, but even in this context, it is relatively uncommon. Patients who sustain higher energy injuries (fracture-dislocations) (Fig. **9–17**)

and those with associated head injuries or burns are at a greater risk of heterotopic ossification with both nonoperative and operative treatment. Additional factors associated with the development of heterotopic ossification include repeated closed reductions and delayed operative management.[46] Operative management more than 2 weeks following surgery seems to increase the risk of heterotopic ossification. This is most likely due to disturbance of the fracture site during the period of

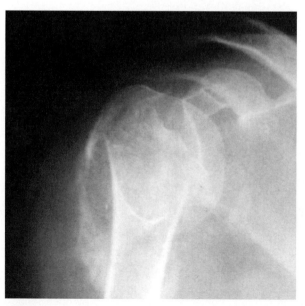

FIGURE 9–17 This 38-year-old man developed heterotopic ossification 4 weeks following closed reduction of a fracture-dislocation.

fracture hematoma organization and early callus formation.

When heterotopic ossification is present, it is not necessarily associated with significant functional disability.[47] Limited heterotopic bone anteriorly, posteriorly, or laterally will not significantly decrease range of motion. However, extensive heterotopic ossification, particularly when there is bridging bone across the subacromial space or the glenohumeral joint, has a major impact on range of motion. In these situations, excision should be considered to improve motion. Resection of heterotopic bone has to be carefully planned with a clear understanding of the location of the heterotopic bone. A preoperative CT scan is helpful in delineating the location and the amount of bone present. Heterotopic bone in medial and inferior locations requires careful microvascular dissection because of the proximity of the neurovascular structures.[48,49] This is usually performed in conjunction with a microvascular surgeon using either magnifying loupes or the operating microscope. Bridging heterotopic bone located anteriorly, laterally, or posteriorly also requires careful dissection. It is often located within the rotator cuff or deltoid muscles. Resection may compromise the integrity of the rotator cuff tissue, requiring repair of any full-thickness defects. In addition, any bone that interferes with the subacromial space should be removed to restore unobstructed gliding.

■ Complications Following Humeral Head Replacement

Complications following humeral head replacement for acute proximal humeral fractures include infection, neurologic injury, periprosthetic fracture, instability, tuberosity malunion and nonunion, rotator cuff tear, heterotopic ossification, glenoid erosion, and stiffness. The incidence of these complications based on a review of the literature is shown in Table 9–1.[3,47,50–57] Although the incidence of any specific complication is relatively low, the cumulative incidence represents 15% or more. For each of these complications we will discuss those factors that predispose to their occurrence, the treatment options available, and the preventive measures that can be considered to minimize the risk.

Infection

The incidence of infection or wound healing problems for this procedure is ~4% (Table 9–1). This includes acute postoperative infections (within 30 days of the surgery) and subacute or delayed presentation within 6 months of the procedure. Both presentations generally represent infection that develops at the time of surgery.

A late infection (more than 6 months after the procedure) more commonly represents hematogenous seeding of the surgical site as a result of an infection at another site (urinary tract infection, dental infection, etc.). The factors that increase the risk of infection include a second operation performed within a short period of time, for example, early failed internal fixation revised to humeral head replacement. Immunocompromised patients are also at increased risk for infection. This at-risk group includes patients with chronic renal failure on dialysis, patients with nutritional deficiencies, patients receiving chemotherapy, and diabetic patients.

The treatment is determined, in part, by the time of presentation. An acute postoperative infection can be treated with urgent irrigation and debridement. Every effort should be made to maintain the security of the tuberosity fixation. For acute infections, one attempt at saving the implant is reasonable. Following debridement, the patient should be placed on intravenous antibiotics as determined by the results of culture and sensitivity testing. We also encourage consultation with an infectious disease specialist to optimize the choice of antibiotics. The success of this approach is difficult to determine because of the small number of patients reported. It is more likely to be successful when the organism involved has a high sensitivity to standard intravenous antibiotics. It is less likely to be successful when gram-negative organisms or those with a limited sensitivity spectrum are involved. If the initial attempt at debridement is not successful and a second debridement is necessary, it should include removal of the implant and cement, and insertion of an antibiotic-impregnated cement spacer. At the same time, the tuberosities should be secured to the shaft in anticipation of potential reimplantation at a later time. Delayed infections should be treated by debridement with removal of the implant and insertion of an antibiotic impregnated cement spacer (Fig. 9–18). These infections are more likely to involve the bone–cement interface and require implant removal. Treatment of late hematogenous infections can be variable. A patient who develops an "acute" infection 5 days following a urinary tract infection or periodontal infection can be treated as an acute infection as long as the x-rays do not show evidence of involvement of the bone–cement interface or other findings that suggest a chronic component; however, if the initial debridement is not successful, a more extensive debridement with prosthesis removal is necessary.

Prevention of infection following humeral head replacement for fracture requires meticulous attention to surgical prepping and draping, particularly because of the potential contamination from the axilla. Perioperative antibiotics should be utilized. Meticulous handling of soft tissues is important, particularly in the context of an acute injury. The fact that these injuries occur more commonly

TABLE 9–1 Complications of Humeral Head Replacement (HHR) for Acute Proximal Humeral Fractures

Series	Number of Fractures	Average Follow-Up (months)	Tuberosity Migration or Cuff Deficiency	Superficial Infection	HO Formation	Instability	Deep Infection	Periprosthetic Fracture	Neurodeficit	Symptomatic Loosening	Contracture	Total
Neer 1970	43	58	2(5%)				1(2%)		1(2%)			4(9.3%)
Kraulis 1976	11	36			4(36%)		2(18%)	1(9%)	2(18%)			9(81.8%)
Willems 1986	10	30										0(0%)
Moeckell 1992	22	36	1(5%)			1(5%)						2(9.1%)
Green 1993	24	37	1(4%)								1(4%)	2(8.3%)
Hawkins 1993	20	40				3(15%)						5(25%)
Compito 1994	64	33	4(6%)				1(2%)		1(5%)	1(5%)	1(2%)	6(9.4%)
Goldman 1995	22	30		1(5%)	3(14%)	1(3%)						4(18.2%)
Dimakopoulos 1997	38	37	2(5%)		2(5%)	3(2%)	2(1%)	3(2%)		1(1%)		5(13.2%)
Robinson 2003	138	76	3(2%)	9(7%)								21(15.2%)
Total	392		13(3.3%)	10(2.6%)	9(2.3%)	8(2.0%)	6(1.5%)	4(1.0%)	4(1.0%)	2(0.5%)	2(0.5%)	58(14.8%)

HO, heterotopic ossification

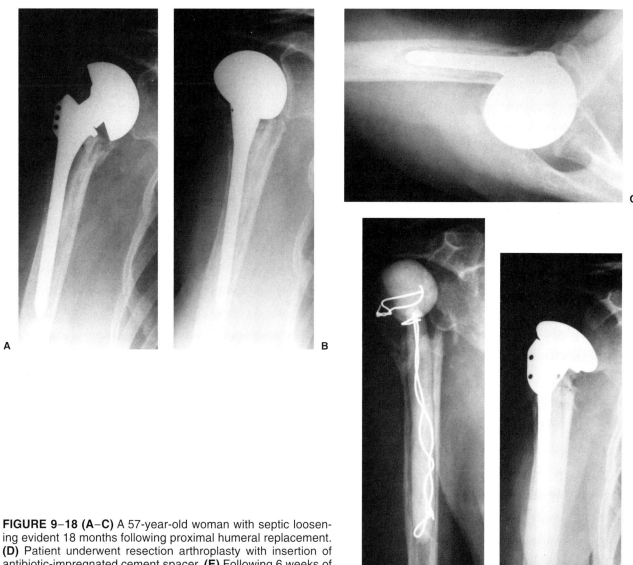

FIGURE 9–18 (A–C) A 57-year-old woman with septic loosening evident 18 months following proximal humeral replacement. **(D)** Patient underwent resection arthroplasty with insertion of antibiotic-impregnated cement spacer. **(E)** Following 6 weeks of intravenous antibiotics, reimplementation was performed.

in elderly patients, whose tissues are more sensitive to injury and surgery, further emphasizes its importance.

Nerve Injury

The incidence of neurologic injury in association with this type of surgery is difficult to determine. The literature indicates the incidence to be on the order of 1% (Table 9–1). As noted earlier, the incidence of neurologic injury associated with proximal humeral fractures is reported to be higher, particularly when electrodiagnostic studies have been utilized. Differentiating a neurologic injury that occurs as a result of the injury from one that occurs as a result of the subsequent surgery is very important for different reasons, including patient management and potential medicolegal issues. A complete neurologic evaluation preoperatively is essential to

identify those deficits associated with the injury. Consequently, a complete neurologic exam postoperatively is also essential to identify any procedure-related deficits.

Operative management of proximal humeral fractures carries a risk for nerve injury. For the axillary nerve, this can occur as it passes in an anterior to posterior direction just below the glenohumeral joint. Retraction in this area, particularly in the subacute setting, can result in axillary nerve injury, which is usually a neuropraxia. However, passage of sutures in this area should be performed carefully and with clear visualization to avoid direct injury to the nerve. The musculocutaneous nerve may be injured by retraction of the conjoined tendon muscles, particularly if the traction is applied more distally. There is also a risk of injury to the suprascapular nerve, although this is less common. It can occur during the treatment of chronic fracture cases in which significant mobilization of the tuberosities and rotator cuff is necessary.[12,58,59] Release of the capsule at the glenoid rim may result in direct injury to the nerve if mobilization exceeds more than 1 cm medial to the glenoid margin.[60]

An axillary nerve deficit that occurs following humeral head replacement should be evaluated carefully. If there is concern about a direct nerve injury (i.e., possible laceration), somatosensory evoked potentials (SSEPs) should be performed following the surgery to confirm the continuity of the nerve. If continuity is confirmed, then observation is the preferred approach, as described earlier. If the SSEPs indicate a disruption of the nerve, early exploration and repair should be considered[36]; however, experience with this approach is limited and is based on the general approach to nerve injuries of this type.

Certainly the best method of treating neurologic injuries is with prevention. At the time of operative management, careful dissection and exposure minimize the risk of nerve injury.[61] Excessive retraction, particularly on the conjoined tendon muscles, should be avoided. Palpation of the axillary nerve during the procedure facilitates continuous awareness of its location, with the goal of avoiding injury.

Periprosthetic Fractures: Intraoperative and Postoperative

Fractures of the proximal humerus can occur intraoperatively during humeral head replacement or postoperatively as a result of fall or other injury mechanism. Intraoperative fractures can occur as a result of extension of the proximal fracture into the shaft or from propagation through the drill holes that are placed through the humeral cortex to facilitate tuberosity reattachment. Forceful manipulation of the humerus during the procedure, particularly to gain exposure, can result in propagation of the proximal fracture. Cementing of the humeral stem with excessive pressurization can also result in fracture when the bone is very osteopenic.

Treatment of fractures that occur intraoperatively depends on their location and the degree of extension.[62–64] Fractures of the proximal portion of the shaft that do not extend beyond the level of the humeral stem can usually be treated with cerclage fixation. With this technique, care must be taken to prevent extravasation of cement into and through the fracture site during cementing of the implant. If the fracture extends distal to the humeral stem, a long stem component with cerclage fixation should be utilized. If a long stem component is not available, then a plate or a strut graft across the junction of the stem and fracture

should be utilized. The plate should be cerclaged in place to avoid the need for screw fixation. If a fracture occurs during cementing with extravasation of the cement through a distal fracture, the area should be explored and the cement removed. There have been reports of nerve injury associated with extravasation of cement from the humeral shaft. This usually represents a thermal injury from the cement, which is particularly problematic because thermal injuries have a poor prognosis for recovery.

Intraoperative fractures can be prevented with careful meticulous technique. Forced manipulation of the shaft should be avoided. Insertion of the humeral component requires the humerus to be placed in extension. This may be difficult if the patient is not properly positioned on the operating table. Therefore, proper positioning prior to the start of surgery is important to assure adequate exposure. The drill holes for passage of sutures for tuberosity fixation should be distal enough to the fracture to minimize the possibility of propagation. Fractures that occur during cementing with pressurization can be avoided with careful technique. Some have recommended avoiding the use of cement restrictors to minimize the pressurization; however, we feel use of a cement restrictor is important for proper cementing technique. With these approaches, the possibility of an intraoperative humeral shaft fracture should be minimized.

Periprosthetic fractures that occur postoperatively are usually the result of a fall either onto the outstretched upper extremity or directly onto the humerus. Evaluation of these fractures should focus on the location of the fracture in relation to the implant and whether the implant stability is compromised by the fracture. Although the treatment of each patient should be individualized based on an evaluation of fracture factors and patient factors, there are general principles that should be followed.

Treatment of isolated tuberosity fractures depends on the degree of displacement and the presence of instability. Significant displacement of the greater or lesser tuberosity, particularly when instability results, requires ORIF, usually with tension band suture fixation. The procedure is easier to perform within 3 weeks after the injury; longer delays makes mobilization and reattachment difficult.

Periprosthetic humeral shaft fractures usually extend distal to the tip of the implant. It is very uncommon to encounter a proximal shaft fracture that is limited to the length of the implant that did not occur intraoperatively.

Factors to consider when treating periprosthetic fractures that extend beyond the distal end of the implant include (1) the stability of the implant within the canal,

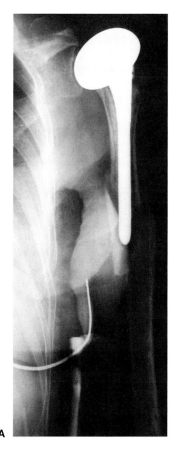
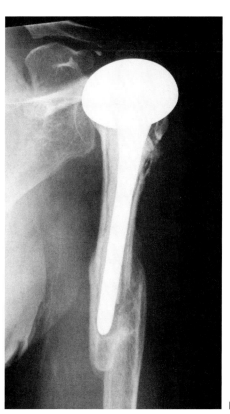

A   B

FIGURE 9–19 (A,B) A 56-year-old woman sustained a periprosthetic fracture following a fall that was treated with a fracture orthosis, resulting in a healed fracture with acceptable alignment.

(2) presence of a cementless or cemented implant, (3) the degree of comminution, (4) bone quality, (5) position of the stem with respect to the distal humeral canal, (6) overall alignment of the humerus, and (7) the impact of a period of immobilization on the function of the proximal humeral replacement. In general, if the implant is aligned with the distal shaft and the overall alignment is acceptable, nonoperative management with a fracture orthosis can be considered (Fig. **9–19**). When the implant cannot be aligned with the distal portion of the shaft and early mobilization is a necessity, operative treatment is indicated consisting of ORIF. Fixation options include plate fixation utilizing a combination of screws distally and cerclage cables/wires proximally. Cortical strut grafts with cerclage can also be used. We frequently utilize a combination of plate fixation with a cortical strut oriented 90° to each other (Fig. **9–8**). Although long stem implants can be used for intraoperative fractures, they are not used for distal periprosthetic fractures because of the difficulty anticipated during removal of the stem, particularly when cemented fixation has been used. Even with noncemented implants, the risk of further compromising the thin humeral cortical bone during implant removal is significant; therefore, our preference is to fix the fracture

as described. If implant loosening becomes a symptomatic problem subsequently, revision can be accomplished more easily in the presence of an intact, well-aligned humeral shaft.

Instability

The incidence of instability following humeral head replacement is most likely underreported. The definition of instability can be quite variable, which affects the reported incidence of this problem. For example, does superior subluxation represent a problem of instability or a rotator cuff problem? How this problem is interpreted affects the incidence of the specific complications being considered. Nonetheless, even in the context of variable reporting, there are important factors that predispose to development of instability following this surgery, including component malposition, rotator cuff compromise, and tuberosity problems.[61]

An important predisposing factor is component malposition. If the component is placed in an incorrect amount of version (Fig. **9–20**) and, if proper restoration of humeral length is not achieved (Fig. **9–21**), the risk of instability is greater.[55,61] Insertion of the component in proper version relies on utilization of consistent

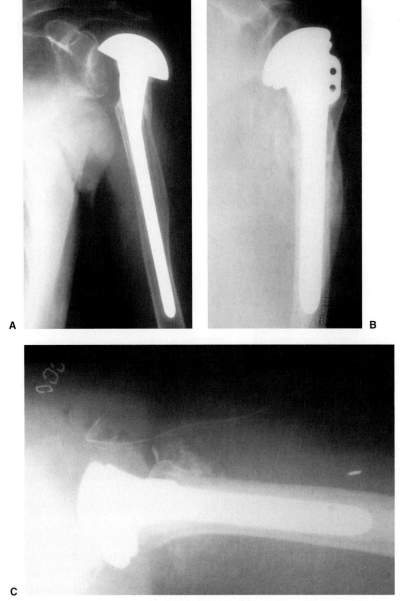

FIGURE 9–20 (A) A 73-year-old woman with pain and limited motion associated with excessive retroversion of a noncemented monobloc humeral head replacement. **(B,C)** Revision to a modular cemented component resulted in resolution of pain and improved range of motion.

landmarks. The goal of placing the component in 20° to 40° of retroversion should be consistently attained. Obtaining the proper version and length during cementing can be difficult because of the absence of metaphyseal bone support. It is very important to maintain the component in the proper amount of retroversion and height during cementing and to maintain this position until the cement has completely hardened. Prevention of these problems should be based on the surgeon having a reliable method to both obtain and maintain position during insertion.[65] Although some authors have described techniques that do not utilize cement, we feel that cemented insertion is mandatory to maintain proper position, particularly in the absence of metaphyseal bone support. If proper position is not obtained at the time of surgery and there is a significant risk of instability, then the component should be revised. If instability develops postoperatively and is felt to be secondary to component position, revision surgery should also be considered. This is more likely to be considered in patients who present with significant pain and weakness associated with the instability.

Rotator cuff compromise can cause instability and usually develops as a result of tuberosity compromise.[61,66] The importance of secure tuberosity fixation and proper position cannot be overemphasized.[14,55,59,67] When tuberosity detachment occurs, particularly early following the procedure, instability can often result.

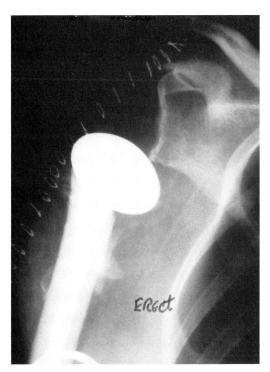

FIGURE 9–21 A 66-year-old woman with inferior instability following humeral head replacement secondary to inadequate restoration of humeral length and postoperative deltoid atony.

Detachment of the lesser tuberosity compromises the anterior support and can result in anterior instability (Fig. **9–22**). Detachment of the greater tuberosity can result in significant superior instability as well as anterior instability (Fig. **9–23**). Although posterior instability can occur, it is less commonly encountered.

The factors that predispose to instability from tuberosity detachment are inadequate tuberosity fixation or the patient's noncompliance with a rehabilitation program designed to avoid early active range of motion.[14,55,66,68] Certainly, secure tuberosity fixation and reattachment using the principles discussed previously will decrease the risk of fixation failure. The use of a supervised, structured rehabilitation program can limit the potential for lack of patient compliance.

The treatment for instability following tuberosity failure can be difficult. If the tuberosity detachment is identified early, then reattachment should be considered. Tuberosity detachment that is recognized more than 6 months after the surgery is more problematic. Mobilization and reattachment of the tuberosities in this situation can be quite difficult. Even with proper mobilization, healing is by no means certain. Nonetheless, in patients who are having significant pain, weakness, and instability, tuberosity reattachment should be considered.[61]

Tuberosity Nonunion

Failure to obtain union of the tuberosities is a significant complication following humeral head replacement for acute fractures. Some authors have documented a very high incidence of tuberosity migration, which can certainly predispose to nonunion (Table **9–1**). The factors that predispose to nonunion are related to the method of reattachment, particularly the ability to obtain proper reduction and secure fixation.[14,68] In addition, bone quality and soft tissue quality are factors that also compromise fixation.[14] The significance of a tuberosity nonunion can be quite variable. The degree of migration and displacement is important. Limited amounts of migration and displacement frequently result in weakness and limitation in range of motion but not in instability. With significant displacement, however, there will be weakness and limitation motion, as well as instability and pain (Fig. **9–22**). In this clinical setting, operative management should be considered.[61] The goal of this surgery is to mobilize the tuberosities and obtain a secure reattachment. This can be difficult because the factors that resulted in the nonunion are the same factors that impact the ability to obtain healing with revision surgery. Nonetheless, in selected patients with significant symptoms, this revision surgery should be undertaken.

The best approach to prevent tuberosity nonunion is utilization of an optimal method of reattachment. We have described the combination of longitudinal fixation to obtain contact between the tuberosity and the shaft and transverse/cerclage fixation to maintain contact of the tuberosities with each other and the shaft. Multiple sutures should be used to maximize the security of the repair. We also recommend the use of cancellous bone grafting from the removed humeral head to enhance the healing potential.[65]

Tuberosity Malunion

Malunion of the greater or lesser tuberosity can occur, although probably with less frequency than nonunion.[61] Malunion usually occurs as a result of either inadequate reduction at the time of surgery or inadequate fixation that allows migration of the fragment with healing in a malunited position[14]; however, the amount of migration is not sufficient to result in nonunion. The significance of the malunion is determined by the location and degree of displacement. Malunion of the lesser tuberosity is usually into a more medial position. This may limit internal rotation but is usually not a significant functional problem. Malunion of the greater tuberosity is of greater significance. If the tuberosity heals in a relatively superior position above the proximal extent of the prosthetic surface, it will interfere with the subacromial space

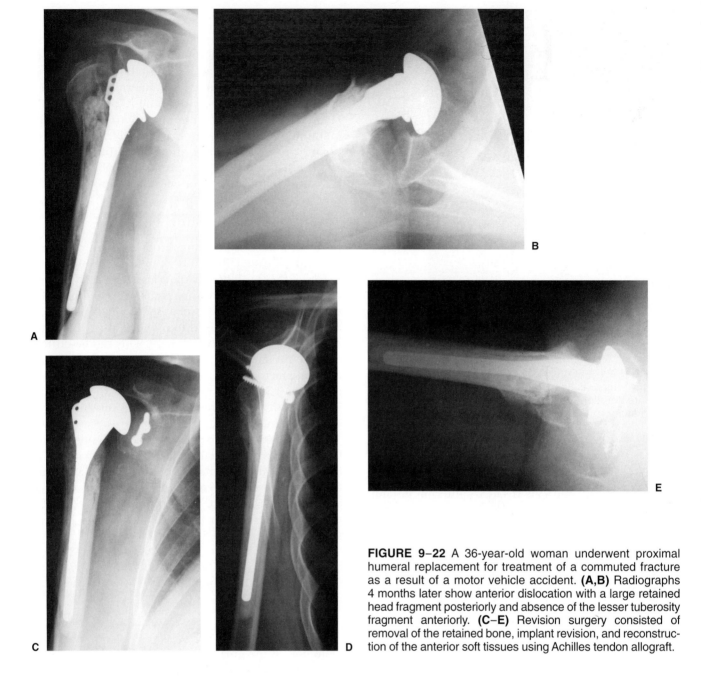

FIGURE 9–22 A 36-year-old woman underwent proximal humeral replacement for treatment of a commuted fracture as a result of a motor vehicle accident. **(A,B)** Radiographs 4 months later show anterior dislocation with a large retained head fragment posteriorly and absence of the lesser tuberosity fragment anteriorly. **(C–E)** Revision surgery consisted of removal of the retained bone, implant revision, and reconstruction of the anterior soft tissues using Achilles tendon allograft.

and limit forward elevation and abduction. When the tuberosity heals in a more posterior position, external rotation will be limited (Fig. **9–24**).[69]

The treatment of tuberosity malunion is dependent on the functional significance. If there is significant pain and limitation of motion, which can be attributed to the tuberosity malunion, operative management can be considered; however, it is important to accurately assess whether the malunion is the primary source of the symptoms and particularly the limitation of motion. When the malunion is judged to be the primary problem, treatment should consist of osteotomy, mobilization, and

reattachment to a more anatomic position. This procedure is difficult for a variety of reasons. First, mobilization can be difficult but is essential not only to reattaching the fragment in a more anatomic position but also to minimizing the tension on the fragment.[10] Second, the reattachment can also be difficult because the presence of the prosthesis can interfere with placement of transosseous fixation. If a modular humeral component is present, it may be possible to use a smaller size head to reduce the tension on the tuberosities[14]; however, this has to be considered carefully to avoid a suboptimal length–tension relationship on the intact tuberosity

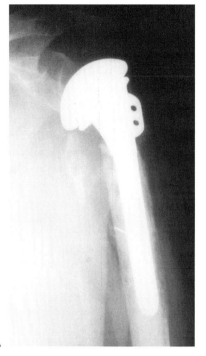

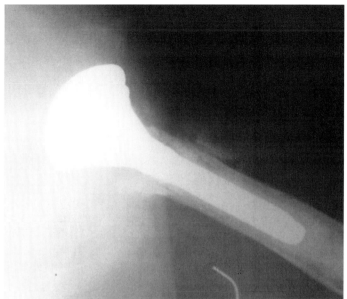

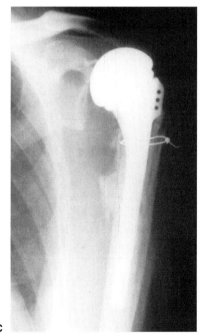

FIGURE 9–23 (A) Anterior instability following humeral head replacement resulting from displacement of the lesser tuberosity shown on an anteroposterior (AP) projection. **(B)** The anterior position of the humeral head in relation to the glenoid is evident on the axillary view. **(C)** Superior instability develops in this case as a result of postoperative displacement of the greater tuberosity.

and the attached soft tissues. In some patients with superior position of the greater tuberosity, subacromial decompression can be considered; however, this does not correct the underlying deformity and should be considered only in selective cases in which the degree of superior displacement is limited and in which osteotomy, mobilization, and reattachment would be difficult to achieve.[10] Another concern about an acromioplasty in this setting is the concomitant detachment of the coracoacromial ligament and loss of integrity of the

coracoacromial arch. This may compromise anterosuperior restraint with the development of anterosuperior instability.

Humeral Component Loosening

Humeral component loosening following treatment of proximal humeral fractures is an uncommon problem. This may be, in part, because the patient population tends to be older with limited activity requirements.

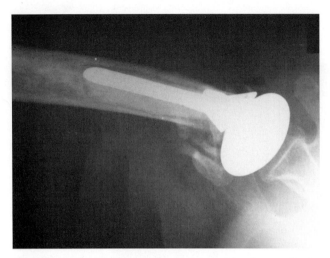

FIGURE 9–24 Displacement of the greater tuberosity in a posterior position results in a mechanical obstruction to external rotation.

In the series of humeral head replacements reported for acute proximal humeral fractures, humeral component loosening has been infrequent (Table **9–1**). Prostheses inserted without the use of cement will be more likely to loosen.[54,55,61] It is very difficult to achieve sufficient component stability without the use of cement primarily because the lack of metaphyseal bone compromises rotational stability and length support. The cementing technique used at the time of insertion is also important. The goal should be to have an appropriate cement mantle for secure fixation. We prefer the use of a cement restrictor at the time of implantation for pressurization that enhances the cement mantle.

The diagnosis of humeral component loosening should be associated with progressive radiolucency at the bone–cement interface. This should be at least 1.5 mm in diameter in multiple zones around the humeral component (Fig. **9–25**).[61] Because there are

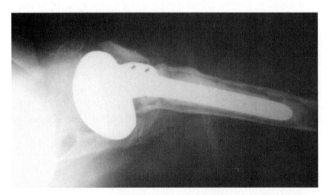

FIGURE 9–25 A 73-year-old woman with shoulder and arm pain 2 years after proximal humeral replacement for fracture. There is a 2-mm continuous radiolucent line at the bone cement interface consistent with loosening.

multiple causes of discomfort following this procedure, it is essential that the symptoms being attributed to the humeral component loosening also be carefully considered for other possible causes. If humeral component loosening is the primary source of symptoms, revision should be considered. This procedure can be technically challenging for several reasons, including the difficulty of cement removal, the position of the tuberosities, and the compromised bone quality. If possible, all cement should be removed and a revision prosthesis inserted, with careful attention to cementing technique. If there is significant endosteal bone compromise, a long stem component should be considered. Although it may be reasonable to consider a noncemented implant at the time of revision, this has to be considered carefully primarily because of the continued lack of metaphyseal bone support. In addition, the bone–prosthesis interface is not optimal for cementless fixation because of the changes that occurred in association with the loosening and the compromise of the "interference fit" fixation.

Rotator Cuff Tears

Rotator cuff compromise following proximal humeral replacement is a relatively common problem (Table **9–1**).[61] This is usually manifested as lack of recovery of range of motion or gradual loss of motion after initial recovery. Uncommonly, a patient who had regained very good range of motion and function may sustain a fall that results in a rotator cuff tear. The primary cause of rotator cuff compromise following this procedure is progressive failure of the rotator cuff that occurs during the first few years following the procedure. This may be evident on standard radiographs as superior migration of the humeral head within the subacromial space. Even in this context, it is difficult to determine whether rotator cuff compromise is a result of progressive degeneration or secondary to compromise of tuberosity fixation with associated displacement of the rotator cuff tendons that allows superior migration. Because it is difficult to determine the exact mechanism of the rotator cuff compromise, it is also difficult to determine the appropriate treatment.

If an acute injury occurs in a patient who was previously doing well with very good range of motion and function, the possibility of acute rotator cuff tear could be considered. Diagnosis should be based on clinical examination with confirmation by radiographic studies. Our experience is that an arthrogram has been the most reliable method of evaluation. Although magnetic resonance imaging (MRI) has been utilized for this purpose,[70] the interpretation is difficult and requires considerable expertise and experience. An arthrogram shows the presence or absence of a full-thickness tear.

If a full-thickness tear is confirmed, operative repair should be considered; however, it is important to emphasize that this should only be considered in a patient who has been doing well and sustained a specific injury that resulted in loss of active motion. This procedure should consist of arthroscopic evaluation to confirm the presence of the tear. Based on these findings, the decision to proceed with open repair should be based on the size of the tear and whether it is felt to be repairable. There is little, if any, experience in the literature that documents treatment outcomes for this clinical situation[61]; therefore, treatment approaches should be individualized and based on established principles.

The more common clinic scenario is a gradual, progressive loss of active range of motion, which is usually consistent with progressive rotator cuff compromise. When this occurs, operative management is generally not considered because of the progressive nature of the failure and the anticipated irreparable nature of the defect. Nonoperative management, including pain management, a limited therapy program, and supportive care is the preferred approach, although significant improvement is not anticipated.[61]

Heterotopic Ossification

Heterotopic ossification following proximal humeral replacement for acute fractures is relatively common, although it is generally not clinically significant.[47,50,56] It can be difficult to differentiate between small areas of heterotopic ossification and reactive bone that occurs in association with the fracture. In general, bone that develops within the rotator cuff tendons, within the subacromial space, or bone bridging from the acromion to the proximal humerus represents heterotopic ossification. The factors that predispose to clinically significant heterotopic ossification include higher energy injuries (fracture-dislocations) and operative delays beyond 10 to 14 days after the acute injury.[3] In our experience, heterotopic ossification can also develop when the procedure is performed after an early failure of internal fixation (Fig. **9−26**). The second procedure, particularly when it is performed 2 to 4 weeks after the initial procedure, carries a significant increased risk of heterotopic ossification.

Most heterotopic ossification is not clinically significant in that it does not contribute to loss of motion; however, when heterotopic bone forms within the subacromial space or bridges across the subacromial space or glenohumeral joint, range of motion can be significantly affected. If there are significant functional limitations, surgical excision should be considered. This should not be undertaken until the ossification process has matured, which is usually at least 6 months following the

surgery. In addition, the exact location of the bone should be identified. Standard radiographs should be combined with a CT scan for accurate localization. Bone within the subacromial space or bridging the subacromial space is more easily excised than bone anterior and inferior to the glenohumeral joint. Bone in this area can be in close proximity to the axillary artery and its branches and the brachial plexus and requires a careful dissection usually with the assistance of a microvascular surgeon. When bone forms within the rotator cuff, excision may significantly compromise the integrity of the rotator cuff tendons, which will require repair of any full-thickness defects.[48,49,71]

Whenever possible, it is important to take measures to prevent the formation of heterotopic bone. At the time of the initial surgery, meticulous technique to minimize soft tissue trauma is important. The timing of surgery is also important. Whenever possible, the "at-risk" period should be avoided. For those patients who are felt to be at high risk for development of heterotopic bone, prophylactic measures should be considered. This would include use of antiinflammatory medications postoperatively and/or the use of single-dose radiation therapy. The use of the preventive measures has to be balanced with the potential to interfere with tuberosity healing. In addition, following excision of heterotopic bone, these measures should be used to prevent recurrence.

Glenoid Complications

Glenoid wear and loss of articular cartilage requiring revision surgery is an uncommon complication (Fig. **9−27**).[55,61] This is probably due in part, to the relatively low activity level in this older patient population. When there is evidence of glenoid articular cartilage loss, it is important to confirm that the patient's symptoms are due to the degenerative changes and not other factors that can cause pain following this procedure. We have found that an intraarticular lidocaine injection can be helpful in confirming that the glenoid changes are the cause of symptoms.

The factors that contribute to the development of the glenoid wear can include preexisting degenerative changes that were relatively minor at the time of surgery but progressed postoperatively, unrecognized injury or additional injury at the time of surgery, and the activity level of the patient (although this is generally not a significant factor). The duration of follow-up is also important. With longer follow-up, glenoid complications are more likely to occur.

The treatment of glenoid articular cartilage loss is generally determined by the symptoms. If the symptoms are mild or moderate, antiinflammatory medications and modification of activity would be beneficial; however,

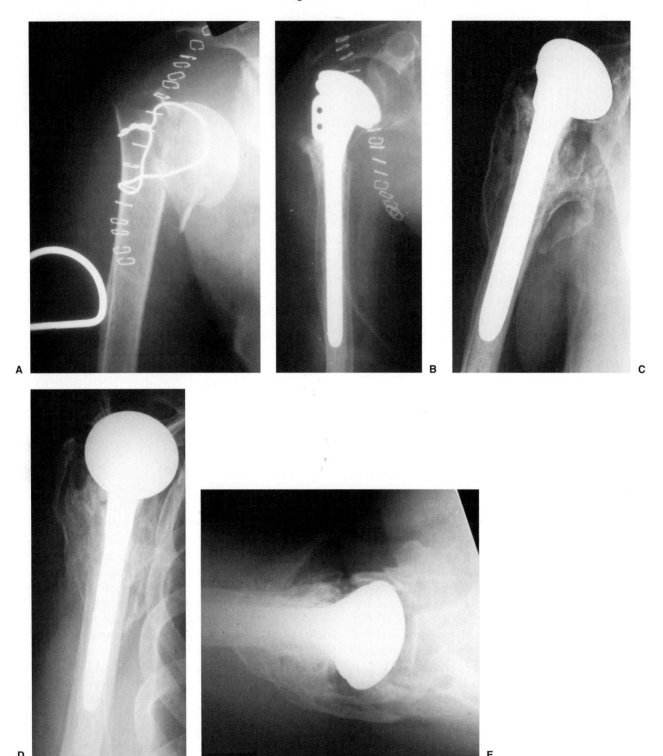

FIGURE 9–26 A 68-year-old woman underwent tension band wire fixation of a three-part fracture. **(A)** Ten days following the procedure follow-up radiographs showed loss of fixation. **(B)** Revision to proximal humerus replacement was performed 1 week later **(C–E)** Heterotopic ossification developed, and 8 months following the procedure there is bridging bone across the subacromial space and the glenohumeral joint, resulting in ankylosis.

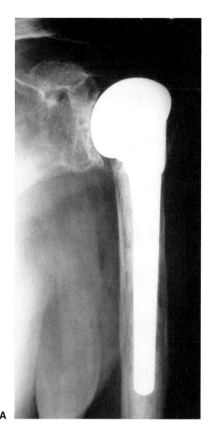
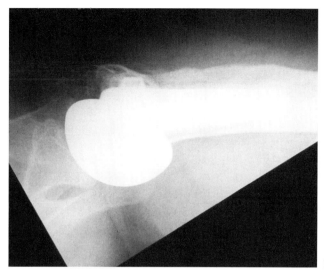

FIGURE 9–27 (A,B) A 61-year-old man 5 years following proximal humeral replacement PHR with mild pain associated with glenoid erosion.

if significant symptoms of pain and disability are associated with glenoid articular cartilage loss, revision with insertion of a glenoid component should be considered.[71] Glenoid bone stock should be evaluated preoperatively to be certain that adequate bone is present to support a glenoid component. If the humeral component is not modular, it will require removal to insert the glenoid component. This revision-type surgery can be technically challenging and requires proper preoperative planning.

Stiffness

It is difficult to determine the incidence of stiffness (i.e., loss of active motion) following this procedure. Many of the complications previously discussed result in loss of active motion. For our purpose, stiffness should be considered loss of active and passive motion that significantly compromises function. Patients who have limitation of active motion but good passive motion most likely have musculotendinous or tuberosity problems as discussed previously; however, there are some patients who undergo this procedure and fail to regain active and passive range of motion, and their radiographs do not indicate any other abnormalities. In this uncommon situation, soft tissue releases should be considered (Fig. **9–28**). These can be performed either arthroscopically or as an open procedure; however, the arthroscopic approach is preferred to minimize the soft tissue dissection. Capsular

release should be performed intraarticularly, including the anterior capsule and the posterior capsule. The subacromial space should be mobilized with complete bursectomy to restore the gliding motion between the rotator cuff and the acromion. We also perform a coracoacromial ligament release and limited acromioplasty because scarring in this area usually contributes to the stiffness. When the releases are completed, a gentle manipulation should be performed to gain additional range of motion. The range of motion obtained in the operating room represents the postoperative goal. A structured, supervised postoperative rehabilitation program is essential to maintain any improvements. We prefer to admit patients to the hospital for 2 to 3 days to initiate this therapy program. Patients receive an interscalene block on the first and second postoperative days so that they can perform the stretching exercises without being limited by postoperative pain. In our experience, this approach can be successful, but patient selection is a very important factor in obtaining a successful outcome.

The complications that can occur following treatment of proximal humeral fractures are many and varied. Complications can occur as a result of the injury itself and the treatment provided. Avoiding complications is an important goal for the orthopaedic surgeon treating fractures of the proximal humerus; however, when complications do occur, prompt recognition, evaluation,

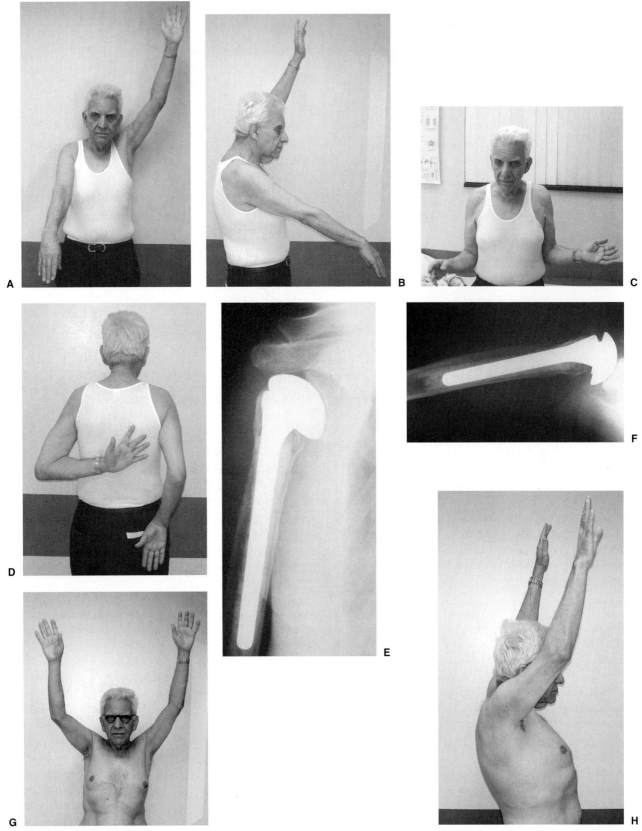

FIGURE 9–28 (A–D) A 75-year-old man 1 year following PHR with significant stiffness. **(E,F)** Radiographs showed a well-positioned component without evidence of tuberosity malposition. **(G–J)** Arthroscopic capsular releases were performed, and 1 year later his range of motion has improved significantly.

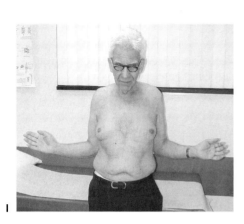
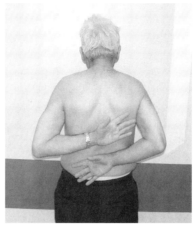

I   J   **FIGURE 9–28** (Continued)

and determination of an appropriate treatment plan is essential to minimize their impact.

REFERENCES

1. Zuckerman JD, Flugstad DL, Teitz CC, King HA. Axillary artery injury as a complication of proximal humerus fractures. Two case reports and a review of the literature. Clin Orthop 1984;189: 234–237

2. Janecki CJ, Barnett DC. Fracture-dislocation of the shoulder with biceps tendon interposition. J Bone Joint Surg Am 1979;61:142–143

3. Neer CS II. Displaced proximal humeral fractures. J Bone Joint Surg Am 1970;52:1077–1103

4. Norris TR, Turner JA, Boville DF. Nonunion of the upper humerus: an analysis of the etiology and treatment in 28 cases. In: Post M, Hawkins RJ, Morrey BF, eds. Surgery of the Shoulder. St Louis: CV Mosby, 1990:63–67

5. Cuomo F, Flatow EL, Maday MG, et al. Open reduction and internal fixation of two- and three-part displaced surgical neck fractures of the proximal humerus. J Shoulder Elbow Surg 1992;1:287–295

6. Duralde XA, Flatow EL, Pollock RG, Nicholson GP, Self EB, Bigliani LU. Operative treatment of nonunions of the surgical neck of the humerus. J Shoulder Elbow Surg 1996;5:169–180

7. Norris TR. Prosthectic arthroplasty in nonunions and malunions of the proximal humerus. Semin Arthroplasty 1997;8:304–307

8. Simpson NS, Jupiter JB. Reconstruction of nonunion of the proximal humerus with a custom blade plate: result of 17 consecutive cases. J Shoulder Elbow Surg 1997;6:182

9. Morris ME, Kilcoyne RF, Shuman W, et al. Humeral tuberosity fractures: evaluation by CT scan and managent of malunion. Orthop Trans 1987;11:242

10. Beredjiklian PK, Iannotti JP, Norris TR, Williams GR. Operative treatment of malunion of a fracture of the proximal aspect of the humerus. J Bone Joint Surg Am 1998;80:1484–1497

11. Solonen KA, Vastamaki M. Osteotomy of the neck of the humerus for traumatic varus deformity. Acta Orthop Scand 1985;56:79–80

12. Norris TR, Green A, McGuigan FX. Late prosthetic shoulder arthroplasty for displaced proximal humerus fractures. J Shoulder Elbow Surg 1995;4:271–280

13. Antuna SA, Sperling JW, Sanchez-Sotelo J, Cofield RH. Shoulder arthroplasty for proximal humeral malunions: long-term results. J Shoulder Elbow Surg 2002;11:122–129

14. Boileau P, Krishnan SG, Tinsi L, Walch G, Coste JS, Mole D. Tuberosity malposition and migration: reasons for poor outcomes after hemiarthroplasty for displaced fractures of the proximal humerus. J Shoulder Elbow Surg 2002;11:401–412

15. Gerber C, Schneeberger AG, Tho-Son Vinh TS. The arterial vascularization of the humeral head: an anatomical study. J Bone Joint Surg Am 1990;72:1486–1494

16. Laing PG. The arterial supply to the adult humerus. J Bone Joint Surg Am 1956;38:1105–1116

17. Kristiansen BK, Christiansen SW. Proximal humerus fractures. Acta Orthop Scand 1987;58:124–127

18. Lee CK, Hansen HR. Posttraumatic avascular necrosis of the humeral head in displaced proximal humerus fractures. J Trauma 1981;21:788–791

19. Leyshon RL. Closed treatment of fractures of the proximal humerus. Acta Orthop Scand 1984;55:48–51

20. Resch H, Povacz P, Frohlich R, Wambacher M. Percutaneous fixation of three- and four-part fractures of the proximal humerus. J Bone Joint Surg Br 1997;79:295–300

21. Sturzenegger M, Fornaro E, Jakob RP. Results of surgical treatment of multifragmented fractures of the humeral head. Arch Orthop Orthop Trauma Surg 1982;100:249–259

22. Jakob RP, Miniaci A, Anson PS, Jaberg H, Osterwalder A, Ganz R. Four-part valgus impacted fractures of the proximal humerus. J Bone Joint Surg Br 1991;73:295–298

23. Resch H, Beck E, Bayley I. Reconstruction of the valgus-impacted humeral head fracture. J Shoulder Elbow Surg 1995;4:73–80

24. Hagg O, Lundberg BJ. Aspects of prognostic factors of comminuted and dislocated proximal humerus fractures. In: Bateman JE, Welsh RP, eds. Surgery of the Shoulder. Philadelphia: BC Decker, 1984:51–59

25. Wijgman AJ, Rookler W, Patt TW, Raaymakers EL, Marti RK. Open reduction and internal fixation of three and four-part fractures of the proximal part of the humerus. J Bone Joint Surg Am 2002; 84:1919–1925

26. Gerber C, Hersche O, Berberat C. The clinical relevance of posttraumatic avascular necrosis of the humeral head. J Shoulder Elbow Surg 1998;7:586–590

27. Berry H, Bril V. Axillary nerve palsy following blunt trauma to the shoulder region: a clinical and electrophysiological review. J Neurol Neurosurg Psychiatry 1982;45:1027–1032

28. Blom S, Dahlback LO. Nerve injuries in dislocations of the shoulder joint and fractures of the neck of the humerus. A clinical and electromyographic study. Acta Chir Scand 1970;136: 461–466

29. Leffert RD, Seddon H. Infraclavicular brachial plexus injuries. J Bone Joint Surg Br 1965;47:9–22

30. Seddon HJ. Nerve lesion complicating certain closed bone injuries. JAMA 1974;135:11–15

31. Visser CP, Coene LN, Brand R, Tavy DL. Nerve lesions in proximal humerus fractures. J Shoulder Elbow Surg 2001;10:421–427

32. Visser CP, Coene LN, Brand R, Tavy DL. The incidence of nerve injury in anterior dislocation of the shoulder and its influence on functional recovery. A prospective clinical and EMG study. J Bone Joint Surg Br 1999;81:679–685

33. Visser CP, Tavy DL, Coene LN, Brand R. Electromyographic findings in shoulder dislocations and fractures of the proximal humerus: comparison with clinical neurological examination. Clin Neurol Neurosurg 1999;101:86–91

34. de Laat EA, Visser CP, Coene LN, Pahlplatz PV, Tavy DL. Nerve lesions in primary shoulder dislocations and humeral neck fractures: a prospective clinical and EMG study. J Bone Joint Surg Br 1994;76:381–383

35. Alnot JY. Traumatic brachial plexus palsy in the adult. Retro- and infraclavicular lesions. Clin Orthop 1988;237:9–16

36. Steinmann SP, Moran EA. Axillary nerve injury: diagnosis and treatment. J Am Acad Orthop Surg 2001;9:328–335

37. Coene LN, Narakas AO. Operative management of lesions of the axillary nerve, isolated or combined with other nerve lesions. Clin Neurol Neurosurg 1992;94(suppl):S64–S66

38. Alnot JY, Valenti P. Surgical repair of the axillary nerve: apropos of 37 cases. Int Orthop 1991;15:7–11

39. Petrucci FS, Morelli A, Raimondi PL. Axillary nerve injuries—21 cases treated by nerve graft and neurolysis. J Hand Surg Am 1982;7:271–278

40. Mikami Y, Nagano A, Ochiai N, Yamamoto S. Results of nerve grafting for injuries of the axillary and suprascapular nerves. J Bone Joint Surg Br 1997;79:527–531

41. Alnot JY. Infraclavicular lesions. Clin Plast Surg 1984;11:127–131

42. McQuillan MW, Nolan B. Ischemia complicating injury. J Bone Joint Surg Br 1968;50:482–492

43. Smyth EH. Major arterial injury in closed fracture of the neck of the humerus: report of a case. J Bone Joint Surg Br 1969;51:508–510

44. Theodorides T, de Keizer C. Injuries of the axillary artery caused by fractures of the neck of the humerus. Injury 1976;8:120–123

45. Hayes MJ, Van Winkle N. Axillary artery injury with minimally displaced fracture of the neck of humerus. J Trauma 1983;23:431–433

46. Schlegel TH, Hawkins RJ. Displaced proximal humerus fractures: evaluation and treatment. J Acad Orthop Surg 1994;2:54–66

47. Goldman RT, Koval KJ, Cuomo F, Gallagher MA, Zuckerman JD. Functional outcome after humeral head replacement for acute three- and four-part humeral fractures. J Shoulder Elbow Surg 1995;4:81–86

48. Garland DE. Surgical approaches for resection of heterotopic ossification in traumatic brain-injured adults. Clin Orthop 1991;263:59–70

49. Warner JJP, Ejnisman B, Akpinar S. Surgical management of heterotopic ossification of the shoulder. J Shoulder Elbow Surg 1999;8:175–178

50. Kraulis J, Hunter G. The results of prosthetic replacement in fracture dislocations of the upper end of the humerus. Injury 1976;8:129–131

51. Willems WJ, Lim TEA. Neer arthroplasty for humerus fractures. Acta Orthop Scand 1985;56:394–395

52. Moeckel BH, Dines DM, Warren RF, Altchek DW. Modular hemiarthroplasty for fractures of the proximal part of the humerus. J Bone Joint Surg Am 1992;74-A:884–889

53. Green A, Barnard WL, Limbird RS. Humeral head replacement for acute, four-part proximal humerus fractures. J Shoulder Elbow Surg 1993;2:249–254

54. Hawkins RJ, Switlyk P. Acute prosthetic replacement for severe fractures of the proximal humerus. Clin Orthop 1993;289:156–160

55. Compito CA, Self EB, Bigliani LU. Arthroplasty and acute shoulder trauma: reasons for success and failure. Clin Orthop 1994;307:27–36

56. Dimakopoulos P, Potamitis N, Lambiris E. Hemiarthroplasty in the treatment of comminuted intraarticular fractures of the proximal humerus. Clin Orthop 1997;341:7–11

57. Robinson CM, Page RS, Hill RM, Sanders DL, Court-Brown CM, Wakefield AE. Primary hemiarthroplasty for treatment of proximal humeral fractures. J Bone Joint Surg Am 2003;85:1215–1223

58. Dines DM, Warren RF, Altchek DW, Moeckel B. Posttraumatic changes of the proximal humerus: malunion, nonunion, and osteonecrosis—treatment with modular hemiarthroplasty or total shoulder arthroplasty. J Shoulder Elbow Surg 1993;2:11–21

59. Tanner MW, Cofield RH. Prosthetic arthroplasty for fractures and fracture-dislocations of the proximal humerus. Clin Orthop 1983;179:116–128

60. Warner JJP, Krushell RJ, Masquelet A, Gerber C. Anatomy and relationships of the suprascapular nerve: anatomical constraints to mobilization of the supraspinatus and infraspinatus muscles in the management of massive rotator-cuff tears. J Bone Joint Surg Am 1992;74:36–45

61. Muldoon MP, Cofield RH. Complications of humeral head replacement for proximal humeral fractures. Instr Course Lect 1997;46:15–24

62. Cameron B, Iannotti JP. Periprosthetic fractures of the humerus and scapula: management and prevention. Orthop Clin North Am 1999;30:305–318

63. Campbell JT, Moore RS, Iannotti JP, Norris TR, Williams GR. Periprosthetic humeral fractures: mechanisms of fracture and treatment options. J Shoulder Elbow Surg 1998;7:406–413

64. Worland RL, Kim DY, Arredondo J. Periprosthetic humeral fractures: management and classification. J Shoulder Elbow Surg 1999;8:590–594

65. Zuckerman JD, Cuomo F, Koval KJ. Proximal humeral replacement for complex fractures: indications and surgical technique. Instr Course Lect 1997;46:7–14

66. Prakash U, McGurty DW, Dent JA. Hemiarthroplasty for severe fractures of the proximal humerus. J Shoulder Elbow Surg 2002;11:428–430

67. Frankle MA, Greenwold DP, Markee BA, Ondrovic LE, Lee WE. Biomechanical effects of malposition of tuberosity fragments on the humeral prosthetic reconstruction for four-part proximal humeral fractures. J Shoulder Elbow Surg 2001;10:321–326

68. Frankle MA, Ondrovic LE, Markee BA, Harris ML, Lee WE. Stability of tuberosity reattachment in proximal humeral hemiarthroplasty. J Shoulder Elbow Surg 2002;11:413–420

69. Norris TR. Complications of proximal humerus fractures: diagnosis and management. In: Iannotti JP, Williams GR, eds. Disorders of the Shoulder: Diagnosis and Management. Philadelphia: Lippincott Williams & Wilkins, 1999:692–693

70. Sperling JW, Potter HG, Craig EV, Flatow E, Warren RF. Magnetic resonance imaging of painful shoulder arthroplasty. J Shoulder Elbow Surg 2002;11:315–321

71. Mighell MA, Kolm GP, Collinge CA, Frankle MA. Outcomes of hemiarthroplasty for fractures of the proximal humerus. J Shoulder Elbow Surg 2003;12:569–577

10

Clavicle Fractures

ERIK N. KUBIAK, KENNETH J. KOVAL, AND JOSEPH D. ZUCKERMAN

Clavicle fractures account for 2.6 to 12% of all fractures, and 44 to 66% of fractures about the shoulder.[1,2] The annual incidence of these injuries is around 50 per 100,000.[3] These fractures often occur as a result of an indirect mechanism, specifically a fall onto an outstretched upper extremity, usually resulting in a middle-third fracture. The direct mechanism, a fall directly onto the shoulder, occurs much less commonly and is usually associated with a fracture of the lateral end of the clavicle.[4] Postacchini et al[1] in 2002 reported on 535 clavicle fractures and observed that 68% of clavicle fracture occurred in males, and most fractures occurred in individuals younger than 20 years old; 81% of the fractures occurred in the middle third of the clavicle, 48% were displaced, and 19% were comminuted. Overall, middle-third fractures account for 80% of all clavicle fractures, whereas fractures of the lateral and medial third of the clavicle account for 15% and 5%, respectively. The prevalence of displaced clavicle fractures increases with age. In adults, clavicle fractures are more disabling and carry a higher incidence of complications because of the greater force required to produce them.[2,4]

■ History

The most common mechanism of injury for this fracture is a fall onto the outstretched hand or a direct blow to the clavicle (Fig. 10–1). Most of these injuries are the result of moderate to high-energy trauma in adolescents and adults; in elderly patients they are often the result of low-energy trauma. The clavicle most commonly fails in compression as a result of axial forces that occur as the patient falls onto the point of the shoulder or the outstretched hand.[5] Stanley et al[5] found that of 150 consecutive patients with clavicle fractures, 122 specifically recalled falling onto an outstretched upper extremity or directly onto the shoulder.

Patients who present with clavicle fractures as a result of high-energy trauma should be evaluated by the protocol advocated by the American College of Surgeons; in all cases, life-threatening injuries must take precedence over the clavicle injury. Most patients, regardless of the mechanism of injury, describe pain in the area of the fracture and increased pain with any attempted shoulder or upper extremity motion.

■ Clinical Evaluation

Clavicle fractures can usually be identified by visual inspection because of its subcutaneous location, its prominence in forming the contour of the shoulder girdle, and the prevalence of the displaced pattern. Most patients present with swelling and tenderness about the area of the fracture. They typically resist shoulder movement and tend to maintain the upper extremity at the side in an adducted, "protected" position. Fracture displacement is usually evident, and the ends of the fracture fragments are frequently palpable. The condition of the overlying skin must be carefully evaluated to be certain the fracture is closed or that there is no impending skin compromise as a result of displaced fragments. Open fractures are very uncommon and require emergency management. Tenting of the skin is most often found in association with displaced middle-third and lateral-third fractures. For middle-third fractures, the superiorly displaced medial fragment (as a result of the pull of the sternocleidomastoid muscle) can stretch the overlying skin (Fig. 10–2); comminuted fragments, especially if rotated, can cause further skin compromise. For lateral-third fractures the superior displacement of the medial fragment can tent the skin

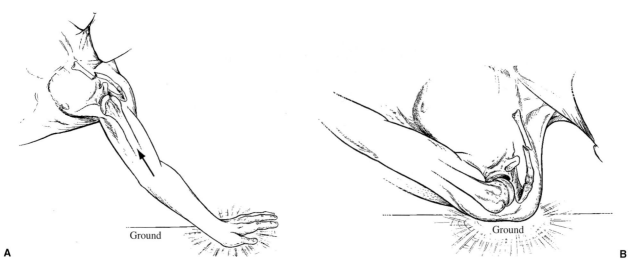

FIGURE 10-1 Clavicle fractures can occur as a result of an indirect **(A)** or direct **(B)** mechanism.

(Fig. **10-3A**). This is further compromised by the skin abrasion that is often found in association with these injuries when the fractures result from a fall off a bicycle or motorcycle (Fig. **10-3B**).

Medial-third fractures are usually nondisplaced and, consequently, are not as evident on examination as

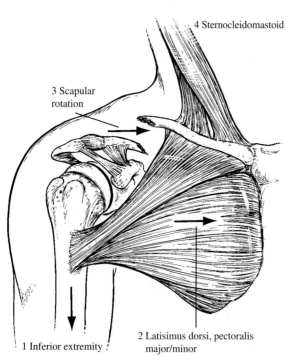

FIGURE 10-2 Midshaft clavicle fractures typically result in prominence at the fracture site, which corresponds to the lateral end of the medial fragment. The lateral fragment is usually displaced inferiorly by the weight of the upper extremity (1) and medially by the pull of the latissimus dorsi and pectoralis muscles (2) and the unopposed rotation of the scapula (3). The medical fragment is displaced superiorly by the unopposed pull of the sternocleidomastoid (4).

displaced lateral- or middle-third fractures. As a result, skin compromise is not usually a concern.

Palpation of the area of the fracture produces tenderness. Active shoulder range of motion is significantly limited by pain. Assisted or passive range of motion is painful and can produce crepitus at the fracture site. The proximity of the clavicle to the neurovascular structures makes a thorough neurovascular examination mandatory (Fig. **10-4**). This is particularly true of middle-third fractures and those that occur as a result of high-energy trauma. A thorough assessment of the brachial plexus and the distal pulses (brachial artery, ulnar artery, and radial artery) should be performed and the results documented. If there is a concern about vascular compromise, a prompt vascular consult should be obtained. The remainder of the upper extremity should be carefully examined to identify other injuries. In addition, the possibility of an associated thoracic injury (rib injuries, pneumothorax, and hemothorax), although very uncommon, should be considered based on the mechanism of the injury and the clinical findings.

Radiographic Evaluation

Initial evaluation of the patient with a suspected clavicle fracture should include a standard trauma series. The anteroposterior (AP) chest radiograph should include the entire clavicle and acromioclavicular (AC) and sternoclavicular (SC) joints. It should be carefully evaluated for evidence of a thoracic cage injury.

Standard AP radiographs are generally sufficient to confirm the presence of a clavicle fracture and the degree of fracture displacement (Fig. **10-5A**). The film should include the AC joint and the SC joint, as well as the proximal humerus and apices of the lung. Special views can assist in the identification and characterization

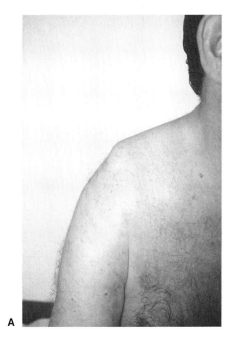
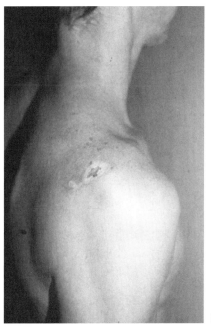

FIGURE 10–3 Lateral-third clavicle fractures have a characteristic appearance that can resemble complete acromioclavicular joint separations **(A)**. When the mechanism of injury involves a fall onto the shoulder, a skin abrasion often results **(B)**.

of clavicle fractures. A 20 to 60° cephalad tilt view provides an image without the overlap of the thoracic anatomy (Fig. **10–5B**).[6,7] An apical oblique view can be helpful in diagnosing minimally displaced fractures, especially in children. This view is taken with the involved

shoulder angled 45° toward the x-ray source, which is angled 20° cephalad. Standard radiographs may be inadequate to properly identify medial-third clavicle fractures and intraarticular lateral-third fractures. In these situations, a computed tomography (CT) scan should be obtained (Fig. **10–6**), not only to identify the presence of the fracture but also to understand the fracture pattern and the degree of intraarticular involvement.

■ Classification

In 1967 Allman[8] described the following classification system for all clavicle fractures based on location:

Group I represented fractures of the middle third, which was the most frequent site of fracture (80%). The proximal and distal ends of the clavicle are secured by the intact ligamentous and muscular attachments. These fractures can then be further described based on fracture pattern, degree of shortening (overriding), and the degree of displacement, although these parameters were not part of Allman's original description. Displacement and comminution are important parameters that should be included in the description of middle-third fractures because of their implications for treatment and prognosis.

Group II represented fractures of the lateral third. These were further subclassified by Neer into three types based on the degree of displacement and the location of the fracture with respect to the coracoclavicular ligaments (Fig. **10–7**):

Type I: minimal displacement; these fractures occur between the conoid and trapezoid ligaments or

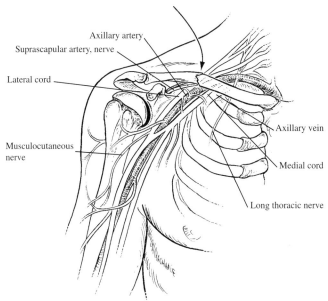

FIGURE 10–4 The clavicle lies in close proximity to the neurovascular structures that supply the ipsilateral upper extremity.

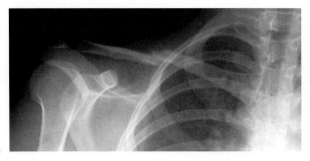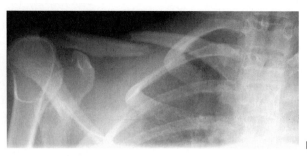

A   B

FIGURE 10–5 (A) An anteroposterior radiograph is usually sufficient to identify the majority of clavicle fractures. **(B)** A 20 to 60° cephalic tilt view provides a clearer image by minimizing overlap with thoracic anatomy.

between the coracoclavicular and AC ligaments; the intact ligaments maintain the fragments in position, thereby limiting displacement

Type II: displaced; these fractures occur medial to the coracoclavicular ligaments, thereby allowing the medial fragment to displace superiorly

Type III: intraarticular; these fractures involve the articular surface of the lateral clavicle

Subsequent to Neer's description, Rockwood further subclassified type II fractures into two subtypes:

Type II A: conoid and trapezoid ligaments remain attached to the distal fragment

Type II B: conoid ligament disrupted and the trapezoid ligament remains attached to distal fragment

Group III fractures, as described by Allman, represented medial-third fractures. These were the least common sites of clavicle fracture.

Craig described a classification (Table **10–1**) that combined the Allman and Neer fracture types and expanded the description of the fractures and included less common injuries (i.e., epiphyseal separations). This system is particularly useful to describe and classify medial- and lateral-third fractures; however, it does not provide a detailed classification of middle-third fractures.

In 1998, after reviewing 1000 consecutive clavicle fractures, Robinson proposed a new classification system (Table **10–2**) that incorporated important prognostic factors including displacement, comminution, and intraarticular involvement (Fig. **10–8**). Although this classification system includes almost all clavicle fractures, it has not yet been used extensively. This may be due, in part, to the numbering system, which is different from that described by Allman and Neer. In the Robinson system, lateral-third fractures are type III, middle-third fractures are type II, and medial-third fractures are type I.

In 1991 the Orthopaedic Trauma Association (OTA) adopted the AO/Association for the Study of Internal Fixation (ASIF) comprehensive fracture classification system originally described in the 1970s and expanded it to include fractures of the spine and distal extremities. Fractures of the clavicle are included in this comprehensive system and are classified based on location and

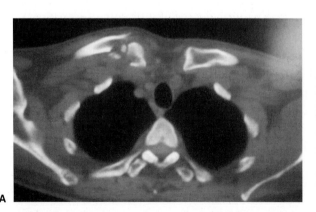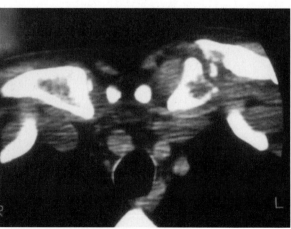

A   B

FIGURE 10–6 (A,B) Computed tomography (CT) scans aid in the diagnosis of intraarticular fractures of the medial third of the clavicle as shown here in these two examples.

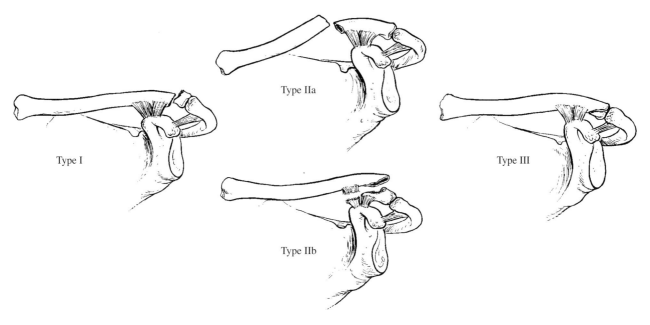

FIGURE 10–7 The Neer classification of lateral clavicle fractures.

displacement. Regardless of the classification system utilized, it is essential to understand the fracture pattern and anatomy and to effectively describe the fracture so that treatment outcomes can be accurately documented and compared.

Table 10–1 Craig Classification of Clavicle Fractures

Group I: Fractures of the middle third	
Group II: Fractures of the distal third	
Type I	Minimal displacement (interligamentous)
Type II	Displaced secondary to fracture line medial to the coracoclavicular ligaments (A) Conoid and trapezoid attached (B) Conoid torn, trapezoid attached
Type III	Fractures of the articular surface
Type IV	Periosteal sleeve fracture (children)
Type V	Comminuted with ligaments attached neither proximally or distally, but to an inferior comminuted fragment
Group III: Fractures of the proximal third	
Type I	Minimal displacement
Type II	Displaced (ligaments ruptured)
Type III	Intraarticular
Type IV	Epiphyseal separation (children and young adults)
Type V	Comminuted

Treatment

The vast majority of clavicle fractures can be successfully treated nonoperatively with some form of immobilization. Various methods of immobilization have been described including: an arm sling (Fig. **10–9A**), a sling and a swath (Fig. **10–9B**), a figure-of-eight bandage

Table 10–2 Robinson Classification of Clavicle Fractures

Type 1: Medial	
A	Nondisplaced
A1	Extraarticular
A2	Intraarticular
B	Displaced
B1	Extraarticular
B2	Intraarticular
Type 2: Middle	
A	Cortical alignment
A1	Nondisplaced
A2	Angulated
B	Displaced
B1	Simple or single butterfly fragment
B2	Comminuted or segmental
Type 3: Distal	
A	Nondisplaced
A1	Extraarticular
A2	Intraarticular
B	Displaced
B1	Extraarticular
B2	Intraarticular

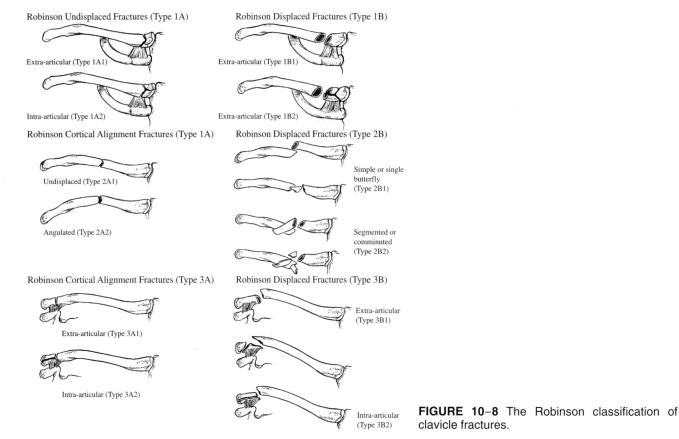

Robinson Undisplaced Fractures (Type 1A)

Extra-articular (Type 1A1)

Intra-articular (Type 1A2)

Robinson Cortical Alignment Fractures (Type 1A)

Undisplaced (Type 2A1)

Angulated (Type 2A2)

Robinson Cortical Alignment Fractures (Type 3A)

Extra-articular (Type 3A1)

Intra-articular (Type 3A2)

Robinson Displaced Fractures (Type 1B)

Extra-articular (Type 1B1)

Extra-articular (Type 1B2)

Robinson Displaced Fractures (Type 2B)

Simple or single butterfly (Type 2B1)

Segmented or comminuted (Type 2B2)

Robinson Displaced Fractures (Type 3B)

Extra-articular (Type 3B1)

Intra-articular (Type 3B2)

FIGURE 10–8 The Robinson classification of clavicle fractures.

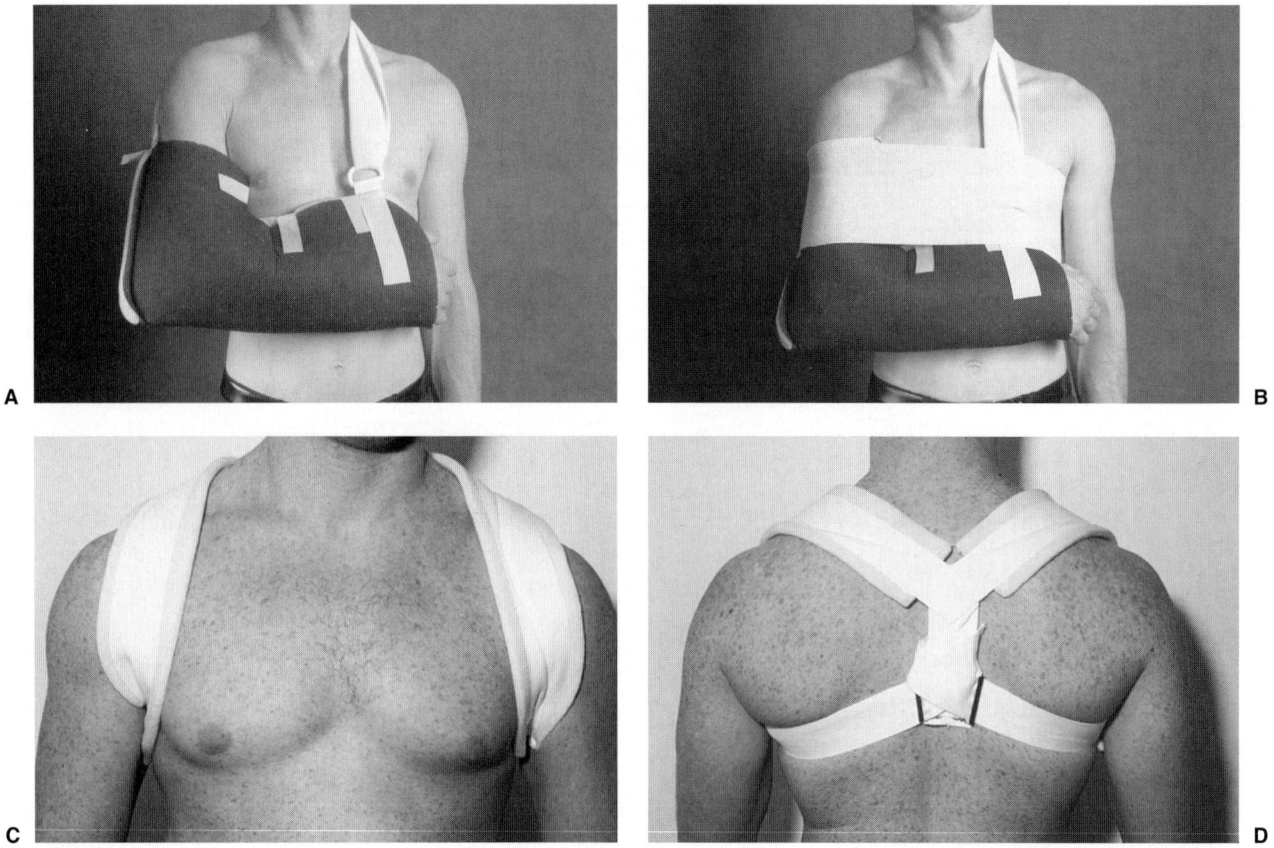

FIGURE 10–9 Immobilization methods include simple sling **(A)**, sling and swath **(B)**, and figure-of-eight bandage **(C,D)**.

(Fig. **10–9C,D**), or shoulder spica.[9,10] The goals of the various methods of immobilization are to (1) support the shoulder girdle, raising the lateral fragment in an upward, outward and backward direction; (2) depress the medial fragment; (3) maintain some degree of fracture reduction; and (4) allow for the patient to use the ipsilateral hand and elbow. Regardless of the method of immobilization utilized, some degree of shortening and deformity are the usual sequelae. We prefer to immobilize most clavicle fractures with a simple sling (and swath if necessary), accepting that some degree of deformity is very unlikely to lead to long-term sequelae (these are discussed later, in the section on complications). A figure-of-eight bandage is sometimes helpful for reducing displaced fractures that are associated with skin problems; however, the location of the padded bandage must not be over the area of potential skin compromise.

In general, the method of immobilization is utilized for 4 to 6 weeks until there has been sufficient progression of clinical and radiographic healing. During the period of immobilization, active range of motion of the elbow, wrist, and hand should be initiated immediately. We institute passive range of motion of the shoulder within 7 to 10 days as discomfort subsides. To minimize clavicular rotation, we may limit forward elevation to 90° for the initial 2 to 3 weeks. The goal is to regain nearly the full passive range of motion by the time the immobilization is discontinued and an active range-of-motion program is begun.

In 1981 Zenni et al,[11] after reviewing the literature, described the following indications for open reduction and internal fixation of clavicle fractures: (1) neurovascular compromise due to posterior displacement and impingement of the bony fragments on the brachial plexus, subclavian vessels, or even the common carotid artery; (2) widely displaced fracture of the lateral third of the clavicle with disruption of the AC ligaments; (3) severe angulation or comminution of a fracture in the middle third of the clavicle; (4) the patient's inability to tolerate prolonged immobilization; and (5) symptomatic nonunion following nonoperative treatment.

Lateral-Third Fractures

Nonoperative treatment of lateral-third clavicle fractures is appropriate for type I and type III injuries. Type II injuries are analogous to AC joint separations. Closed treatment should be reserved for those injuries with limited displacement and no evidence of skin compromise. The method of treatment appropriate for these fractures depends on the location of the fracture relative to the AC ligaments. This was the impetus for Neer's classification system and treatment recommendations.

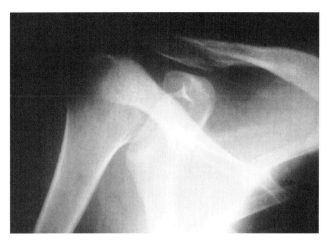

FIGURE 10–10 Type I lateral clavicle fracture showing minimal displacement.

Type I

The ligaments are intact in type I clavicle fractures, and displacement is therefore generally minimal (Fig. **10–10**). We treat these patients with a sling for comfort and begin mobilization as pain permits. Patients typically require a sling for 3 to 4 weeks. Active assisted range of motion of the shoulder is started as the patient is able to tolerate; forward elevation of the shoulder is limited to less than 90° for the first 2 weeks and then advanced as described previously.

Type II

The most important parameter determining the treatment of type II lateral clavicle fractures is the degree of displacement. Some authors have indicated that all type II fractures require operative management. In our experience, all type II fractures do not require operative treatment. We have found that if the bone ends are in contact, healing can be expected even if there is some degree of displacement. In this situation, nonoperative management consisting of sling immobilization and progressive range of motion as described can result in healing of the fracture with a satisfactory functional outcome (Fig. **10–11**). When there is significant displacement such that the bone ends are not in contact, operative management is indicated. Of course, the decision to proceed with operative management is made based on a careful consideration of patient factors as well. In most situations, however, when there is wide displacement of type II lateral clavicle fractures, operative management is indicated.

A variety of techniques have been described for the operative management of type II lateral clavicle fractures, which primarily consist of reducing the medial fragment to the lateral fragment. This is accomplished by using either coracoclavicular fixation (Fig. **10–12**) or

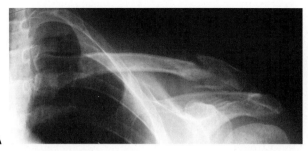
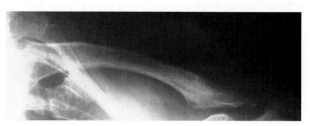

A   B

FIGURE 10–11 (A) A 63-year-old with type II lateral clavicle fracture. The fracture fragments remain in close proximity. **(B)** Nonoperative management resulted in healing and an excellent functional outcome.

fixation across the AC joint, through the lateral fragment, and into the medial fragment (Fig. **10–13**). Although both AC and coracoclavicular techniques have been used successfully, we prefer the coracoclavicular method primarily because it avoids compromise of the AC joint and does not require a second procedure for hardware removal.

Coracoclavicular type fixation with Mersilene tape or sutures, wires,[12] and screws has been described. When planning fixation, four forces that potentiate displacement of the medial fragment must be overcome: (1) the weight of the arm, which pulls the lateral fragment downward; (2) the pectoralis major, pectoralis minor, and latissimus dorsi, which medialize the lateral segment and cause overriding; (3) scapular rotation; and (4) the trapezius muscle, which tends to displace the medial fragment posteriorly and superiorly.[12]

Our preferred approach consists of an open reduction combined with coracoclavicular fixation using suture material (Figs. **10–12** and **10–14**). The procedure is generally performed with regional or general anesthesia. The patient is positioned in a semi-sitting position with

appropriate support. The entire forequarter and upper extremity should be prepped and draped free to allow full mobility of the upper extremity. A superior strap incision is made directly over the AC joint area. This incision should begin ~1 cm posterior to the clavicle and extend ~2 cm anterior to the clavicle. After dividing the skin and subcutaneous tissues, medial, lateral, and anterior/posterior flaps are developed to expose the deeper tissues. The displaced clavicle will usually be located in the subcutaneous tissue. Some of the deltoid and trapezius attachments to the clavicle have usually been stripped as a result of the injury. It is important to expose both sides of the fracture site by elevating the deltoid fascia anteriorly and the trapezius fascia posteriorly. Care should be taken to avoid any disruption of the AC joint. The exposure and dissection does not need to extend as far laterally as the AC joint. Only a limited amount of the lateral fragment requires exposure. The medial portion of the fracture requires about 2 to 3 cm of exposure. The deltoid should be split anteriorly in line with the fibers directly over the coracoid process. The base of the coracoid can be palpated and the soft

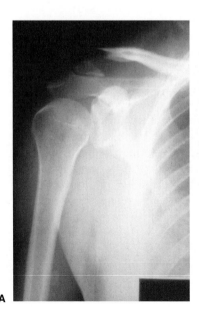
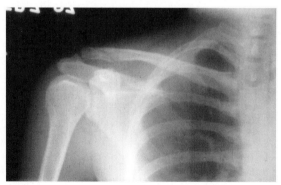

A   B

FIGURE 10–12 A 32-year-old with widely displaced type II lateral clavicle fracture **(A)** treated by open reduction and coracoclavicular fixation using No. 5 nonabsorbable sutures **(B)**.

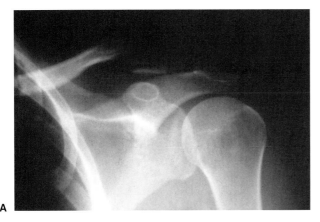

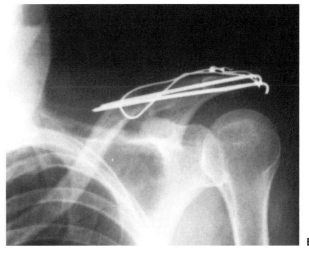

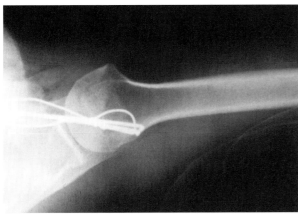

FIGURE 10–13 A 58-year-old with type II lateral clavicle fracture **(A)** treated with acromioclavicular fixation, consisting of two longitudinal Kirschner wires (K-wires) and a tension band wire **(B,C)**.

tissue overlying this area should be elevated on both its medial and lateral aspect. A curved periosteal elevator should be used for this dissection. At this point, we utilize a curved suture passer to pass a No. 5 Mersilene tape around the base of the coracoid. This is placed in a medial to lateral direction because of the location of the neurovascular structures. When the Mersilene tape has

been passed around the base of the coracoid, the suture passer is removed. The Mersilene tape can then be used to pass three to five No. 5 Mersilene sutures or No. 2 Fiberwire™ (Arthrex) sutures around the coracoid. These sutures are used for fracture fixation.

The fixation of the medial fragment is performed by placing a drill hole through the midportion of the clavicle

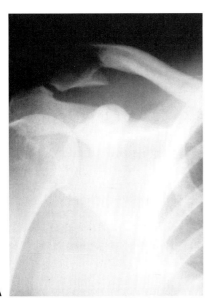

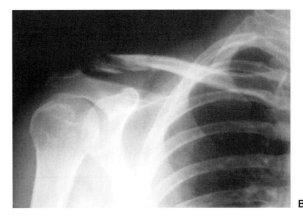

FIGURE 10–14 A 38-year-old man with displaced type II lateral clavicle fracture **(A)** treated by open reduction and internal fixation (ORIF) using coracoclavicular suture fixation **(B)**.

about 1.5 to 2 cm medial to the fracture site. This drill hole should be placed far enough from the fracture site to minimize the potential for propagation into the fracture site. The drill hole can be prepared with a 2.0- or 2.7-mm drill. It should be placed at the junction of the posterior two thirds and anterior one third of the clavicle. The sutures passed around the medial portion of the coracoid base are then passed through the drill hole in an inferior to superior direction. Both ends of the suture are then pulled over the top of the medial fragment to evaluate the reduction. This usually results in satisfactory apposition of the medial and lateral fragments. The sutures are passed through a drill hole on the lateral clavicle rather than around it to avoid excessive anterior translation of the medial fragment. Excessive anterior translation compromises the desired bony contact needed to obtain fracture healing. Pulling on each individual suture allows the individual sutures to be separated. The fracture is held in reduced position by placing upward traction on the arm and downward traction on the medial fragment. Each suture is tied individually. The knots are translated anteriorly so that they can be covered by the anterior deltoid. We have found that at least three individual sutures should be used and, based on the size of the individual and the security of the fixation, up to five sutures may be necessary. We have used No. 5 Mersilene most commonly. Recently, we have used No. 2 Fiberwire successfully. The relative strengths of the two sutures are comparable.

After fracture fixation is obtained, the arm should be supported to avoid excessive downward traction. The fracture reduction should bring the superior surface of the medial clavicle and lateral clavicle to the same level with good apposition of the fracture surfaces. The split in the deltoid is closed first. The deltoid-trapezius fascia is then repaired directly over the clavicle. This provides soft tissue coverage of the sutures. The subcutaneous tissue and the skin are closed in standard fashion. A single AP radiograph is obtained in the operating room to confirm the reduction.

Postoperatively, the patient is maintained in a sling for 4 to 6 weeks. Active range of motion of the elbow, wrist, and hand is begun the first postoperative day, with care taken to maintain proper support of the upper extremity when the exercises are being performed. Follow-up x-rays are obtained 10 to 14 days following the surgery at the time of suture removal. At that point, assisted range of motion of the shoulder can be started. We generally limit forward elevation to 90° to limit any rotational stress on the fracture site. External rotation can be performed, as well as internal rotation to the chest. At 4 to 6 weeks, x-rays generally show adequate healing to allow immobilization to be discontinued and progression to an active range-of-motion program with stretching to increase the overall range. Isometric strengthening can

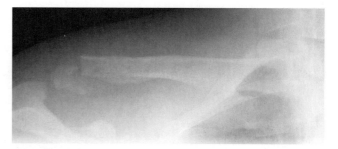

FIGURE 10–15 Type III lateral clavicle fracture with intraarticular component.

be started at this time. Resistive strengthening can be started at 8 to 10 weeks. We avoid heavy downward pulling on the upper extremity until 10 to 12 weeks following surgery.

Type III

Minimally displaced type III fractures, that is, fractures with less than 2 mm of articular step-off, are treated nonoperatively with sling immobilization for 3 to 4 weeks. Early range of motion is initiated as previously described.

Although it has been suggested that intraarticular step-off of greater than 2 mm should be treated operatively, we prefer nonoperative management for virtually all type III fractures (Fig. **10–15**). The exception would be intraarticular fracture in association with a displaced type II fracture. Type III fractures are at risk for the development of posttraumatic arthritis of the AC joint; however, based on our experience, the risk is small and can be adequately treated by lateral clavicle resection if nonoperative management proves to be ineffective.

Middle-Third Clavicle Fractures

We prefer to use a simple arm sling sometimes combined with a swath for immobilization of middle-third clavicle fractures. For the most part reduction maneuvers cause excessive discomfort, are unnecessary, and generally cannot be maintained. Sling immobilization provides enough support to maintain the patient's comfort, which usually subsides in 10 to 14 days. Patients should be followed closely during this time period to be certain that fracture displacement does not compromise the overlying skin. Sling immobilization is customarily continued for 6 weeks. Active range of motion of the hand, wrist, and elbow is initiated immediately. Passive shoulder range of motion is initiated as patient comfort subsides. This consists of forward elevation, external rotation, and internal rotation to the chest. Forward elevation is limited to less than 90° for the first 2 to 3 weeks. After 3 to 4 weeks active-assisted exercises are started, including internal rotation behind the back. The sling can be discontinued in 4 to 6 weeks based on patient comfort

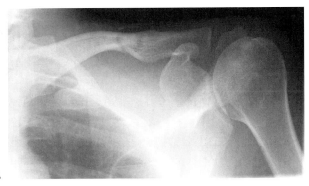
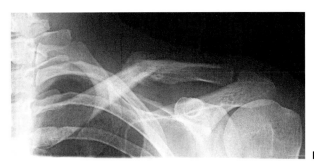

A   B

FIGURE 10–16 (A) A 26-year-old man with displaced middle-third fracture from a fall while skiing. **(B)** Nonoperative management with a sling immobilization resulted in clinical and radiographic union.

and clinical and radiographic evidence of healing. Radiographic signs of healing are usually evident by 4 to 6 weeks (Fig. **10–16**). Most patients take 3 to 4 months to return to their preinjury functional status.

Clinical series indicate that the majority of patients with middle-third clavicle fractures do well with sling immobilization and have excellent functional outcomes.[13–18] Nordqvist et al[17] in 1998 retrospectively reviewed the results of nonoperative and operative treatment in 225 of a possible 492 patients at an average of 17 years postinjury and found that 82% were asymptomatic; only one patient had a poor clinical rating, and this patient had been diagnosed with thoracic outlet syndrome prior to the fracture. Within the follow-up group, 197 patients were treated with figure-of-eight immobilization for 3 weeks with no attempt at reduction, and 24 patients were allowed immediate free shoulder mobilization with no impact on outcomes.

Indications for the operative treatment of acute middle-third clavicle fractures include (1) associated neurovascular compromise, (2) open fractures, and (3) impending skin compromise. Significant displacement or shortening of more than 2 cm has been described as a relative indication for surgery, although universal agreement on this indication is lacking. When open reduction is indicated, internal fixation should be performed. Intramedullary fixation[15,19–21] and compression plates and screws[22–27] have been used for the treatment of these fractures. The use of an intramedullary device has the advantage of a limited exposure and avoids the potential problems with prominent hardware (Fig. **10–17**). The modified Hagie pin has been used successfully for these fractures. The Rockwood clavicle pin is a similar implant that has a blunt tip to decrease the risk of violation of the cortex. Both implants utilize a "nut" at the lateral end to minimize the risk of migration and to enhance compression at the fracture site. It should be noted that the use of intramedullary fixation requires (1) frequent radiographic follow-up to monitor the possibility of hardware migration; and (2) a second procedure for hardware removal. Plate

and screw fixation require a more extensive exposure than intramedullary devices but has the advantage of more secure fixation (Fig. **10–18**). Plate and screw fixation is more likely to be prominent. If removal is required, the screw holes become stress risers that have an increased risk of refracture, which has been reported.[23,28] In general, intramedullary fixation can be used in fractures without comminution or when a butterfly fragment is present. More extensive comminution generally requires plate and screw fixation to obtain adequate stability.

Surgical Technique

The operation is performed under general anesthesia, with the patient in the semi-sitting beach chair position utilizing an appropriate positioner. A rolled towel should be placed between the patient's scapulae. The entire forequarter and upper extremity should be prepped and draped so that the upper extremity can be used to mobilize the lateral fragment to aid in reduction. A linear incision is made directly over the clavicle fracture site along Langer's lines; the length of the incision varies based on the technique utilized. For intramedullary fixation a 3- to 4-cm incision is needed, whereas for plate and screw fixation a longer incision is required. This incision is carried through the dermis. The fibers of the platysma are then splint longitudinally to prevent the disruption of the supraclavicular nerve branches, which can lead to the formation of painful neuromas. The remaining soft tissue including the periosteum is incised sharply over the clavicle and adjacent to the fracture site. The ends of the fracture are mobilized with a minimum amount of soft tissue stripping. The fracture ends are meticulously cleaned of hematoma and fibrinous material with small curettes as necessary. Reduction can be obtained with the help of bone clamps on each fragment, with care taken to avoid further comminution.

When modified Hagie pin intramedullary fixation is used, only a limited exposure of the fracture site is

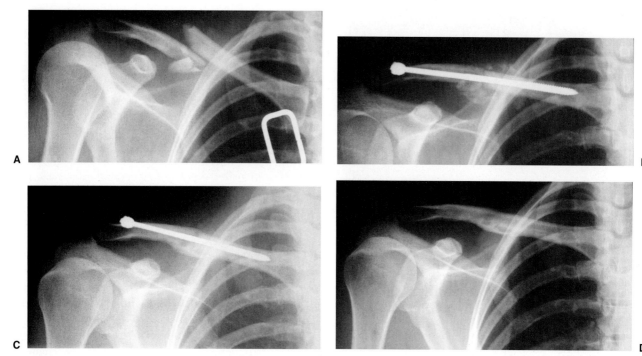

FIGURE 10–17 A 31-year-old with displaced, comminuted middle-third fracture **(A)** with significant tenting of the skin. Following ORIF with modified intramedullary Hagie pin fixation **(B)**, fracture alignment is restored. Ten weeks later **(C)**, the fracture is healed and the pin was removed **(D)**.

required. With the fracture site exposed, small drills should be used to enter the medullary canal of the medial fragment. The small drills are used in a similar fashion to enter the medullary canal of the lateral fragment. In acute fractures, this can be performed quite easily. The size of the drills to be used to enlarge the canals depends on the size of the intramedullary pin to be used.

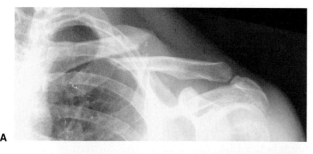

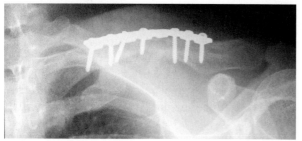

FIGURE 10–18 A 26-year-old with comminuted middle-third fracture **(A)** treated by ORIF using a plate and screws **(B)**.

This should be based on the manufacturer's guidelines. After the medial and lateral fragments are prepared, the intramedullary pin can be inserted. It is first passed in retrograde fashion through the lateral fragment. Because of the S shape of the clavicle, the pin exits the posterior aspect of the lateral fragment. After it is passed through the clavicle, it is palpable underneath the skin. A small skin incision should be made and the pin should be advanced retrograde through this incision. When a sufficient length of pin is exposed posterolaterally, it should be advanced from its lateral end so that the end of the pin is completely within the lateral fragment. At this point, the fracture should be reduced anatomically and held reduced as the pin is then advanced into the medial fragment. The pin is advanced until it engages the cortex but should not be passed beyond the cortex. A nut is then placed on the protruding lateral portion of the pin and tightened directly down to the cortex of the lateral clavicle. This provides further protection against migration. The pin is then cut close to the nut to avoid any prominence that can result in irritation of the soft tissues. When there is limited comminution at the fracture site, we have found it helpful to reduce large fragments and maintain as much bony contact as possible. A single butterfly fragment can usually be reduced after passage of the intramedullary pin and held in place with either suture or cerclage wire fixation; however, when there is excessive comminution, this technique should not be utilized. Rather, plate and screw fixation would

Rokito et al[18] reviewed 3
operatively and 14 treated
were seven nonunions in
were no differences in t
scores between the grou]
clude that operative man
not absolutely indicated. I
nonoperative treatment (
which went on to nonuni
the three with nonunio
level of activity. These ai
operative treatment of ty]
cated. Nonoperatively tr(
retrospective series, have
this does not preclude s:
in these patients.

■ Complications

Malunion

Malunion, to some degree
treated nonoperatively.
is overriding shortening
(Fig. **10–16**).[36] This re
with little, if any, functio
jority of cases and speci
Shortening greater thar
dysfunction and pain in
formity is present in the
compromise, operative r
however, it is essential
dysfunction. In these ver
correction of the deforn

Nonunion

The incidence of nonui
ranges from 0.1 to 13.0%
nonunions occurring i
incidence of nonunions
uted to the fact that 80%
the middle third. Asymp
common and require n(
erally either hypertrop
nonunions tend to be n
cated in the developme
are (1) inadequate peri
ture, (3) severity of initi
ment of fracture fragme
and (6) primary open
treatment.[19,20,22–27,38–42]

The first step in the (
clavicle nonunion is to
toms and disability as:

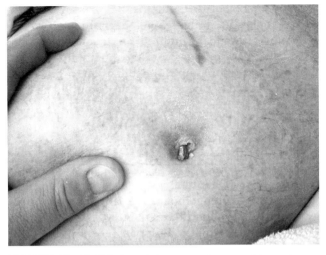

FIGURE 10–19 Skin breakdown can be a problem when an intramedullary pin is prominent posterolaterally. In this patient, the pin became exposed 3 weeks after insertion. It remained in place until 6 weeks after insertion when fracture healing had progressed. In spite of the exposed pin, infection did not develop.

be preferred. Closure of the soft tissues over the fracture site should provide adequate soft tissue coverage. This is followed by closure of the subcutaneous tissues and skin. The posterior incision can be closed in standard fashion. It is important to avoid prominence of the pin in this area because it can cause skin irritation and breakdown (Fig. **10–19**).

When plate and screw fixation is preferred, a somewhat more extensive exposure is needed. A 3.5-mm

pelvic reconstruction plate can be used (Fig. **10–18**) because this allows appropriate contouring in two planes, which will allow the plate to fit the **S** shape of the clavicle. In addition, precontoured plates designed specifically for the clavicle are also now available (Fig. **10–20**). These can be potentially beneficial in comminuted fractures to aid in restoration of anatomic alignment. If precontoured plates are not available to treat comminuted fractures, it may be helpful to contour a 3.5-mm reconstruction plate preoperatively using a clavicle bone model. When using plate and screw fixation, fracture reduction should be as anatomic as possible. Butterfly fragments should be fixed with interfragmentary fixation either separately or with screws passed through the plate. With noncomminuted fractures, depending on the obliquity of the fracture, it may be possible to place an interfragmentary screw across the fracture site. This improves reduction and fixation. With the fracture reduced, the plate is applied to the clavicle and secured to the medial and lateral fragment with bone reduction forceps. The plate is then fixed to the clavicle using the appropriate-size drill and tap preparation for the screw. Depending on the degree of comminution, one or two screws can be placed in compression mode. Care must be used while drilling to prevent compromise of the neurovascular structures located inferior to the clavicle. We find it helpful to place an elevator below the inferior surface of the clavicle to prevent unintentional advancement of the drill. When placement of the screws has been completed, the stability of the construct should be assessed with range of motion of the

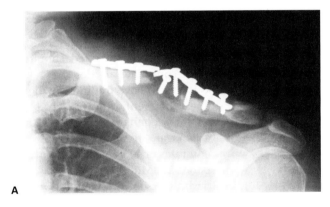

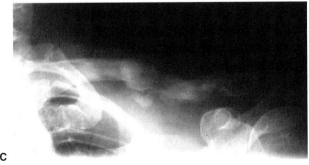

FIGURE 10–20 (A) A 47-year-old woman who underwent plate and screw fixation of a middle-third clavicle nonunion that did not heal, resulting in plate breakage. **(B)** The plate was removed, but the patient remained very symptomatic with an atrophic nonunion. **(C)** Open reduction and fixation with a precontoured plate and iliac crest bone grafting was performed with healing evident 3 months later.

upper extremity
rehabilitation pr

Following cor
formed. Once ag
closed over the
nence and the
skin is closed wit
An AP x-ray is ob
proper placemer

The upper ext
6 weeks followin
of the elbow, wri
operative day. \
assisted range o
time. We prefer
the first 2 to 3
that point, assis
grees can be pe
internal rotation
postoperative da
operatively to as
be discontinued
followed by mor
at approximately

Medial-Third |

Medial-third fra
nonoperatively
mobilization pr
dle-third and la
displaced medi
immobilization
fractures may
6 weeks. With an
cle, an evaluatio
This should inclu
the presence of
Any compromis
thoroughly evalu

Operative ma
is indicated for
placement resu
These situation:
tive managemer
fractures using
taneous tissues
rior and inferio
over the lateral
ture site. The r
fashion. Manipu
fracture to be r
fixation. A drill
direction throu
through the me

---

fragment and then antegrade into the medial fragment. It is essential that the bone ends are well opposed, with the maximum amount of contact. Bone grafting is an important part of the procedure. For hypertrophic nonunions, bone graft can be taken from the fracture site. Trimming the ends of the bone also decreases the possibility of the compression of the underlying neurovascular structures. In addition to drilling the intramedullary canals, the edges of the bone should be rongeured to a bleeding surface to enhance healing potential. If additional bone graft is necessary, we prefer to use cancellous autograft. An iliac crest graft is preferred; however, if a small amount is necessary, the proximal humerus can be used by opening a small window in the lateral humeral cortex and removing cancellous bone. A separate incision is needed, combined with a deltoid splitting approach.

We generally prefer plate and screw fixation for atrophic nonunions, although it has also been used successfully for hypertrophic nonunions. The ends of the fragments should be carefully exposed. A small osteotome should be used to "shingle" the ends of the bone to expose bleeding surfaces. Whenever possible, interfragmentary screw fixation should be used to enhance the fixation. A 3.5-mm pelvic reconstruction plate (Fig. **10–22**) can be used as described previously. In addition, the precontoured clavicle plates (Fig. **10–20**) are particularly beneficial in this setting because they allow the clavicular anatomy and contour to be restored. Bone grafting should also be performed as described.

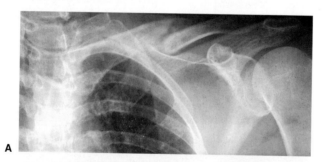

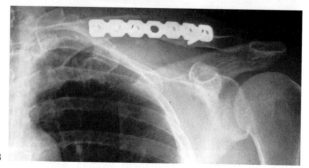

FIGURE 10–22 A 43-year-old with nonunion of a middle-third clavicle fracture (**A**) treated by ORIF with a reconstruction plate placed in an anterior and inferior position (**B**) combined with iliac crest bone graft.

Middle-third nonunions are frequently associated with some degree of bone loss. For bone loss less than 1 cm, the previously described techniques can be utilized. When the bone loss is more significant, particularly 2 cm or greater, consideration should be given to an intercalary structural bone graft to restore clavicular length. A tricortical iliac crest bone graft should be obtained and interposed between the fracture fragments to restore the length. The ends of the fracture fragments should be prepared as described. Plate and screw fixation is necessary to obtain secure fixation. It should span from the medial and lateral fragments across the bone graft with compression if possible.

Postoperative rehabilitation following internal fixation of middle-third nonunions progresses more slowly than following internal fixation of acute clavicle fractures. Sling immobilization is utilized for 6 to 8 weeks postoperatively. We prefer to limit exercise to active range of motion of the elbow, wrist, and hand for the first 3 weeks following surgery. At that point, a limited assisted range-of-motion program of the shoulder is performed with forward elevation limited to 90°, external rotation out to the side, and internal rotation to the chest. Full passive and active-assisted range of motion is allowed at 6 weeks. Active range of motion begins when the sling is discontinued. Follow-up radiographs are obtained at 3 weeks to confirm that there has been no change in the fixation or alignment of the fracture. Radiographs at 6 weeks are evaluated for early evidence of healing. It frequently requires 3 months or longer for radiographic confirmation of healing. During this time, follow-up x-rays should be obtained to evaluate whether there has been a change in position of the fixation or bony alignment. When there is clinical and radiographic evidence of healing, the patient can return to full activities with the exception of contact sports or strenuous manual labor. The activities can be started approximately 6 months postoperatively.

The treatment of lateral-third nonunions is also dependent on the associated symptoms. As noted previously, many lateral-third nonunions are asymptomatic, so these nonunions require operative management much less frequently than middle-third nonunions (Fig. **10–23**). For symptomatic patients, there are two treatment options to consider. When the lateral fragment is small, it may be reasonable to consider resection of the lateral fragment combined with coracoclavicular fixation of the medial fragment, possibly combined with coracoacromial ligament transfer. This approach is similar to that used for operative repair of a chronic AC joint dislocation. When the lateral fragment is large, open reduction and fixation should be performed. We prefer coracoclavicular fixation as previously described for fixation of an acute lateral-third fracture. In this situation, it is essential to prepare the ends of the bone and expose bleeding surfaces to encourage healing. Coracoclavicular

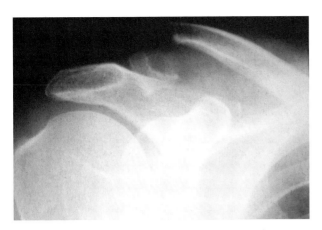

FIGURE 10–23 A 51-year-old man 18 months following type II lateral fracture with asymptomatic nonunion.

fixation should be passed through a drill hole in the medial fragment. The reduction should maximize the bony contact between the surfaces. Bone graft is an important component of the procedure. It can be obtained either from the iliac crest or from the proximal humerus as described. Plate and screw fixation has also been utilized for lateral third nonunions. If the lateral fragment is large enough, it can be applied only to the clavicle; however, if the lateral fragment is relatively small, the fixation must traverse the AC joint. This necessitates removal when healing is complete. Tension band wire fixation has also been described with Kirschner wires (K-wires) placed across the AC joint, through the lateral fragment, and into the medial fragment, combined with tension band wire fixation. There is very limited experience with these techniques, but both have been used successfully. The disadvantage is that a second procedure is required for removal of the implant and it involves fixation of the uninvolved acromion and AC joint.

Results of operative treatment of clavicle nonunions have generally been excellent. Boyer and Axelrod[24] reported on seven midshaft nonunions treated with compression plating. All nonunions healed at an average of 9 weeks following the procedure, and no patients had functional disabilities based on Disability of the Arm, Shoulder, and Hand (DASH) scores. Ballmer et al[22] reported on the treatment of 37 clavicular nonunions treated with decortication and osteosynthesis. Cancellous autograft was used in 24 patients with atrophic nonunions. Tricortical autogenous corticocancellous graft was used in nine patients with greater than 15 mm of bone loss. At an average of 8.6 years follow-up, 35 fractures had united and 32 patients exhibited a painless full range of motion of the ipsilateral shoulder. Laursen et al[26] reported union in all 16 middle-third clavicular nonunions after treatment with compression plating and autogenous bone grafting. Twelve patients underwent clinical review at an average of 54 months, and 11 patients had excellent Constant scores (greater than 70)

and 9 of 12 returned to their previous level of activity. Bradbury et al[25] reviewed the results of plate fixation with autograft for clavicular nonunion in 32 patients, at an average of 8 years' follow-up; 31 fractures had united and there were no fixation failures. Reconstruction plates and dynamic compression plates performed equally with average Constant scores of 82 and 87, respectively.

Boehme et al[19] reported on 21 patients with middle-third nonunions treated by intramedullary fixation with Hagie pins and bone grafting. Twenty of 21 nonunions healed at an average time of 22 weeks; 14 patients were completely asymptomatic, four patients had mild symptoms, two patients continued to have pain and functional limitations, and one patient died of an unrelated medical problem. In a similar series of 14 middle-third fracture nonunions, Capicotto et al[20] reported that all nonunions had united at an average of 4 years when operative fixation was performed using threaded Steinmann pins and autogenous corticocancellous bone graft. Two patients had shoulder pain at latest follow-up, and all patients had excellent shoulder range of motion.

Neurovascular Compromise

Neurovascular compromise is uncommon and can result from either the initial injury or secondary to compression of adjacent structures by callus or residual deformity. Acute vascular injuries are potentially life threatening and require prompt evaluation by a vascular specialist. Open reduction and internal fixation is indicated for cases of acute neurovascular compromise. Late vascular compromise that occurs secondary to compression of vascular structures by fracture deformity or callus is treated by resection of the fracture callus and osteotomy with correction of the impinging deformity.

REFERENCES

1. Postacchini F, Gumina S, De Santis P, Albo F. Epidemiology of clavicle fractures. J Shoulder Elbow Surg 2002;11:452–456
2. Robinson CM. Fractures of the clavicle in the adult. Epidemiology and classification. J Bone Joint Surg Br 1998;80:476–484
3. Nowak J, Mallmin H, Larsson S. The aetiology and epidemiology of clavicular fractures. A prospective study during a two-year period in Uppsala, Sweden. Injury 2000;31:353–358
4. Nordqvist A, Petersson CJ. Incidence and causes of shoulder girdle injuries in an urban population. J Shoulder Elbow Surg 1995;4:107–112
5. Stanley D, Trowbridge EA, Norris SH. The mechanism of clavicular fracture. A clinical and biomechanical analysis. J Bone Joint Surg Br 1988;70:461–464
6. Herscovici D Jr, Sanders R, DiPasquale T, Gregory P. Injuries of the shoulder girdle. Clin Orthop 1995;318:54–60
7. Sharr JR, Mohammed KD. Optimizing the radiographic technique in clavicular fractures. J Shoulder Elbow Surg 2003;12:170–172
8. Allman FL Jr. Fractures and ligamentous injuries of the clavicle and its articulation. J Bone Joint Surg Am 1967;49:774–784

9. Golser K, Sperner G, Thoni H, Resch H. [Early and intermediate results of conservatively and surgically treated lateral clavicular fractures] Aktuelle Traumatol 1991;21:148–152

10. Rowe CR. An atlas of anatomy and treatment of midclavicular fractures. Clin Orthop 1968;58:29–42

11. Zenni EJ Jr, Krieg JK, Rosen MJ. Open reduction and internal fixation of clavicular fractures. J Bone Joint Surg Am 1981;63:147–151

12. Neer CS II. Fractures of the distal third of the clavicle. Clin Orthop 1968;58:43–50

13. Edwards SG, Whittle AP, Wood GW II. Nonoperative treatment of ipsilateral fractures of the scapula and clavicle. J Bone Joint Surg Am 2000;82:774–780

14. Egol KA, Connor PM, Karunakar MA, Sims SH, Bosse MJ, Kellam JF. The floating shoulder: clinical and functional results. J Bone Joint Surg Am 2001;83-A:1188–1194

15. Grassi FA, Tajana MS, D'Angelo F. Management of midclavicular fractures: comparison between nonoperative treatment and open intramedullary fixation in 80 patients. J Trauma 2001;50: 1096–1100

16. Deafenbaugh MK, Dugdale TW, Staeheli JW, Nielsen R. Nonoperative treatment of Neer type II distal clavicle fractures: a prospective study. Contemp Orthop 1990;20:405–413

17. Nordqvist A, Petersson CJ, Redlund-Johnell I. Mid-clavicle fractures in adults: end result study after conservative treatment. J Orthop Trauma 1998;12:572–576

18. Rokito AS, Zuckerman JD, Shaari JM, Eisenberg DP, Cuomo F, Gallagher MA. A comparison of nonoperative and operative treatment of type II distal clavicle fractures. Bull Hosp Jt Dis 2002–2003; 61:32–39

19. Boehme D, Curtis RJ Jr, DeHaan JT, Kay SP, Young DC, Rockwood CA Jr. The treatment of nonunion fractures of the midshaft of the clavicle with an intramedullary Hagie pin and autogenous bone graft. Instr Course Lect 1993;42:283–290

20. Capicotto PN, Heiple KG, Wilbur JH. Midshaft clavicle nonunions treated with intramedullary Steinmann pin fixation and onlay bone graft. J Orthop Trauma 1994;8:88–93

21. Hoe-Hansen CE, Norlin R. Intramedullary cancellous screw fixation for nonunion of midshaft clavicular fractures. Acta Orthop Scand 2003;74:361–364

22. Ballmer FT, Lambert SM, Hertel R. Decortication and plate osteosynthesis for nonunion of the clavicle. J Shoulder Elbow Surg 1998;7:581–585

23. Bostman O, Manninen M, Pihlajamaki H. Complications of plate fixation in fresh displaced midclavicular fractures. J Trauma 1997;43:778–783

24. Boyer MI, Axelrod TS. Atrophic nonunion of the clavicle: treatment by compression plate, lag-screw fixation and bone graft. J Bone Joint Surg Br 1997;79:301–303

25. Bradbury N, Hutchinson J, Hahn D, Colton CL. Clavicular nonunion. 31/32 healed after plate fixation and bone grafting. Acta Orthop Scand 1996;67:367–370

26. Laursen MB, Dossing KV. Clavicular nonunions treated with compression plate fixation and cancellous bone grafting: the functional outcome. J Shoulder Elbow Surg 1999;8:410–413

27. Leupin S, Jupiter JB. LC-DC plating with bone graft in posttraumatic nonunions in the middle third of the clavicle. Swiss Surg 1998;4:89–94

28. Poigenfurst J, Rappold G, Fischer W. Plating of fresh clavicular fractures: results of 122 operations. Injury 1992;23:237–241

29. Chu CM, Wang SJ, Lin LC. Fixation of mid-third clavicular fractures with Knowles pins: 78 patients followed for 2–7 years. Acta Orthop Scand 2002;73:134–139

30. Neer CS II. Nonunion of the clavicle. JAMA 1960;172:1006–1011

31. Edwards DJ, Kavanagh TG, Flannery MC. Fractures of the distal clavicle: a case for fixation. Injury 1992;23:44–46

32. Yamaguchi H, Arakawa H, Kobayashi M. Results of the Bosworth method for unstable fractures of the distal clavicle. Int Orthop 1998;22:366–368

33. Ballmer FT, Gerber C. Coracoclavicular screw fixation for unstable fractures of the distal clavicle. A report of five cases. J Bone Joint Surg Br 1991;73:291–294

34. Mall JW, Jacobi CA, Philipp AW, Peter FJ. Surgical treatment of fractures of the distal clavicle with polydioxanone suture tension band wiring: an alternative osteosynthesis. J Orthop Sci 2002;7:535–537

35. Kona J, Bosse MJ, Staeheli JW, Rosseau RL. Type II distal clavicle fractures: a retrospective review of surgical treatment. J Orthop Trauma 1990;4:115–120

36. Edelson JG. The bony anatomy of clavicular malunions. J Shoulder Elbow Surg 2003;12:173–178

37. McKee MD, Wild LM, Schemitsch EH. Midshaft malunions of the clavicle. J Bone Joint Surg Am 2003;85-A:790–797

38. Simpson NS, Jupiter JB. Clavicular nonunion and malunion: evaluation and surgical management. J Am Acad Orthop Surg 1996;4:1–8

39. Kloen P, Sorkin AT, Rubel IF, Helfet DL. Anteroinferior plating of midshaft clavicular nonunions. J Orthop Trauma 2002;16:425–430

40. Ring D, Barrick WT, Jupiter JB. Recalcitrant nonunion. Clin Orthop 1997;340:181–189

41. Martell JR Jr. Clavicular nonunion. Complication with the use of Mersilene tape. Am J Sports Med 1992;20:360–362

42. Momberger NG, Smith J, Coleman DA. Vascularized fibular grafts for salvage reconstruction of clavicle nonunion. J Shoulder Elbow Surg 2000;9:389–394

43. Kitsis CK, Marino AJ, Krikler SJ, Birch R. Late complications following clavicular fractures and their operative management. Injury 2003;34:69–74

11

Scapula Fractures

GERARD K. JEONG AND JOSEPH D. ZUCKERMAN

Fractures of the scapula are relatively uncommon injuries representing about 0.5 to 1.0% of all fractures and only 3 to 5% of shoulder fractures.[1] Due to the uncommon nature of these injuries, experience in the management of scapula fractures has been limited. Scapula fractures are usually the result of high-velocity blunt trauma and often present in the setting of polytrauma. Peak incidence is in males between the ages of 30 and 40 years.[2-7] Scapula fractures are commonly the result of motor vehicle accidents (MVAs) and high-energy falls.[2-8] The most common location of scapula fractures is the body, followed by the neck, glenoid, and then acromion.[2-7] Thirty percent of fractures may have intraarticular involvement.[9]

Three important factors—soft tissue coverage, mobility, and location—enable the scapula to be relatively resistant to fracture. A significant amount of protection is provided by the thick, muscular, soft tissue envelope surrounding the scapula (see Fig. 2–8 in Chapter 2). The scapular and periscapular muscles provide a soft tissue cover that helps dissipate forces imparted to the scapula by the specific mechanisms of injury. The mobility provided by the scapulothoracic articulation enables injury forces to be dissipated to adjacent structures. Its axial location, as opposed to an appendicular location, posterior to the thoracic cage further adds to its relative resistance to injury. In this location, it is not subjected to bending or torsional forces, which are the most common mechanisms of fracture in the appendicular skeleton.

Due to its relatively protected anatomy and mobility of the scapula, injuries to the scapula require a high-energy mechanism and frequently occur as part of a constellation of injuries of the ipsilateral thoracic cage that can include rib fractures and severe pulmonary injuries. The most important aspect in the management of scapular fractures is the prompt recognition of associated injuries to the ipsilateral lung, chest wall, thoracic cage, and shoulder girdle, which are reported to occur in greater than 80% of scapular fractures.[2-6,8] Concomitant injuries include intrathoracic and thoracic wall injuries, brachial plexus injuries, vascular injuries, and scapulothoracic dissociation (Table 11–1). A scapular fracture with a concomitant first rib fracture is a particularly serious injury pattern because of its association with pulmonary and neurovascular compromise.[3]

The most extreme example of an ipsilateral shoulder girdle injury is a scapulothoracic dissociation, which warrants special mention. It is the anatomic equivalent of a closed forequarter amputation and is the result of violent, high-energy, blunt trauma that disrupts all static and dynamic stabilizers of the shoulder girdle (Fig. 11–1).[10] Osseous or ligamentous injuries lead to disruption of the acromioclavicular (AC) and sternoclavicular joints. The dynamic stabilizers are injured due to complete or near-complete tears of the deltoid, pectoralis, and periscapular musculature. Vascular disruption and brachial plexus avulsion is common.[11] The extremity is often flail, insensate, and pulseless. Fortunately, this devastating, life- and limb-threatening injury is rare. These associated injuries have far greater significance than the scapula fracture in the initial evaluation and management of these patients.

■ Relevant Anatomy

The scapula is a flat, triangular bone enveloped in layers of muscle. The scapula and the complex of muscles that surround it provide a critical role in the mechanics and kinematics of the shoulder girdle. It is the origin of the rotator cuff muscles, deltoid muscle, biceps, and the long head of the triceps. It also is the site of insertion for the trapezius, levator scapulae, rhomboids, serratus

TABLE 11–1 Injuries Associated with Scapular Fractures

Associated Injuries	Incidence (%)
Rib fractures	27–54
Pulmonary contusion	11–54
Clavicle fractures	23–39
Pneumothorax	11–38
Brachial plexus injuries	5–13
Vascular injuries (usually subclavian or axillary vessels)	1
Scapulothoracic dissociation	<1

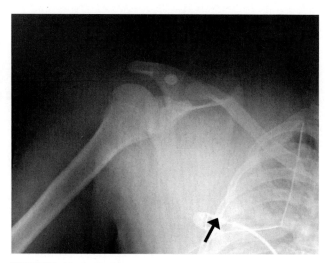

FIGURE 11–1 Anteroposterior (AP) chest radiograph of a scapulothoracic dissociation. The arrow demonstrates the widened medial border of the laterally displaced scapula. Note the associated clavicle fracture. The lateral fragment of the clavicle cannot be visualized because of the significant lateral displacement.

anterior, and pectoralis minor, all of which hold the contoured scapula against the posterior chest wall (see Fig. 2–1 in Chapter 2). Through its three true joints and one muscular articulation, it is not only the sole link between the upper extremity and the axial skeleton, but also a mobile platform upon which the proximal humerus is balanced as the upper extremity moves. Various ligaments originating from the scapula serve as important static stabilizers of the shoulder girdle. The coracoclavicular (CC) ligaments prevent superior migration of the distal clavicle to stabilize the AC articulation. The joint capsule, glenohumeral ligaments, and coracohumeral ligaments stabilize the glenohumeral joint in various directions and arm positions, whereas the coracoacromial ligament serves as a superior static restraint to humeral head stability.

Goss[12] has introduced the concept of the superior shoulder suspensory complex (SSSC) to emphasize the function of the scapula in maintaining the normal stable relationship between the shoulder girdle/upper extremity and the axial skeleton. The scapula is suspended from the lateral end of the clavicle by the CC and AC ligaments. These are the only fixed attachments of the

scapula to the axial skeleton. The SSSC is a ring composed of the glenoid, coracoid process, CC ligaments, distal clavicle, AC joint, and acromial process. The superior strut is the middle clavicle, and the inferior strut is the lateral scapular body and spine (Fig. 11–2).

A disruption of one part of the ring (i.e., scapular neck fracture, glenoid fracture, or clavicle fracture) still maintains the structural integrity of the shoulder girdle complex with the axial skeleton (Fig. 11–3A); however, a double disruption of the SSSC (i.e., associated scapular neck fracture and clavicle fracture) produces an inherently unstable relationship between the shoulder girdle complex and the axial skeleton and has been

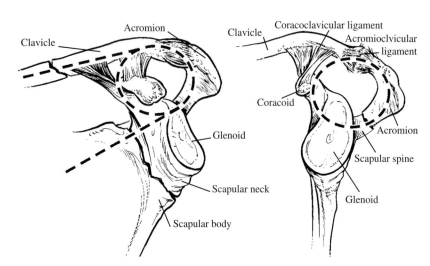

FIGURE 11–2 The diagrams demonstrate the oblique and lateral views of the two struts and the one ring of the superior suspensory shoulder complex (SSSC). The two struts consist of the clavicle and scapular neck. The ring consists of the distal clavicle, acromioclavicular ligaments, acromial process, glenoid fossa, coracoid, and coracoclavicular ligaments.

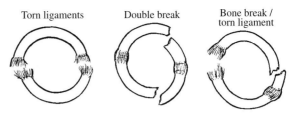

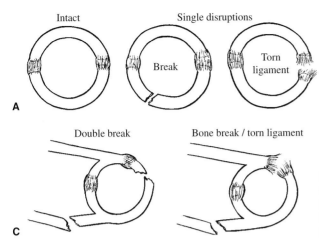

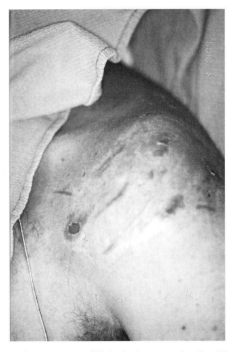

FIGURE 11–3 The diagrams demonstrate an intact ring, a single disruption, and double disruption of the SSSC. **(A)** A single disruption maintains stability of the shoulder girdle. **(B,C)** A double disruption of the SSSC represents an inherently unstable shoulder girdle.

termed "the floating shoulder" (Fig. **11–3B,C**).[12] Double disruptions may take a variety of forms from purely osseous or ligamentous disruptions to a combination of both. Double disruptions may also range from pure ring or strut injuries to a combination of both. Williams et al[13] have disputed the concept of shoulder instability following a double disruption of the SSSC in biomechanical testing of sequentially sectioned cadaveric shoulders. They found that pure strut injuries (ipsilateral clavicle and scapular neck fractures) did not produce an unstable shoulder without an additional ligamentous disruption of the ring (coracoacromial or AC ligaments).

Several important neurovascular structures lie in close proximity to the scapula (see Fig. **2–11** in Chapter 2). Due to the mobility of the scapula and the lack of fixed attachments of the scapula to the axial skeleton, neurovascular structures are at risk for injury. The brachial plexus and axillary artery are in close contact with the undersurface of the coracoid and lie deep to the pectoralis minor tendon. In high-energy mechanisms of injury, these structures may be tethered as they course from the thoracic outlet, past the anterior aspect of the shoulder girdle, and into the upper extremity. The suprascapular neurovascular structures pass through the incisura scapula, or scapular notch. The notch is bridged by the transverse scapular ligament, and the suprascapular artery and nerve pass over and under this ligament, respectively. The suprascapular nerve is especially vulnerable both to direct injury due to an extension of a scapular neck fracture into the scapular notch and to indirect injury due to traction caused by fracture displacement. Similarly, the axillary nerve may sustain direct or indirect injury due to a displaced scapular neck fracture. Finally, the dorsal scapular and accessory nerves found in association with the branches of the transverse cervical artery along the medial border of the scapula are vulnerable to injury in displaced fractures of scapular body.

■ Clinical Evaluation

The most important aspect of the initial clinical evaluation of the patient with a scapular fracture is the prompt recognition and management of any associated injuries. Given the high association of concomitant injuries (80 to 95%) to the thorax, neurovascular structures, and shoulder girdle, an isolated fracture of the scapula is diagnosis of exclusion. Full Advanced Trauma Life Support (ATLS) evaluation is routinely performed. The mechanism of injury, level of consciousness, and Glasgow Coma Scale score are all documented.

FIGURE 11–4 Clinical photograph of a 38-year-old man who sustained a displaced left scapular body fracture, demonstrating the soft tissue injury associated with this high-energy mechanism.

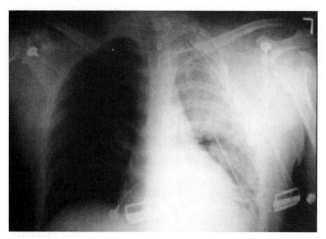

FIGURE 11–5 Chest radiograph of a displaced left scapular body fracture with an ipsilateral pulmonary contusion.

The clinical assessment begins with a systematic and careful examination for associated injuries, which may be potentially life threatening or limb threatening. Detailed examination of the mediastinum and thorax is performed to evaluate pulmonary contusions, tension pneumothorax, and rib fractures.

A focused examination of the shoulder is then performed. Physical findings can be subtle with minimal deformity, as in a nondisplaced fracture of the acromion process, to obvious with gross deformity, as in a potentially life- and limb-threatening scapulothoracic dissociation. Careful assessment and documentation of soft tissue injury including abrasions, open wounds, closed degloving injuries, and muscular trauma is critical. Skin surface abrasions lead to bacterial contamination and

may delay or preclude surgical intervention (Fig. 11–4). Deeper soft tissue injury can also lead to wound healing problems after surgery. Patients typically present with the upper extremity in an adducted, immobile position, and supported by the contralateral hand. There is usually diffuse tenderness and swelling about the shoulder girdle with limited, painful range of motion. Crepitus in the scapula is difficult to elicit, given the significant soft tissue coverage; however, crepitus and a palpable step-off in the clavicle may be obvious based on its subcutaneous location and should be specifically evaluated.

A comprehensive neurologic examination is performed to identify any brachial plexus pathology. Not only is the function of the musculocutaneous, radial, median, and ulnar nerves tested, but also particular attention is paid to the axillary and suprascapular nerves due to their close anatomic relationship with the scapula. It is often difficult to evaluate the function of these nerves in the acutely injured patient; however, serial exams should be performed after the initial evaluation to identify a potential deficit. A careful examination is conducted also to detect any vascular injury and to assess limb viability. Although easily performed in the awake patient, this evaluation is more difficult in the patient with a significant head injury.

Radiographic Evaluation

The trauma series consisting of an anteroposterior (AP) chest radiograph, lateral cervical spine radiograph, and AP pelvis radiograph is standard in the evaluation of the polytrauma patient with a scapular fracture. Often, the scapular fracture is first identified on the AP chest radiograph (Fig. 11–5). The chest radiograph should be

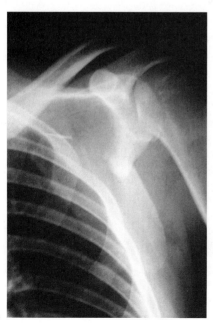

A

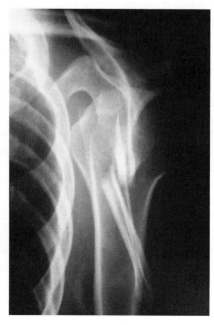

B

FIGURE 11–6 Anteroposterior **(A)** and scapular lateral **(B)** of a displaced scapular body fracture.

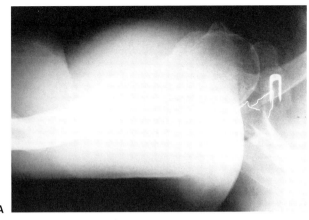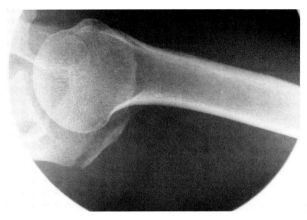

A
B

FIGURE 11-7 Axillary radiographs of a displaced glenoid (A) demonstrating anterior subluxation of the humeral head and (B) a fracture of the posterior portion of the acromion.

considered an essential part of the evaluation because of the high incidence of associated injuries to the thorax and its contents. Scapulothoracic dissociation can also be diagnosed on the chest radiograph when the nonrotated film demonstrates significant lateral displacement of the scapula as measured by the distance from the sternal notch to the medial border of the scapula or to the glenoid margin.[14]

The radiographic evaluation specific to scapula fractures includes the standard shoulder trauma series of the shoulder, consisting of not only AP and lateral views of the affected shoulder in the plane of the scapula (Fig. 11-6), but also an axillary view. The axillary view can be particularly helpful in identifying acromial fractures or in determining glenohumeral subluxation associated with an intraarticular glenoid fracture (Fig. 11-7). Further radiographic images that may be helpful in certain situations include oblique views to better delineate fracture lines of the scapula, a 45° caudal tilt view to better identify fractures of the clavicle, and a 45° cephalic tilt view to better identify fractures of the coracoid (Fig. 11-8).

A computed tomography (CT) scan with two-dimensional reconstruction in the sagittal and coronal planes can provide additional anatomic detail and can better delineate the personality of the scapula fracture. It is especially important in intraarticular glenoid fractures to assess the amount of intraarticular involvement as well as the degree of displacement of the humeral head (Fig. 11-9). It is also especially helpful in preoperative planning when considering operative management. CT scan with three-dimensional reconstruction provides excellent reproductions of fracture patterns and may provide important information in complex cases (Fig. 11-10); however, their direct benefits in determining a treatment plan have yet to be determined.

■ Classification

Scapular fractures are commonly described according to the anatomic location (Fig. 11-11). Scapular body fractures are most commonly encountered, accounting for 50 to 60% of scapular fractures in most series. Scapular neck fractures occur in about 25% of cases, followed by glenoid, acromion, spine, and coracoid fractures, in decreasing order of frequency.[2–8,15] In many cases, fractures represent some combination of these different types. The most common combinations include body fractures with extraarticular extension into the neck, and intraarticular glenoid fractures with extraarticular extension into the neck and body. Ada and Miller[2] introduced an anatomic classification based upon their review of fracture patterns in 116 scapular fractures. Scapular fractures were divided into four types and classified according to the anatomic location of the fracture (Table 11-2).

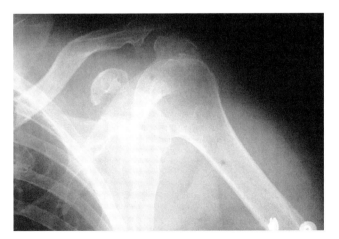

FIGURE 11-8 Additional radiographic view with a 45° cephalic tilt to identify a fracture of the base of the coracoid.

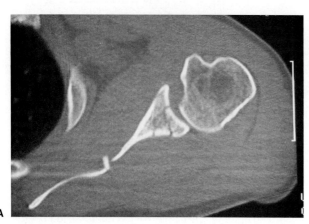 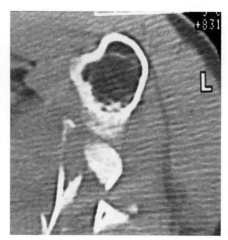

FIGURE 11–9 Computed tomography (CT) scan of a scapular body fracture with a nondisplaced intraarticular component **(A)** and a scapular body fracture with a comminuted and displaced glenoid component **(B)**.

Other classification systems have focused on specific fracture locations. Eyres et al[16] classified coracoid fractures according to the degree of extension of the fracture into the base of the coracoid. Types I, II, and III do not involve the body of the scapula and can be treated nonoperatively. Type IV fractures involve the body of the scapula, and type V involve the glenoid fossa. Operative management is indicated for types IV and V fractures. Kuhn et al[17] introduced a classification system of acromial fractures. Acromial fractures were divided into three types: nondisplaced (type I), displaced (type II), and displaced with subacromial impingement (type III). Surgical treatment was recommended only for type III fractures.

Ideberg[18] introduced a classification system specifically for intraarticular fractures of the glenoid and based on fracture pattern (Fig. 11–12). Five types have been described and are classified according to the location of the exiting fracture line (Table 11–3). In type I fractures, there is an avulsion fracture of the anterior rim of the glenoid. In type IIA fractures there is a transverse fracture through the glenoid fossa exiting inferiorly, and in type IIB there is an oblique fracture through the glenoid fossa exiting inferiorly. In type III there is an oblique fracture through the glenoid that exits superiorly and is often associated with an AC joint injury. In type IV fractures there is a transverse fracture exiting the medial border of the scapula. Type V fractures represent a combination of type II and type IV injury patterns. Goss[19] added a modification to the Ideberg classification and included a type VI glenoid fracture to differentiate severely comminuted glenoid fractures.

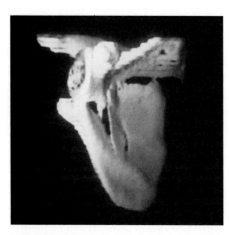

FIGURE 11–10 Three-dimensional CT reconstruction of a displaced scapular neck and body fracture.

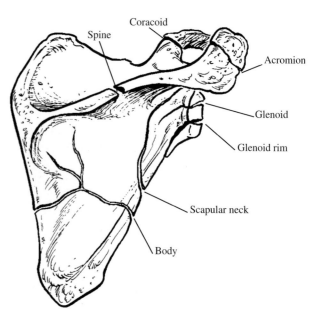

FIGURE 11–11 The anatomic classification of scapular fractures.

TABLE 11–2 Ada and Miller Anatomic Classification of Scapula Fractures

Type I	Acromion, scapular spine, coracoid process fractures
Type II	Scapular neck fractures
Type III	Glenoid fractures
Type IV	Scapular body fractures

The Orthopaedic Trauma Association (OTA) has introduced the most comprehensive classification of scapular fractures (Table **11–4**).[20] Fractures are classified into either extraarticular (Fig. **11–13A**) or intraarticular involvement (Fig. **11–13B**). Extraarticular (type A) fractures are further subclassified into fractures of the scapular processes (A1), body (A2), and complex (A3). Intraarticular (type B) fractures are subclassified into impacted glenoid (B1), nonimpacted glenoid (B2), and complex glenoid (B3) fractures. The clinical utility of this slightly cumbersome classification scheme is based on the fact that nearly all scapular fractures can be classified. Double disruptions of the SSSC, or "floating shoulder" injuries, can be classified under extraarticular complex (A3) injuries. Intraarticular glenoid fractures with extraarticular extension into the

TABLE 11–3 Ideberg Classification of Glenoid Fractures

Glenoid Fractures	Exiting Fracture Line(s)	Description
Type 1	Anterior to glenoid fossa	Avulsion fracture of glenoid rim
Type 2	Inferior to glenoid fossa	Type 2A: Transverse Type 2B: Oblique
Type 3	Superior to glenoid fossa	Usually oblique fracture Often associated with acromioclavicular (AC) joint injury
Type 4	Medial border of scapula	Transverse fracture
Type 5	Inferior to glenoid fossa *and* medial border of scapula	Combination of types 2 and 4
Type 6		Severe comminution Modification of original classification

neck or body can be classified under intraarticular complex (B3) injuries.

A simple, user-friendly, yet comprehensive classification system of scapular fractures that is useful not only in guiding management but also in predicting outcomes is still lacking. The difficulty in developing such a classification

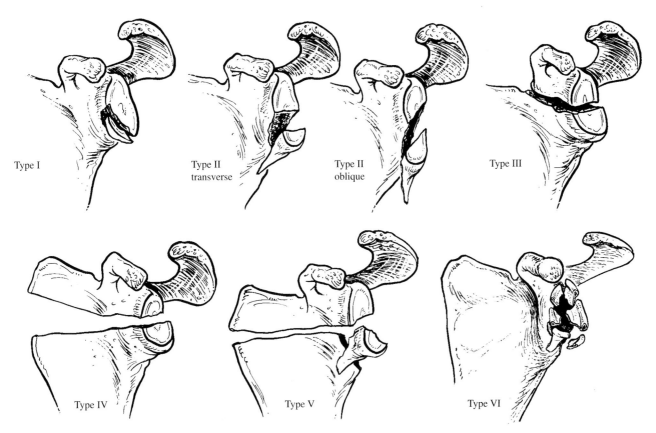

FIGURE 11–12 The Ideberg Classification of glenoid fractures. Type VI fractures were an addition to the original classification and represents a severely comminuted glenoid fracture.

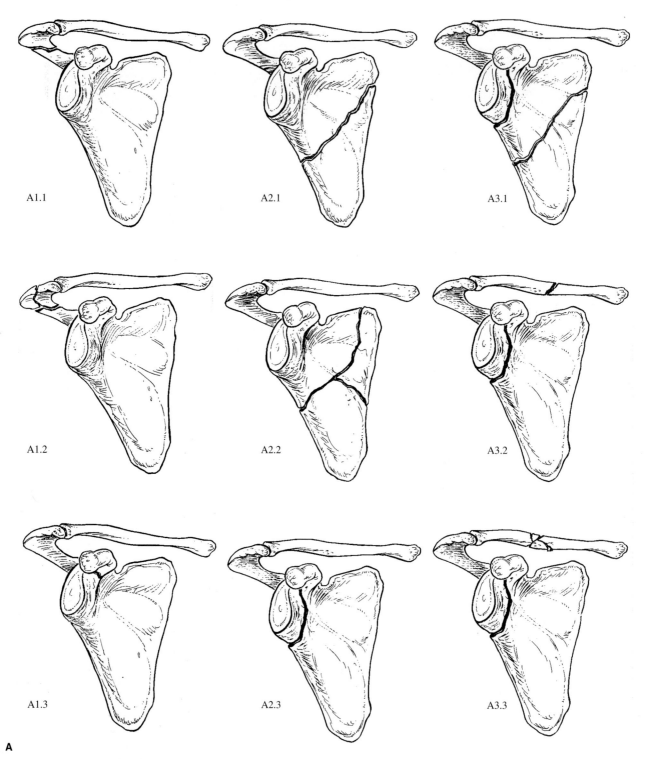

A1.1   A2.1   A3.1

A1.2   A2.2   A3.2

A1.3   A2.3   A3.3

A

FIGURE 11–13 The Orthopaedic Trauma Association (OTA) classification of scapular fractures. Fractures are classified based on either extraarticular **(A)** or intraarticular **(B)** involvement. Extraarticular (type A) fractures are subclassified into fractures of

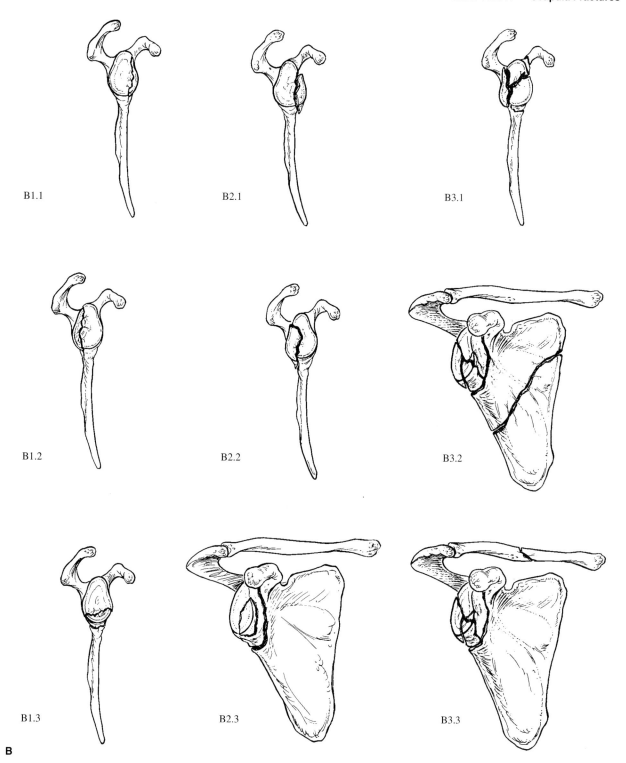

B1.1

B2.1

B3.1

B1.2

B2.2

B3.2

B1.3

B2.3

B3.3

B

FIGURE 11–13 *(Continued)* the scapular processes (A1), body (A2), and complex (A3). Intraarticular (type B) fractures are subclassified into impacted glenoid (B1), nonimpacted glenoid (B2), and complex glenoid (B3) fractures.

TABLE 11–4 Orthopaedic Trauma Association (OTA) Classification of Scapular Fractures

Type	Subtype	Modifier
Type A: Extraarticular scapula	A1: Scapular processes	A1.1: Acromion, simple A1.2: Acromion, multifragmentary A1.3: Coracoid process
	A2: Scapular body	A2.1: Simple A2.2: Multifragmentary A2.3: Glenoid neck
	A3: Complex	A3.1: Glenoid neck and body A3.2: Glenoid neck and clavicle (simple) A3.3: Glenoid neck and clavicle (multifragmentary)
Type B: Intraarticular glenoid	B1: Impacted glenoid	B1.1: Anterior rim B1.2: Posterior rim B1.3: Inferior rim
	B2: Nonimpacted glenoid	B2.1: Anterior rim, free fragment B2.2: Posterior rim, free fragment B2.3: Anterior/posterior rim with glenoid neck
	B3: Complex glenoid	B3.1: Multifragmentary, intraarticular B3.2: Multifragmentary with glenoid neck and/or body B3.3: Multifragmentary with associated clavicle fracture

scheme may be due to the complex and unique anatomy of the scapula, the uncommon nature of these injuries, and the relatively few outcome studies directly comparing the nonoperative and operative management of these injuries.

■ Treatment

Nonoperative

Although there has been increasing interest in the surgical management of scapular fractures, the majority of scapular fractures can be successfully managed nonoperatively with a period of brief immobilization in a sling followed by early range-of-motion exercises as soon as comfort permits. Initially, ice is applied to the affected shoulder to decrease swelling, and a sling is used to support the ipsilateral upper extremity. Early passive range of motion is initiated as soon as discomfort subsides. This approach is useful for both intra- and extraarticular fractures. Fractures that might be displaced by immediate or early passive motion, such as glenoid fossa, scapular

neck, or scapular spine fractures, can be immobilized for 2 to 3 weeks to allow early fracture healing; however, in our experience, early assisted range of motion is unlikely to cause additional displacement in these fracture patterns. Closed reduction of displaced fractures is usually not attempted because the significant soft tissue envelope surrounding the scapula precludes a successful effort.

Numerous series have reported the satisfactory results of nonoperative management of scapular fractures.[3–5,7,21] Caution should be exercised in interpreting the results of closed treatment of scapular fracture because most series contain various types of fracture patterns, including intraarticular, extraarticular, and complex fractures. The importance of identifying the results based on specific fracture patterns cannot be overemphasized. Nevertheless, most series report good-to-excellent results in greater than 70% of patients using the criteria of pain, strength, and range of motion.[3–5,7,21] Extraarticular fractures (body, neck, and spine) were successfully managed using closed treatment in most series.[3,7]

Certain fracture patterns treated nonoperatively have been associated with varying degrees of shoulder disability, such as loss of shoulder motion, painful motion, and limited muscle strength. Poor outcomes with closed management have been found in displaced, incongruent intraarticular glenoid fractures, scapular neck fractures with translational displacement greater than 1 cm, or angulatory displacement greater than 40°, acromial fractures with subacromial impingement, and coracoid fractures with extension into the base or glenoid fossa.[2,9,16,17,19,21–23] As a result, these fractures are more commonly considered for operative management.

Operative

Surgical treatment is reserved only for a minority of scapular fractures. The indications for surgical management remain controversial and continue to evolve as more studies comparing the functional outcomes of nonoperative and operative management are reported. Although universal agreement does not exist concerning surgical indications, there are specific situations when surgical management should be considered. Absolute indications for operative treatment include open scapular fractures and scapular fractures with associated vascular injury, in which skeletal stabilization is warranted to protect the vascular repair; however, the incidence of these types of injuries is exceedingly rare. The remainder of scapular fractures discussed can be considered relative indications for operative treatment (Table 11–5).

Displaced glenoid fractures that involve more than 25% of the articular surface are best managed with open reduction and internal fixation (ORIF) to restore articular

TABLE 11-5 Operative Indications for Scapular Fractures

Operative indications
Absolute indications
   1. Open scapula fractures
   2. Scapula fractures with associated vascular injury
Relative indications
   1. Displaced glenoid fractures involving >25% articular surface
   2. Scapular neck or body fractures >1 cm displacement
   3. Scapular neck fractures >40° angulation
   4. Acromion fractures resulting in subacromial impingement
   5. Coracoid process fractures resulting in functional AC separation
   6. "Floating shoulder": double disruption of the SSSC

congruity.[19,24-26] This is particularly important if the glenoid fracture results in subluxation of the humeral head. Restoration of a stable and congruent glenohumeral joint is an important goal of treatment. Displaced intraarticular glenoid fractures may result in the development of posttraumatic glenohumeral arthritis. Some authors report that as little as 2 mm of articular incongruity can lead to glenohumeral arthritis. Others report that 5 mm displacement of the glenoid fossa and 10 mm displacement of the glenoid rim can result in residual instability.[9,19] In these situations, articular congruity must be restored to ensure stability of the glenohumeral joint and to minimize the possibility of glenohumeral arthritis.

Scapular neck or body fractures with translational displacement of more than 1 cm or angulatory displacement of more than 40° have been associated with poor outcomes when managed nonoperatively and should be considered for operative management (Fig. 11–14).[2,22,23] Open reduction restores the direction and position of the glenoid fossa, and thereby restores the position of the humeral head within the coracoacromial arch. It also restores the anatomic relationship of the rotator cuff musculature and reestablishes the dynamic stabilization of the glenohumeral joint provided by force coupling and concavity-compression. At less than 90° of abduction, the deltoid muscle generates a shear vector in the glenoid fossa. This force is neutralized by the downward-directed vector of the rotator cuff muscles, which creates a stabilizing compressive force across the glenoid. A marked change in the glenoid axis (greater than 40°) caused by fracture displacement alters the lever arm of the rotator cuff muscles and converts the desired compressive force into an undesirable shear or sliding force. Furthermore, medial displacement (greater than 1 cm) of body, spine, and neck fractures compromises rotator cuff function as a result of the shortened lever arm of the rotator cuff muscles.

Operative indications for double disruptions of the SSSC, or "floating shoulder" injuries, are currently

evolving. Long-term functional impairment including muscle weakness, shoulder pain, subacromial impingement, degenerative joint disease, and neurovascular compromise as a result of the loss of structural integrity to the shoulder girdle have been proposed as the indications for operative management (Fig. 11–15).[12,27,28] Other studies have disputed these findings, reporting good functional outcomes with nonoperative treatment (Fig. 11–16).[29-32] Egol et al[31] found that good results could be seen with both operative and nonoperative management and emphasized the importance of individualizing treatment of these injuries.

The results following operative management of "floating shoulder" injuries have been good, whether both injuries or only one injury was addressed.[27,33-35] Leung and Lam[33] reported 93% (14 of 15) good-to-excellent results in patients treated with operative fixation of both injuries, in particular scapular neck and clavicle fractures; however, Rikli et al[34] and Hersovici et al[27] also reported successful management of ipsilateral clavicle and scapular neck fractures with ORIF of the clavicle fracture only (Fig. 11–17). Oh et al[35] found no differences in functional outcome between patients with clavicle fixation only and patients with fixation of both the clavicle and scapula.

Whether a double disruption of the SSSC produces an inherently unstable relationship between the shoulder girdle complex and axial skeleton is still a point of controversy. Despite the good results reported with both operative and nonoperative treatment, most studies have been retrospective series and may introduce a selection bias in which only the more severely displaced fractures underwent surgery. Prospective randomized studies directly comparing the two treatment modalities are needed to provide more definitive indications for surgery.

Acromial fractures are very uncommon and are usually treated nonoperatively with satisfactory results; however, fractures of the anterior or lateral aspects of the acromion with inferior displacement may result in significant compromise of the subacromial space and can lead to rotator cuff impingement, causing pain and restricted motion.[8,17,28] In these cases, elevation of the fragment and internal fixation may be indicated due to the poor results found with nonsurgical treatment.[17] When a rotator cuff tear is found in association with these fractures, surgical repair of the rotator cuff should also be performed.

Although the majority of coracoid fractures are treated nonoperatively, certain coracoid fractures are amenable to operative fixation. Fractures that extend beyond the base of the coracoid and into the glenoid fossa causing articular incongruity are best managed with ORIF.[16] Displaced fractures of the coracoid process that occur in the context of an AC joint separation may

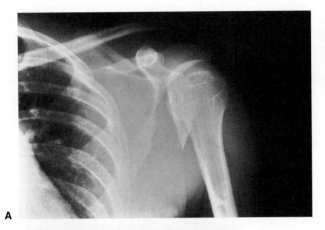

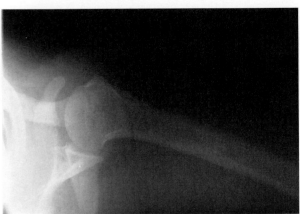

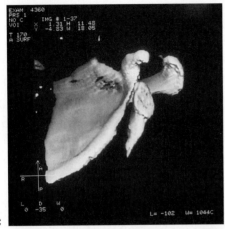

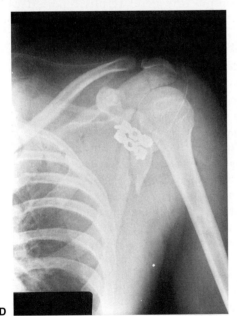

FIGURE 11–14 A displaced scapular neck fracture. **(A)** AP radiograph. **(B)** Axillary view. **(C)** 3D CT reconstruction. The fracture was reduced and fixed with two 3.5-mm reconstruction plates utilizing a posterior approach. Posterior AP **(D)** and axillary **(E)** radiographs show restoration of alignment and orientation of the articular surface.

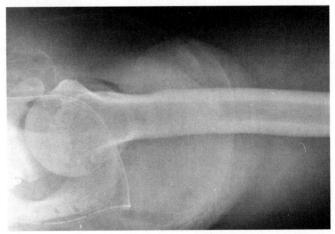

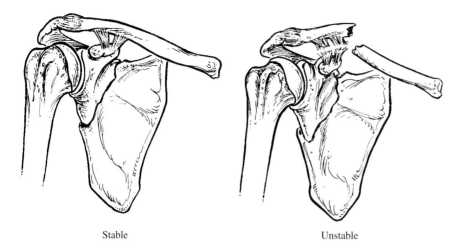

Stable   Unstable

FIGURE 11–15 An isolated scapular neck fracture maintains stability of the shoulder girdle due to the intact clavicular strut. A disruption of both bony struts (scapular body and clavicle) in association with a disruption of the ring (coracoclavicular ligaments) represents an inherently unstable shoulder complex.

also be considered for operative treatment when there is significant shoulder dysfunction or skin compromise.[28,36,37] A complete AC joint dislocation occurs from not only the functional loss of the CC ligaments that are attached to the coracoid process fragment, but also a concomitant disruption in the integrity of the AC ligaments.

Preferred Technique

Preoperative Planning
The more complex, significantly displaced injuries indicated for operative management require a thorough assessment of the personality of the fracture; therefore, careful preoperative planning is of paramount importance in the management of these injuries. High-quality radiographs are necessary for understanding the fracture pattern and the nature of displacement. Frequently, radiographs of the contralateral, uninjured shoulder may be helpful. CT scan with two-dimension reconstructions in the sagittal and coronal planes can provide additional information about intraarticular involvement, size and location of fracture fragments, and humeral head subluxation/displacement. CT scanning with three-dimensional reconstructions may also provide additional information in complex scapular fractures.

The surgical plan is formulated in a systematic fashion by understanding the fracture pattern and fragments of the injured side and comparing it with the

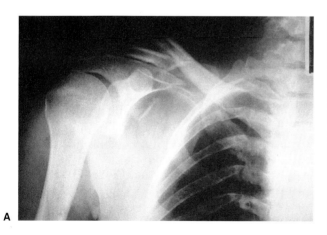

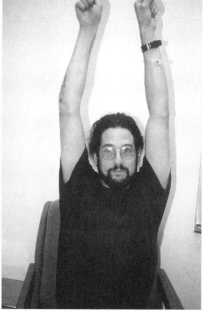

FIGURE 11–16 (A) AP radiograph of double disruption of the SSSC (ipsilateral scapular neck and clavicle fractures). (B) This injury was treated nonoperatively with an excellent functional outcome.

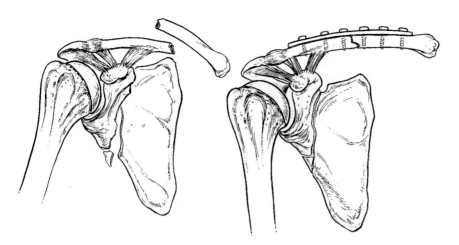

FIGURE 11–17 Fixation of one of the bony struts (clavicle fracture) in a double disruption of the SSSC can indirectly reduce the second disruption (scapular body fracture) when the ligaments remain intact.

"anatomically intact" uninjured side. The position of the patient, incision, and exposure are all determined based on the personality of the fracture. Reduction techniques, reduction instruments, and implants for fixation are anticipated as part of the preoperative plan. The use of preoperative drawings that include the step-by-step operative plan can be helpful. Although intraoperative changes may be necessary due to unrecognized injuries or severity of injury, preparation and a careful preoperative plan eliminate most of the guesswork, reduce operative time, and optimize the operative result.

Surgical Exposure

Due to the numerous neurovascular structures that lie in close proximity to the scapula, surgical management of scapular fractures requires a thorough understanding of the osseous and soft tissue anatomy of the shoulder girdle. The three most commonly utilized approaches are the anterior or deltopectoral approach, the posterior approach, and the superior approach. The location and personality of the fracture determine the operative approach. The anterior approach is recommended for fixation of fractures of the anterior and inferior glenoid and coracoid fractures. The posterior approach is utilized for fractures of the posterior rim of the glenoid, glenoid fossa, scapular neck, body, and spine. The superior approach is used for acromial fractures, and in some situations, coracoid fractures. In some clinical situations, a combination of approaches can be used. For example, a superior approach may be used in conjunction with a posterior approach if there is difficulty in controlling the glenoid fragment associated with a scapular neck fracture.

Anterior Approach

The anterior approach is primarily utilized for intraarticular glenoid fractures in which the displaced fragment is anterior, as well as for coracoid fractures. The patient is placed in the beach chair position with the head stabilized on a headrest to prevent neck hyperextension and traction on the cervical nerve roots or the brachial plexus. A small bolster is often placed behind the scapulae to facilitate exposure to the anterior aspect of the shoulder.

With the arm in neutral rotation, a straight skin incision is utilized that begins just lateral to the coracoid process and is directed distally to the deltoid insertion. The cephalic vein is identified in the deltopectoral interval and is usually retracted laterally because most of its branches enter from the deltoid side. The deltoid is retracted laterally and the pectoralis major medially. The clavicopectoral fascia is identified and divided just lateral to the conjoined tendon muscles, thereby allowing these muscles to be retraced medially. The subscapularis tendon and its insertion into the lesser tuberosity can be identified (Fig. **11–18A**).

When the arm is then externally rotated, the subscapularis tendon becomes more visible. The subscapularis tendon and underlying capsule are divided ~1 cm medial to the lesser tuberosity and retracted medially to expose the glenoid. The subscapularis tenotomy extends from the rotator interval proximally to the anterior humeral circumflex vessels distally. Dissection inferiorly must be meticulous as the neurovascular bundle as the axillary nerve lies just inferior to the subscapularis at its medial portion. A humeral head retractor is then inserted into the glenohumeral joint to displace the humeral head posteriorly and expose the glenoid articular surface (Fig. **11–18B**). When exposure of the coracoid is necessary, the rotator interval should be divided medially to the glenoid margin. This corresponds to the base of the coracoid, which exposes fractures in this area.

Posterior Approach

When the primary component of the fracture is posterior, fractures of the scapular neck, body, spine, and glenoid are best exposed using the posterior approach.

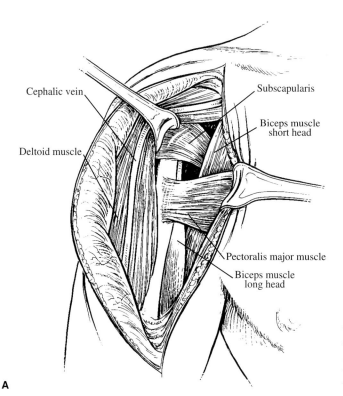

Cephalic vein

Deltoid muscle

Subscapularis

Biceps muscle
short head

Pectoralis major muscle

Biceps muscle
long head

A

FIGURE 11–18 Anterior exposure of the glenohumeral joint (right shoulder) utilizing a deltopectoral approach. Superficially, the deltoid along with the cephalic vein is retracted laterally, while the pectoralis major is retracted medially. **(A)** The clavicopectoral fascia is incised to expose the conjoined tendon and subscapularis. **(B)** After the subscapularis and capsule are incised and elevated off the lesser tuberosity, the glenoid is exposed using an angled retractor to displace the humeral head posteriorly.

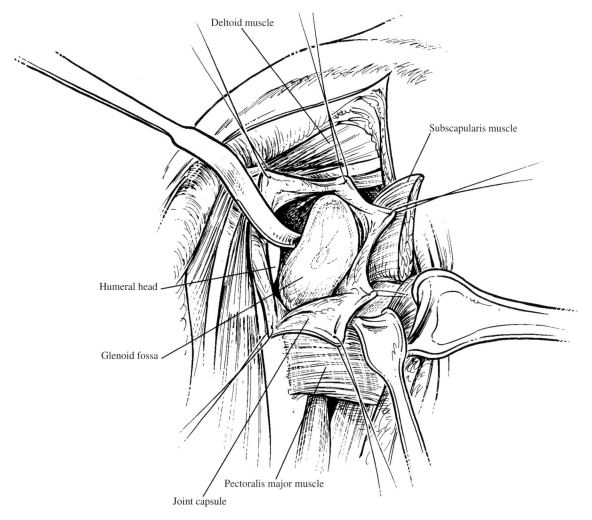

Deltoid muscle

Subscapularis muscle

Humeral head

Glenoid fossa

Pectoralis major muscle

Joint capsule

B

This is performed with the patient in the lateral decubitus position.

The skin incision is placed in the posterior axillary line extending proximally to the acromion and inferiorly to the axilla. Medial and lateral skin flaps are developed to expose the underlying deltoid muscle as well as the scapular spine. The extent of dissection depends on the degree of exposure necessary. For isolated posterior glenoid fractures, a muscle-splitting approach can be utilized; however, when a more extensile approach is necessary, the deltoid should be sharply dissected from the acromion, extending several centimeters along the spine. When elevating the deltoid, caution must be exercised, as the suprascapular nerve is at risk for injury as it courses around the base of the scapular spine. The interval between the posterior and middle deltoid is then developed distally from the posterolateral corner of the acromion. The deeper interval between the infraspinatus and teres minor is then identified and developed. Development of this plane is facilitated by identifying the insertion of the teres minor onto the inferior facet of the greater tuberosity. By staying within this interval and preventing traction inferior to the teres minor, injury to the axillary nerve can be avoided. As the infraspinatus is retracted superiorly and the teres minor inferiorly, the posterior capsule is then exposed (Fig. 11–19A). A longitudinal capsular incision is made to expose the joint. A humeral head retractor can be inserted to expose the glenoid articular surface (Fig. 11–19B). Additional exposure to the scapular body can be obtained

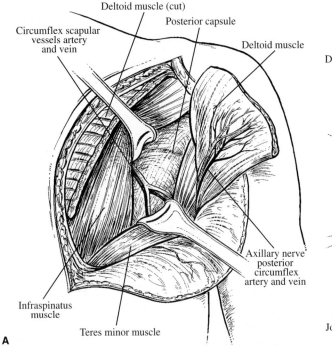

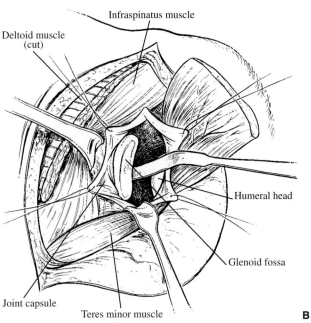

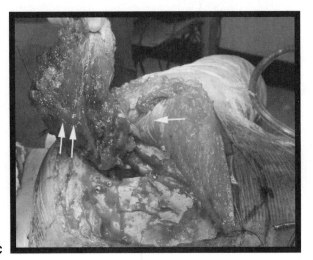

FIGURE 11–19 (A) Posterior exposure of the glenohumeral joint (right shoulder) and/or scapular body through the Judet approach using the internervous plane between the infraspinatus and teres minor. Exposure of the glenoid fossa is accomplished through a posterior capsulotomy. **(B)** An angled retractor is used to displace the humeral head anteriorly. **(C)** Intraoperative photograph demonstrating the posterior deltoid detached from the posterior acromion (single arrow). The deep interval is through the infraspinatus and teres minor. Greater exposure of the scapular body and neck may be accomplished by reflecting the infraspinatus laterally off of the scapula (double arrow).

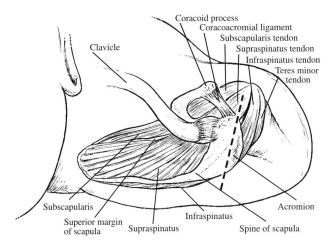

Clavicle
Coracoid process
Coracoacromial ligament
Subscapularis tendon
Supraspinatus tendon
Infraspinatus tendon
Teres minor tendon
Subscapularis
Superior margin of scapula
Supraspinatus
Infraspinatus
Spine of scapula
Acromion

FIGURE 11-20 The superior approach utilizes a strap incision over the acromion placed adjacent to the acromioclavicular joint. The superior approach is usually used for acromial fractures and can be used in conjunction with posterior or anterior approaches.

by elevating the posterior deltoid off the scapular spine and by reflecting the infraspinatus laterally off the scapula (Fig. **11-19C**).

Superior Approach

Acromial fractures and occasionally coracoid fractures are best exposed with the superior approach. It may also be used in combination with a posterior or anterior approach to provide additional exposure to a superiorly displaced glenoid fragment (Fig. **11-20**). A strap incision is centered over the acromion or AC joint, depending on whether the acromion or the coracoid, respectively, is being exposed. If used in combination, an anterior or posterior approach can be extended superiorly to create the strap incision (Fig. **11-21**). Flaps are developed to facilitate exposure of the acromion. For acromial fractures, deltoid detachment is usually not necessary. For coracoid fractures, the anterior deltoid is split in line with its fibers at the AC joint. Blunt dissection allows exposure of the coracoid fracture, which is usually displaced superiorly.

Reduction and Fixation Techniques

Open, direct reduction of fracture fragments as opposed to closed, indirect reduction is generally necessary for most fractures involving the scapula. Indirect reduction of fracture fragments is often difficult to obtain except in the cases of double disruption of the SSSC. In these situations, reduction and stabilization of one of the disruptions often indirectly reduces and stabilizes the other disruption. For example, ORIF of a displaced clavicle fracture frequently indirectly reduces and stabilizes an ipsilateral scapular neck fracture and obviates the need for scapular fixation; however, if the second

disruption cannot be satisfactorily reduced and stabilized indirectly, a direct ORIF may be necessary.

The selection of fixation implants is dependent on the type of fracture, available bone stock, and preference of the operating surgeon. Plates and screws from the AO/Association for the Study of Internal Fixation (ASIF) small fragment and the 4.0- or 4.5-mm cannulated screw set are frequently used. In cases with significant comminution or with fracture fragments too small for screw fixation, suture fixation or Kirschner wire (K-wire) fixation utilizing tension band principles is also an option. Because of the risk of migration, K-wires alone are not recommended for definitive fixation. They can be utilized in combination with tension band wiring to decrease the concerns about wire migration. The 3.5-mm reconstruction plates can be useful in fixation of neck, spine, and some acromial fractures because they can be contoured to fit the scapular anatomy. Fixation of intraarticular glenoid fragments is usually achieved with 4.0-mm cannulated screws.

Stable fixation requires adequate bony purchase. Because much of the scapular body is a thin plate of bone, fracture fixation should utilize the four regions of adequate bone stock. These include the glenoid neck, the coracoid process, the lateral scapular border, and the base of the scapular spine (Fig. **11-22A**). Depending on the type and location of the fracture, at least one of these regions should be incorporated in the fixation (Fig. **11-22B**).

Techniques for Specific Fracture Types
Glenoid Rim Fractures

Rim fractures of the glenoid are usually anteriorly displaced, and so an anterior approach is generally utilized. Large fragments are usually stabilized with 4.0- or 4.5-mm cannulated cancellous screws (Fig. **11-23**). The fracture fragment is reduced and provisionally stabilized with one or two K-wires. The inclination of the glenoid fossa serves as a guide for appropriate position of the K-wires. After intraoperative and fluoroscopic confirmation of anatomic fracture reduction and appropriate K-wire placement, the cannulated drill and appropriately size cancellous screws are placed. There may be an associated labral injury accompanying these fractures. The labral detachment may be reduced using either suture anchors or nonabsorbable sutures through osseous tunnels.

Glenoid Fossa Fractures

Fractures of the glenoid fossa generally involve larger fragments than glenoid rim fractures. Therefore, the humeral head may be subluxated in the direction of the displaced fragment. Although the fracture line is generally transverse, large anterior or posterior fragments may subluxate the humeral head anteriorly or posteriorly, respectively. The location of fracture fragment and

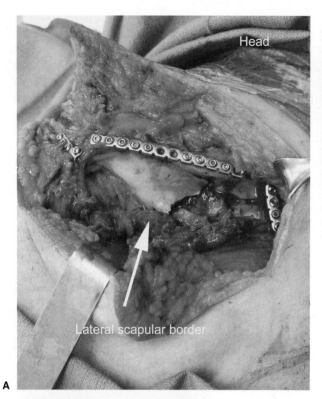

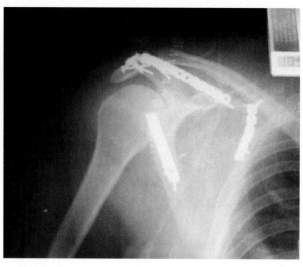

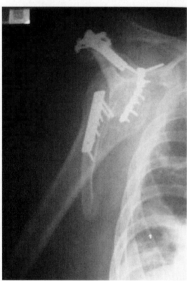

FIGURE 11–21 The superior approach combined with the posterior approach **(A)** was used to reduce and fix the scapular body, scapular spine, and acromion fractures in this case. **(B,C)** The postoperative radiographs demonstrate a near-anatomic reduction as a result, in part, of the extensile nature of the combined approaches.

humeral head determines the surgical approach. An anterior approach is favored for anteriorly displaced fossa fractures; a posterior approach is favored for posteriorly displaced glenoid fossa fractures.

Lag screw fixation using 4.0-mm cancellous or 4.0-mm cannulated screws or compression plating with 3.5-mm limited contact dynamic compression (LCDC) plate is used to stabilize the fragment. The application of a 3.5-mm one-third tubular, LCDC or reconstruction plate with 3.5-mm cortical screws as a neutralization plate to lag screw fixation is also recommended to provide stable

fixation for early active range of motion postoperatively (Fig. 11–24).

Scapular Neck and Body Fractures

Fractures of the scapular neck and body are generally approached posteriorly. It is not uncommon for these fractures to have intraarticular extension into the glenoid fossa. Lag screw fixation or compression plating similar to that used in glenoid fossa fractures is performed for scapular neck fractures. Large fragments of the scapular neck should be buttressed posteriorly with

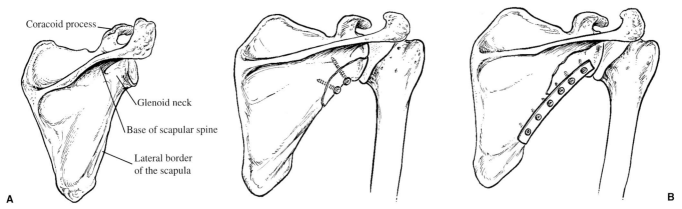

FIGURE 11–22 (A) There are four primary regions of the scapula with adequate bone stock for fixation: the glenoid neck, coracoid process, lateral scapular border, and base of the scapular spine. **(B)** Depending on the type and location of the fracture, fixation (plates, screws) should incorporate at least one of these regions.

a one-third tubular plate or malleable reconstruction plate, compressing the articular fragment against the proximal lateral border of the scapula. The combination of the plate with a 3.5-mm cortical lag screw increases the stability of the fixation. Fractures of the scapular body are reduced directly and stabilized with a contoured reconstruction plate.

Double Disruptions of the Superior Suspensory Shoulder Complex

Ipsilateral scapular neck and clavicle fractures constitute a double disruption of the SSSC. As mentioned, reduction and stabilization of one part of the ring–strut complex usually leads to indirect reduction and stabilization of the other disruption. In this situation, ORIF of the clavicle fracture is generally performed first due to its subcutaneous, easily accessible location. After stabilization of the clavicle with LCDC or reconstruction plate using 3.5-mm cortical screws, the scapular neck is usually reduced adequately and additional fixation of the scapular neck fracture is rarely required (Fig. **11–25**); however, if the scapular neck fracture remains significantly displaced, it may be reduced and stabilized utilizing the posterior approach (Fig. **11–26**).

Acromial Fractures

Displaced acromial fractures with subacromial impingement or AC joint subluxation or dislocation are amenable to ORIF. A superior approach is generally performed. Acromial process fractures are usually too small to allow screw fixation and are fixed with sutures or K-wires using tension band principles. Larger acromial fractures may be amenable to screw fixation (Fig. **11–27**). For fractures at the base of the acromion, 3.5-mm plate and screw fixation is the preferred method for stabilization.

Coracoid Fractures

In coracoid fractures that extend into the base or glenoid, an open reduction through an anterior approach

and internal fixation using 4.0-mm cancellous screws or 4.0-mm cannulated screws is generally performed. In coracoid fractures with concomitant AC joint subluxation or dislocation, the AC joint can be directly reduced using a superior approach and stabilized using CC screw fixation or Steinmann pin fixation across the AC joint. The AC joint can also be indirectly reduced with ORIF of the coracoid fracture.

Postoperative Management and Functional Rehabilitation

A suction drain is often placed intraoperatively to prevent hematoma formation. The patient is initially placed in a sling for comfort. Antibiotics are continued postoperatively for at least 24 hours or until the suction drain has been removed.

The postoperative physical therapy regimen and "safe zones" of motion are determined intraoperatively and are dependent on two factors: (1) the extent of soft tissue exposure utilized, and (2) the stability of fixation. The therapy protocol must be specific and individualized. For example, after an anterior approach with release and repair of the subscapularis, external rotation should be limited to an arc of motion that does not stress the subscapularis repair. On the other hand, after a posterior approach, internal rotation should be limited to an arc of motion that does not stress the external rotators.

Early supervised passive range-of-motion exercises and isometric exercises of the muscles not involved in the surgical exposure are usually begun on the first postoperative day. When the stability of fracture fixation is a concern, the initiation of passive range-of-motion exercises may be delayed to allow some fracture healing to occur; however, almost all patients can be started on at least a limited range of passive motion on the first postoperative day. As fracture healing progresses, the range of motion can be increased. Active-assisted range-of-motion exercises are begun usually at 3 to 4 weeks when some

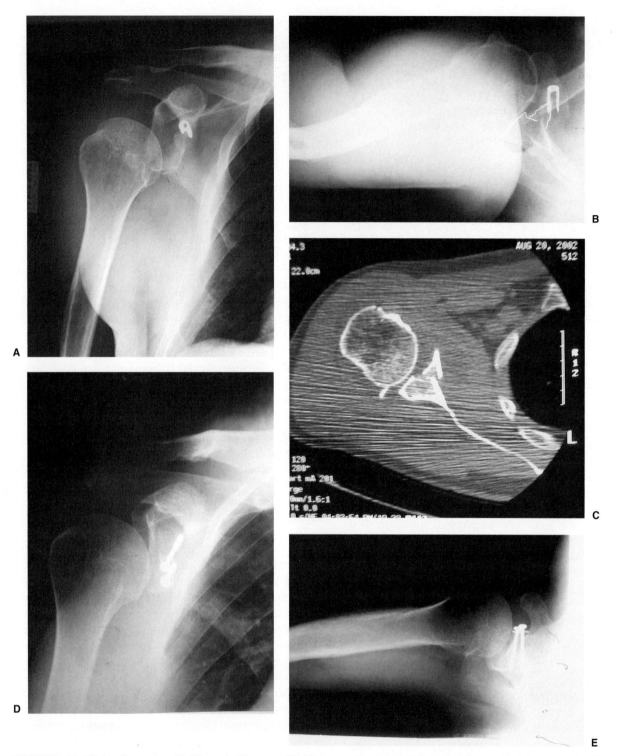

FIGURE 11–23 Radiographs **(A,B)** and CT scan **(C)** of a 52-year-old man with glenohumeral subluxation secondary to a displaced anterior glenoid rim fracture as a result of a fall. The patient had a prior shoulder stabilization procedure for recurrent anterior glenohumeral dislocation. **(D,E)** Postoperative radiographs demonstrate removal of the staple, anatomic reduction of the glenoid, and fixation using two lag screws with washers.

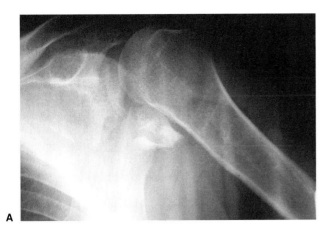

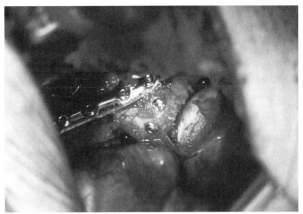

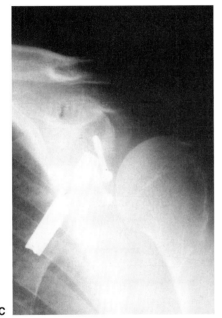

FIGURE 11–24 (A) Radiograph of a 38-year-old man who sustained an intraartic-ular glenoid fracture from a fall off a ladder. (B) A posterior approach was utilized to reduce and fix the glenoid fracture. (C) The postoperative radiograph demon-strates reduction and fixation using two lag screws to reduce the articular surface combined with a neutralization plate. Fixation incorporated the glenoid neck and the lateral border of the scapula, two of the four regions of good bone stock in the scapula.

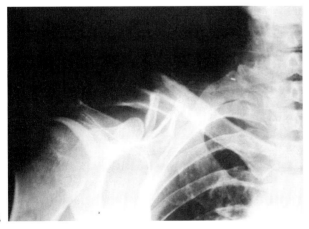

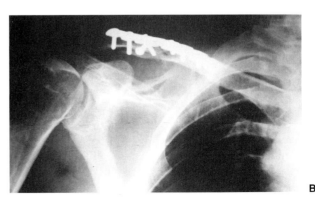

FIGURE 11–25 (A) This 26-year-old man sustained a double disruption of the SSSC consisting of ipsilateral midshaft clavicle and scapular body fractures. (B) Fixation of the clavicle resulted in an indirect reduction of the scapular body fracture and stabilization of the SSSC.

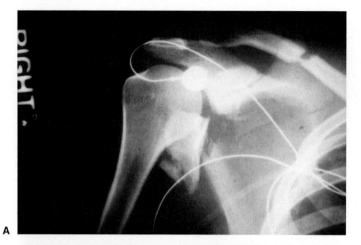

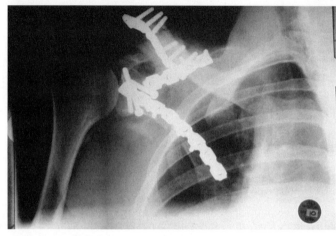

FIGURE 11–26 (A) This 24-year-old man sustained a double disruption of the SSSC consisting of ipsilateral scapula and clavicle fractures. Based on the extent of comminution and intraarticular glenoid involvement, fixation of the clavicle alone would not have resulted in reduction of the glenoid component; therefore, ORIF of the clavicle, glenoid, scapular neck, and scapular body resulted in stabilization of the shoulder girdle and an excellent clinical result **(B)**.

muscle healing has occurred. The patient is progressed to active range-of-motion exercises at about 4 to 6 weeks based on the fracture location. Resistive exercises can be initiated at about 8 to 10 weeks as fracture healing has occurred. Throughout the postoperative rehabilitation program, emphasis should be placed on recovery of the ability to perform activities of daily living.

■ Complications

The most significant complications associated with scapular fractures are those that result from the initial injury. Complications specifically associated with scapular fractures include malunion, nonunion, glenohumeral arthritis, and suprascapular neuropathy; however, the incidence of significant symptoms associated with these complications is small.

Although the vast majority of scapular fractures heal with some degree of malunion, it rarely results in significant shoulder dysfunction. Mild-to-moderate displacement is generally well tolerated. However, patients with severe displacement and substantial malalignment have been shown to have less favorable long-term out-comes compared with patients with scapular fractures in the absence of glenoid malalignment.[38] Thus, malunion of scapular fractures may result in scapulothoracic pain, which can usually be treated with antiinflammatory medications and steroid injections.[24]

Nonunion is extremely uncommon due to the well-vascularized and extensive soft tissue envelope surrounding the scapula. Glenoid fractures are at a greater risk for nonunion due to the intraarticular location and the possibility that synovial fluid can lyse the fracture hematoma and to fracture hematoma and interfere with healing. However, this complication remains primarily a theoretical concern as very few glenoid nonunions have been reported in the literature.

Although late glenohumeral arthritis is an expected complication after displaced intraarticular glenoid fractures, it is rarely reported.[9] If posttraumatic glenohumeral arthritis does occur, it should be treated with the standard measures used to treat glenohumeral arthritis with consideration of prosthetic replacement when nonoperative measures are not effective.

Suprascapular nerve injury can occur in association with body, neck, or coracoid fractures that extend into the suprascapular notch.[24,39,40] The suprascapular nerve

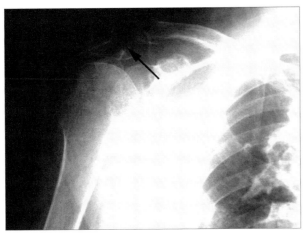 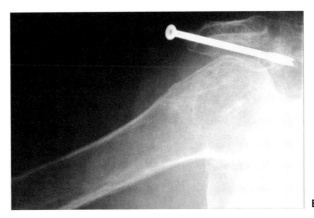

FIGURE 11–27 (A) Radiograph of an acromial neck fracture with inferior displacement into the subacromial space. (black arrow) **(B)** Open reduction and internal fixation was performed using a superior approach and a cannulated screw.

passes through the notch beneath the transverse scapular ligament. Displaced fractures that extend into the notch can decrease the available space within the notch, resulting in a compression neuropathy.[39] The diagnosis requires a high index of suspicion in any patient who has significant loss of active motion and weakness following a scapular body fracture. Electrodiagnostic studies should be performed to confirm the diagnosis. Surgical exploration of the suprascapular notch and release of the transverse scapular ligament may be effective in relieving the symptoms of compression.

■ Summary

Fractures of the scapula are relatively uncommon injuries representing only a small proportion of shoulder fractures; however, scapular fractures may be the most serious injury of all fractures of the shoulder girdle due to their association with high-energy blunt trauma and subsequent life- and limb-threatening injuries, which include pulmonary contusion, pneumothorax, hemothorax, and scapulothoracic dissociation. Prompt recognition and treatment of these potentially life- and limb-threatening injuries are of paramount importance in the management of scapular fractures.

The anatomy of the scapula and its adjacent muscular, ligamentous, and neurovascular structures is unique. A complete appreciation of the complex anatomy of the scapula and its surrounding tissues is critical for appropriate management of these injuries. Due to the uncommon nature of these injuries, experience in the management of scapula fractures is relatively limited. Most scapular fractures are treated nonoperatively with successful functional outcomes. The indications for operative management of scapular fractures, in particular double disruptions of the SSSC, remain

controversial and continue to evolve as more outcome studies of operative and nonoperative management are introduced. Operative management of scapular fractures requires appropriate knowledge of the scapular and periscapular anatomy, a thorough understanding of the personality of the fracture, and a carefully planned surgical approach. Although the functional outcome of the patient is determined in large part by the severity of the initial injury, adequate reduction, stable fixation, meticulous handling of soft tissues, along with the early and appropriate initiation of physical therapy are factors within the control of the orthopaedic surgeon that can improve the surgical result.

REFERENCES

1. Edeland HG, Zachrisson BE. Fracture of the scapular notch associated with lesion of the suprascapular nerve. Acta Orthop Scand 1975;46:758–763
2. Ada JR, Miller ME. Scapular fractures. Analysis of 113 cases. Clin Orthop 1991;269:174–180
3. Armstrong CP, Van der Spuy J. The fractured scapula: importance and management based on a series of 62 patients. Injury 1984;15:324–329
4. McGahan JP, Rab GT, Dublin A. Fractures of the scapula. J Trauma 1980;20:880–883
5. McGinnis M, Denton JR. Fractures of the scapula: a retrospective study of 40 fractured scapulae. J Trauma 1989;29:1488–1493
6. Thompson DA, Flynn TC, Miller PW, Fischer RP. The significance of scapular fractures. J Trauma 1985;25:974–977
7. Wilber MC, Evans EB. Fractures of the scapula. An analysis of forty cases and a review of the literature. J Bone Joint Surg Am 1977;59:358–362
8. Zuckerman JD, Koval KJ, Cuomo F. Fractures of the scapula. Instr Course Lect 1993;42:271–281
9. Bauer G, Fleischmann W, Dussler E. Displaced scapular fractures: indication and long-term results of open reduction and internal fixation. Arch Orthop Trauma Surg 1995;114:215–219
10. Ebraheim NA, An HS, Jackson WT, et al. Scapulothoracic dissociation. J Bone Joint Surg Am 1988;70:428–432

11. Damschen DD, Cogbill TH, Siegel MJ. Scapulothoracic dissociation caused by blunt trauma. J Trauma 1997;42:537–540

12. Goss TP. Double disruptions of the superior shoulder suspensory complex. J Orthop Trauma 1993;7:99–106

13. Williams GR Jr, Naranja J, Klimkiewicz J, Karduna A, Iannotti JP, Ramsey M. The floating shoulder: a biomechanical basis for classification and management. J Bone Joint Surg Am 2001;83-A:1182–1187

14. Kelbel JM, Jardon OM, Huurman WW. Scapulothoracic dissociation. A case report. Clin Orthop 1986;209:210–214

15. Ideberg R, Grevsten S, Larsson S. Epidemiology of scapular fractures. Incidence and classification of 338 fractures. Acta Orthop Scand 1995;66:395–397

16. Eyres KS, Brooks A, Stanley D. Fractures of the coracoid process. J Bone Joint Surg Br 1995;77:425–428

17. Kuhn JE, Blasier RB, Carpenter JE. Fractures of the acromion process: a proposed classification system. J Orthop Trauma 1994;8:6–13

18. Ideberg R. Fractures of the scapula involving the glenoid fossa. In: Bateman JE, Welsh RP, ed. Surgery of the Shoulder. Philadelphia: BC Decker, 1984:63–66

19. Goss TP. Fractures of the glenoid cavity. J Bone Joint Surg Am 1992;74:299–305

20. Orthopaedic Trauma Association. Fracture and dislocation compendium. J Orthop Trauma 1996;10(suppl 1):81–84

21. Zdravkovic D, Damholt VV. Comminuted and severely displaced fractures of the scapula. Acta Orthop Scand 1974;45:60–65

22. Goss TP. Fractures of the glenoid neck. J Shoulder Elbow Surg 1994;3:42–52

23. Nordqvist A, Petersson C. Fracture of the body, neck, or spine of the scapula. A long-term follow-up study. Clin Orthop 1992;283:139–144

24. Butters K. Fractures of the scapula. In: Bucholz RW, Heckman JD, ed. Rockwood and Green's Fractures in Adults. Philadelphia: Lippincott Williams & Wilkins, 2001:1079–1108

25. Schandelmaier P, Blauth M, Schneider C, Krettek C. Fractures of the glenoid treated by operation. A 5- to 23-year follow-up of 22 cases. J Bone Joint Surg Br 2002;84:173–177

26. Kavanagh BF, Bradway JK, Cofield RH. Open reduction and internal fixation of displaced intra-articular fractures of the glenoid fossa. J Bone Joint Surg Am 1993;75:479–484

27. Herscovici D Jr, Fiennes AG, Allgower M, Ruedi TP. The floating shoulder: ipsilateral clavicle and scapular neck fractures. J Bone Joint Surg Br 1992;74:362–364

28. Hardegger FH, Simpson LA, Weber BG. The operative treatment of scapular fractures. J Bone Joint Surg Br 1984;66:725–731

29. Ramos L, Mencia R, Alonso A, Ferrandez L. Conservative treatment of ipsilateral fractures of the scapula and clavicle. J Trauma 1997;42:239–242

30. van Noort A, te Slaa RL, Marti RK, van der Werken C. The floating shoulder. A multicentre study. J Bone Joint Surg Br 2001;83:795–798

31. Egol KA, Connor PM, Karunakar MA, Sims SH, Bosse MJ, Kellam JF. The floating shoulder: clinical and functional results. J Bone Joint Surg Am 2001;83-A:1188–1194

32. Edwards SG, Whittle AP, Wood GW II. Nonoperative treatment of ipsilateral fractures of the scapula and clavicle. J Bone Joint Surg Am 2000;82:774–780

33. Leung KS, Lam TP. Open reduction and internal fixation of ipsilateral fractures of the scapular neck and clavicle. J Bone Joint Surg Am 1993;75:1015–1018

34. Rikli D, Regazzoni P, Renner N. The unstable shoulder girdle: early functional treatment utilizing open reduction and internal fixation. J Orthop Trauma 1995;9:93–97

35. Oh W, Jeon H, Kyung S, Park C, Kim T, Ihn C. The treatment of double disruption of the superior shoulder suspensory complex. Int Orthop 2002;26:145–149

36. Bernard TN Jr, Brunet ME, Haddad RJ Jr. Fractured coracoid process in acromioclavicular dislocations. Report of four cases and review of the literature. Clin Orthop 1983;175:227–232

37. Smith DM. Coracoid fracture associated with acromioclavicular dislocation. A case report. Clin Orthop 1975;108:165–167

38. Romero J, Schai P, Imhoff AB. Scapular neck fracture–the influence of permanent malalignment of the glenoid neck on clinical outcome. Arch Orthop Trauma Surg 2001;121:313–316

39. Solheim LF, Roaas A. Compression of the suprascapular nerve after fracture of the scapular notch. Acta Orthop Scand 1978;49:338–340

40. Ganz R, Noesberger B. [Treatment of scapular fractures]. Hefte Unfallheilkd 1975;126:59–62

Index

Page numbers followed by *f* or *t* refer to figures or tables respectively.